Update on General Medicine

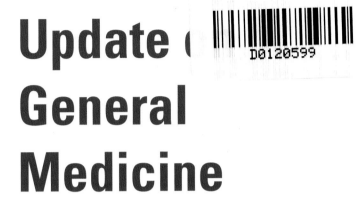

D0120599

Section 1

2012–2013

(Last major revision 2010–2011)

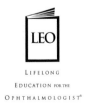

LEO

LIFELONG
EDUCATION FOR THE
OPHTHALMOLOGIST®

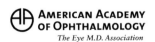

**AMERICAN ACADEMY
OF OPHTHALMOLOGY**
The Eye M.D. Association

The Basic and Clinical Science Course is one component of the Lifelong Education for the Ophthalmologist (LEO) framework, which assists members in planning their continuing medical education. LEO includes an array of clinical education products that members may select to form individualized, self-directed learning plans for updating their clinical knowledge. Active members or fellows who use LEO components may accumulate sufficient CME credits to earn the LEO Award. Contact the Academy's Clinical Education Division for further information on LEO.

The Academy provides this material for educational purposes only. It is not intended to represent the only or best method or procedure in every case, nor to replace a physician's own judgment or give specific advice for case management. Including all indications, contraindications, side effects, and alternative agents for each drug or treatment is beyond the scope of this material. All information and recommendations should be verified, prior to use, with current information included in the manufacturers' package inserts or other independent sources, and considered in light of the patient's condition and history. Reference to certain drugs, instruments, and other products in this course is made for illustrative purposes only and is not intended to constitute an endorsement of such. Some material may include information on applications that are not considered community standard, that reflect indications not included in approved FDA labeling, or that are approved for use only in restricted research settings. **The FDA has stated that it is the responsibility of the physician to determine the FDA status of each drug or device he or she wishes to use, and to use them with appropriate, informed patient consent in compliance with applicable law.** The Academy specifically disclaims any and all liability for injury or other damages of any kind, from negligence or otherwise, for any and all claims that may arise from the use of any recommendations or other information contained herein.

Cover image courtesy of Jason M. Jacobs, MD, and Michael J. Hawes, MD.

Basic and Clinical Science Course

Gregory L. Skuta, MD, Oklahoma City, Oklahoma, *Senior Secretary for Clinical Education*

Louis B. Cantor, MD, Indianapolis, Indiana, *Secretary for Ophthalmic Knowledge*

Jayne S. Weiss, MD, New Orleans, Louisiana, *BCSC Course Chair*

Section 1

Faculty Responsible for This Edition

Eric P. Purdy, MD, *Chair,* Fort Wayne, Indiana
James P. Bolling, MD, Jacksonville, Florida
Anna Luisa Di Lorenzo, MD, Troy, Michigan
Herbert J. Ingraham, MD, Danville, Pennsylvania
Jonathan Walker, MD, Fort Wayne, Indiana
Anne Louise Coleman, MD, PhD, *Consultant,* Los Angeles, California
Gwen Sterns, MD, *Consultant,* Rochester, New York
Harold E. Shaw, MD, Greenville, South Carolina, and
James Mitchell, MD, Edina, Minnesota
    Practicing Ophthalmologists Advisory Committee for Education

The Academy wishes to acknowledge Mary Lou Jackson, MD, *Vision Rehabilitation Committee,* for her review of this edition.

Financial Disclosures

Academy staff members who contributed to the development of this product state that they have no significant financial interest or other relationship with the manufacturer of any commercial product discussed in this course or with the manufacturer of any competing commercial product.

The authors state the following financial relationships:

Dr Coleman: Alcon Laboratories, consultant; Allergan, consultant; National Eye Institute, consultant and grant recipient; Science Based Health, consultant

Dr Walker: Regeneron, grant recipient

The other authors state that they have no significant financial interest or other relationship with the manufacturer of any commercial product discussed in the chapters that they contributed to this course or with the manufacturer of any competing commercial product.

Recent Past Faculty

Roger Kaldawy, MD
Rohit Varma, MD, MPH

In addition, the Academy gratefully acknowledges the contributions of numerous past faculty and advisory committee members who have played an important role in the development of previous editions of the Basic and Clinical Science Course.

American Academy of Ophthalmology Staff

Richard A. Zorab, *Vice President, Ophthalmic Knowledge*
Hal Straus, *Director, Publications Department*
Christine Arturo, *Acquisitions Manager*
Stephanie Tanaka, *Publications Manager*
D. Jean Ray, *Production Manager*
Ann McGuire, *Medical Editor*
Steve Huebner, *Administrative Coordinator*

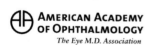

**AMERICAN ACADEMY
OF OPHTHALMOLOGY**
The Eye M.D. Association

655 Beach Street
Box 7424
San Francisco, CA 94120-7424

Contents

General Introduction

The Basic and Clinical Science Course (BCSC) is designed to meet the needs of residents and practitioners for a comprehensive yet concise curriculum of the field of ophthalmology. The BCSC has developed from its original brief outline format, which relied heavily on outside readings, to a more convenient and educationally useful self-contained text. The Academy updates and revises the course annually, with the goals of integrating the basic science and clinical practice of ophthalmology and of keeping ophthalmologists current with new developments in the various subspecialties.

The BCSC incorporates the effort and expertise of more than 80 ophthalmologists, organized into 13 Section faculties, working with Academy editorial staff. In addition, the course continues to benefit from many lasting contributions made by the faculties of previous editions. Members of the Academy's Practicing Ophthalmologists Advisory Committee for Education serve on each faculty and, as a group, review every volume before and after major revisions.

Organization of the Course

The Basic and Clinical Science Course comprises 13 volumes, incorporating fundamental ophthalmic knowledge, subspecialty areas, and special topics:

1 Update on General Medicine
2 Fundamentals and Principles of Ophthalmology
3 Clinical Optics
4 Ophthalmic Pathology and Intraocular Tumors
5 Neuro-Ophthalmology
6 Pediatric Ophthalmology and Strabismus
7 Orbit, Eyelids, and Lacrimal System
8 External Disease and Cornea
9 Intraocular Inflammation and Uveitis
10 Glaucoma
11 Lens and Cataract
12 Retina and Vitreous
13 Refractive Surgery

In addition, a comprehensive Master Index allows the reader to easily locate subjects throughout the entire series.

References

Readers who wish to explore specific topics in greater detail may consult the references cited within each chapter and listed in the Basic Texts section at the back of the book.

These references are intended to be selective rather than exhaustive, chosen by the BCSC faculty as being important, current, and readily available to residents and practitioners.

Related Academy educational materials are also listed in the appropriate sections. They include books, online and audiovisual materials, self-assessment programs, clinical modules, and interactive programs.

Study Questions and CME Credit

Each volume of the BCSC is designed as an independent study activity for ophthalmology residents and practitioners. The learning objectives for this volume are given on page 1. The text, illustrations, and references provide the information necessary to achieve the objectives; the study questions allow readers to test their understanding of the material and their mastery of the objectives. Physicians who wish to claim CME credit for this educational activity may do so by mail, by fax, or online. The necessary forms and instructions are given at the end of the book.

Conclusion

The Basic and Clinical Science Course has expanded greatly over the years, with the addition of much new text and numerous illustrations. Recent editions have sought to place a greater emphasis on clinical applicability while maintaining a solid foundation in basic science. As with any educational program, it reflects the experience of its authors. As its faculties change and as medicine progresses, new viewpoints are always emerging on controversial subjects and techniques. Not all alternate approaches can be included in this series; as with any educational endeavor, the learner should seek additional sources, including such carefully balanced opinions as the Academy's Preferred Practice Patterns.

The BCSC faculty and staff are continuously striving to improve the educational usefulness of the course; you, the reader, can contribute to this ongoing process. If you have any suggestions or questions about the series, please do not hesitate to contact the faculty or the editors.

The authors, editors, and reviewers hope that your study of the BCSC will be of lasting value and that each Section will serve as a practical resource for quality patient care.

Objectives

Upon completion of BCSC Section 1, the reader should be able to

- describe the ophthalmic manifestations of the major systemic diseases covered in this volume

- summarize the most common human pathogens and their manifestations

- discuss the epidemiology, clinical findings, and treatment of HIV infection

- review the newer antiviral, antifungal, and antibacterial agents and their benefits

- classify levels of hypertension by blood pressure measurements

- list the major classes of antihypertensive medications and some of their characteristics and side effects

- describe the various diagnostic procedures used in the evaluation of patients with coronary artery disease

- review the current treatment options for atrial fibrillation, atrial flutter, and ventricular tachycardia

- discuss the indications for dietary and pharmacologic treatment of hypercholesterolemia

- distinguish between obstructive and restrictive, reversible and irreversible, pulmonary diseases, and give examples of each type

- describe the classification, pathophysiology, presentation, and diagnostic criteria for diabetes mellitus

- review the various therapeutic approaches for diabetes mellitus, including new insulins and oral agents

- list the most prevalent types of cancer for men and for women together with the appropriate screening methods for detecting them

- review current concepts about the etiologies of most malignancies

- describe traditional as well as more novel approaches to the treatment of cancers

- summarize the major behavioral disorders and possible therapeutic modalities for these conditions (including the ocular side effects of psychoactive medications)

- list some of the factors associated with a patient's compliance or noncompliance with medical regimens

- explain the rationale for and value of screening programs for various systemic diseases

- summarize the major disease processes affecting most of the adult population, and briefly explain how preventive measures may reduce the morbidity and mortality they cause

- assess medical literature more critically in regard to appropriate study design and validity of conclusions

- explain the importance of the randomized, controlled clinical study in evaluating the effects of new treatments

CHAPTER 1

Infectious Disease

Recent Developments

- Vancomycin-resistant strains of enterococci and staphylococci have emerged in recent years as a cause of life-threatening infection in hospitalized patients.
- DNA probes using polymerase chain reaction (PCR) provide new, more sensitive diagnostic tools for detecting gonorrhea, syphilis, Lyme disease, and infections caused by *Chlamydia,* mycobacteria, fungi, and many viruses.
- The incidence of cytomegalovirus (CMV) retinitis and other opportunistic infections in HIV-infected patients has decreased significantly in the era of highly active antiretroviral therapy (HAART).
- Newer antibiotics, such as meropenem, cefepime, linezolid, quinupristin/dalfopristin, evernimicin, telithromycin, daptomycin, grepafloxacin, and teicoplanin, provide expanded antimicrobial coverage and offer treatment options for multidrug-resistant infections.

General Microbiology

Despite formidable immune and mechanical defense systems, the human body harbors an extensive, well-adapted population of microorganisms on the skin and in the gastrointestinal, vaginal, and upper respiratory tracts. The organisms maintain their foothold on these epithelial surfaces chiefly by adherence, and they indirectly benefit the host by excluding pathogenic bacterial colonization and by priming the immune system. If antimicrobial agents alter this host–microbe interplay by eliminating the normal flora, the host's susceptibility to normally excluded pathogenic microorganisms is increased. When the mechanical defenses of the epithelial layers are breached so as to expose normally sterile areas, or if a critical component of the immune system that usually prevents microbial invasion fails, severe infections can result from the normal microbial flora.

Components of the immune system of multicellular organisms are categorized into innate and adaptive immunity. *Innate immunity* is present in nearly all muticellular organisms and includes humoral and cellular immune receptors that have broad specificity. These receptors recognize many related molecular structures called PAMPs (*pathogen-associated molecular patterns*). PAMPs are polysaccharides and polynucleotides that differ very little among pathogens but are not found in the host. The innate immune response is usually immediate; there is no immune memory of prior exposure.

Adaptive immunity is only found in vertebrates and does involve immune memory of prior exposure. Pathogens are recognized by many randomly generated B-lymphocyte and T-lymphocyte receptors, each of which has a very narrow specificity, able to recognize a particular epitope. Most epitopes are derived from polypeptides and reflect the individuality of each pathogen. Adaptive immune response is initially slower (days), because of the need for proliferation of clones of responding immune cells. After the first encounter, the adaptive immune response is faster and stronger, due to immunologic memory.

However, even when both the mechanical and immune defense systems are intact, pathogenic microbes can cause infections by means of specific virulent characteristics that allow the microbes to invade and multiply. These virulent traits vary among different species.

Following are several mechanisms of virulence:

- *Attachment. Neisseria gonorrhoeae* and *Neisseria meningitidis* breach epithelial barriers by adhering to host epithelial cell surface receptors by means of a ligand on the bacteria's pili. Presence of the cell surface receptors is genetically determined.
- *Polysaccharide encapsulation. Streptococcus pneumoniae, N meningitidis, Haemophilus,* and *Bacteroides* evade phagocytosis in the absence of antibody and complement because of their polysaccharide coating.
- *Blocking of lysosomal fusion.* Intracellular existence, as well as protection from humoral immune mechanisms, is a characteristic of *Chlamydia, Toxoplasma, Legionella,* and *Mycobacterium.*
- *Antigenic surface variation.* Antigenic shifts in the cell wall of *Borrelia recurrentis* incapacitate the humoral immune system, which has a lag time in antibody production. Similar antigenic shifts are found in *Chlamydia* and influenza viruses.
- *IgA protease. Haemophilus influenzae, N gonorrhoeae,* and *N meningitidis* eliminate the IgA antibody normally found on mucosal surfaces, which would otherwise prevent the microbes' adherence.
- *Endotoxin.* A normal constituent of the gram-negative bacterial cell wall, endotoxin produces dramatic systemic physiologic responses ranging from fever and leukocyte margination to disseminated intravascular coagulation and septic shock.
- *Exotoxin.* Exotoxins are a diverse set of proteins with specific actions on target tissues that can cause severe systemic effects in such diseases as cholera or tetanus.
- *Biofilm formation.* Staphylococci have the ability to develop biofilms on various biomaterials, such as catheters and prosthetic heart valves.
- *Multiple mechanisms.* Some organisms, such as coagulase-positive *Staphylococcus aureus,* may possess multiple mechanisms of virulence. Also, it appears that nearly any *S aureus* genotype carried by humans can transform into a life-threatening pathogen, but certain clones are more virulent than others.

The immune system, which makes possible the host's adaptive response to colonization and infection, is classically divided into the humoral and cellular immune systems. The *humoral immune system,* composed of cells derived from the B lymphocytes, is responsible for antibody-mediated opsonization, complement-mediated bacterial killing, antitoxin, and mediation of intracellular infections. The *cellular immune system,* determined by the

T lymphocytes, is responsible for interaction with and stimulation of the humoral immune system, direct cytotoxicity, release of chemical messengers, and control of chronic infections. The successful interplay between the humoral and cellular immune systems mitigates and usually eradicates the infection, allowing for repair and healing. See also Part I, Immunology, in BCSC Section 9, *Intraocular Inflammation and Uveitis*.

Staphylococcus

Staphylococcus aureus colonizes the anterior nares and other skin sites in 15% of community isolates. Of the tertiary-care hospital isolates, over 25% are resistant to all β-lactam antibiotics. Transmission of organisms is usually by direct contact. Resistance of organisms to antimicrobials is usually plasmid determined and varies by institution. The increasing prevalence of methicillin-resistant *S aureus* (MRSA) in tertiary referral hospitals appears to be related to the population of high-risk patients at such centers. Unfortunately, MRSA is now an increasingly more common cause of serious infection in primary care settings as well. The natural history of staphylococcal infections indicates that immunity is of short duration and incomplete. Delayed hypersensitivity reactions to staphylococcal products may be responsible for chronic staphylococcal disease.

Conditions caused by staphylococcal infections include stye, furuncle, acne, bullous impetigo, paronychia, osteomyelitis, septic arthritis, deep-tissue abscesses, bacteremia, endocarditis, enterocolitis, pneumonia, wound infections, scalded skin syndrome, toxic shock syndrome, and food poisoning.

Acute serious staphylococcal infections require immediate intravenous antibiotic therapy. A penicillinase-resistant penicillin or first-generation cephalosporin is normally used, pending the results of susceptibility tests. With the emergence of methicillin-resistant staphylococci, vancomycin has become the drug of choice for treating life-threatening infections, pending susceptibility studies. The increasing emergence of vancomycin-resistant enterococci (VRE) has led to concern about cases of vancomycin-resistant *S aureus* (VRSA) infection, mediated through plasmid transfer.

Since 1997, infections due to strains of *S aureus* with reduced susceptibility to vancomycin (glycopeptide-intermediate *S aureus*) have been identified, with increasing frequency throughout the world. Many of the cases occurred after prolonged inpatient treatment with intravenous vancomycin. Some reported cases have been successfully treated with various forms of combination therapy, including rifampin and trimethoprim-sulfamethoxazole; vancomycin, gentamicin, and rifampin; and vancomycin and nafcillin. Other agents with activity against vancomycin-intermediate *S aureus* (VISA) are ampicillin-sulbactam (Unasyn) and some newer antibiotics: trovafloxacin (Trovan), daptomycin (Cubicin), evernimicin (Ziracin), linezolid (Zyvox), and quinupristin/dalfopristin (Synercid). The first case of true VRSA was reported in July 2002, and 5 additional van-A mutation positive cases have been confirmed in the United States since then. Exposure to vancomycin-intermediate and vancomycin-resistant isolates of *S aureus* has been shown to increase the organism's resistance to vancomycin and other new agents, such as teicoplanin. Most VISA and nearly all VRSA isolates reported to date have arisen from endemic MRSA and, in the case of VRSA, have acquired genes from VRE. Accordingly, the emergence of VISA and VRSA provides strong motivation for containing MRSA and VRE transmission.

Staphylococcus epidermidis is an almost universal inhabitant of the skin, present in up to 90% of skin cultures. It can cause infection when local defenses are compromised. Its characteristic adherence to prosthetic devices makes it the most common cause of prosthetic heart valve infections, and it is a common infectious organism of intravenous catheters and cerebrospinal fluid shunts.

Most isolates are resistant to methicillin and cephalosporins; therefore, the drug of choice is vancomycin, occasionally in combination with rifampin or gentamicin. Unfortunately, there have also been recent reports of vancomycin-resistant infections caused by coagulase-negative staphylococcus. In addition to antibiotic therapy, management usually involves removal of the infected prosthetic device or vascular catheter.

Holmes RL, Jorgensen JH. Inhibitory activities of 11 antimicrobial agents and bactericidal activities of vancomycin and daptomycin against invasive methicillin-resistant Staphylococcus aureus isolates obtained from 1999 through 2006. *Antimicrob Agents Chemother.* 2008;52(2):757–760.

Leonard SN, Cheung CM, Rybak MJ. Activities of ceftobiprole, linezolid, vancomycin, and daptomycin against community-associated and hospital-associated methicillin-resistant Staphylococcus aureus. *Antimicrob Agents Chemother.* 2008;52(8):2974–2976.

Lewis JS II, Ellis MW. Approaches to serious methicillin-resistant Staphylococcus aureus infections with decreased susceptibility to vancomycin: clinical significance and options for management. *Curr Opin Infect Dis.* 2007;20(6):568–573.

Sievert DM, Rudrik JT, Patel JB, McDonald LC, Wilkins MJ, Hageman JC. Vancomycin-resistant Staphylococcus aureus in the United States, 2002-2006. *Clin Infect Dis.* 2008;46(5):668–674.

Streptococcus

Group A β-hemolytic streptococci *(Streptococcus pyogenes)* cause a variety of acute suppurative infections through droplet transmission. The infection is modulated by an opsonizing antibody, which provides a type-specific immunity that lasts for years and is directed against the protein in the cell wall pili. Suppurative streptococcal infections in humans include pharyngitis, impetigo, pneumonia, erysipelas, wound and burn infections, puerperal infections, and scarlet fever. Genetically mediated humoral and cellular responses to certain strains of group A streptococci play a role in the development of the postinfectious syndromes of glomerulonephritis and rheumatic fever, both of which represent delayed, nonsuppurative, noninfectious complications of group A streptococcal infections. Rapid identification with antigen detection tests allows prompt treatment of patients with pharyngitis due to this strain of streptococcus and can reduce the risk of spread of infection.

S pyogenes remains highly susceptible to penicillin G; however, in the presence of allergy, erythromycin or (if no cross allergy exists) a cephalosporin is substituted. In recent years, macrolide-resistant and clindamycin-resistant strains of group A β-hemolytic streptococci have been reported. Antibiotic prophylaxis against bacterial endocarditis is administered for procedures that may result in transient bacteremia. However, such prophylaxis may not prevent acute glomerulonephritis.

Streptococcus pneumoniae organisms are lancet-shaped diplococci that cause α-hemolysis on blood agar. Although 10%–30% of the normal population carry 1 or more serologic types of pneumococci in the throat, the incidence and mortality of pneumococcal pneumonia increase sharply after age 50, with a fatality rate approaching 25%. Pneumococcal virulence is determined by its complex polysaccharide capsule, of which there are more than 80 distinct serotypes.

Conditions caused by *S pneumoniae* include pneumonia, sinusitis, meningitis, otitis media, and peritonitis. Pneumococci are usually highly susceptible to penicillin, other β-lactams, erythromycin, or the newer fluoroquinolones. Routine susceptibility testing should be performed on patients with meningitis, bacteremia, or other life-threatening infections. Penicillin-resistant strains of *S pneumoniae* have been reported with increasing frequency. In several regions of the world, more than 25% of isolates are penicillin resistant; many of these are also resistant to cephalosporins and macrolides. Recently, some cases of ketolide and fluoroquinolone resistance have been reported as well. Treatment of highly resistant strains may require vancomycin or meropenem. Prophylaxis is available through use of the 23-valent vaccine for adults and the 7-valent vaccine for children (see Chapter 13, Preventive Medicine). Interestingly, new drug-resistant strains have evolved in pediatric infections due to the impact of the 7-valent vaccine.

α-Hemolytic streptococci and staphylococci cause the majority of cases of subacute bacterial endocarditis (55% and 30% of cases, respectively). Other pathogens that cause subacute bacterial endocarditis (SBE) include *Enterococcus, Haemophilus,* and fungi. The SBE prophylaxis recommendations changed dramatically in 2007. It is no longer recommended following routine gastrointestinal or genitourinary surgical procedures. Prophylaxis for SBE is usually not considered necessary for routine ocular surgery in an uninfected patient but can be considered for surgery involving the nasolacrimal drainage system or sinuses or for surgical repair of orbital trauma, if the patient has a high-risk cardiac congenital or valvular condition (Table 1-1).

Duesberg CB, Malhotra-Kumar S, Goossens H, et al. Interspecies recombination occurs frequently in quinolone resistance-determining regions of clinical isolates of Streptococcus pyogenes. *Antimicrob Agents Chemother.* 2008;52(11):4191–4193.

Nishimura RA, Carabello BA, Faxon DP, et al. ACC/AHA 2008 guideline update on valvular heart disease: focused update on infective endocarditis. A report of the American College of Cardiology/American Heart Association Task Force on Practice Guidelines. Endorsed by the Society of Cardiovascular Anesthesiologists, Society for Cardiovascular Angiography and Interventions, and Society of Thoracic Surgeons. *Circulation.* 2008;118(8):887–896. Full online text available at: http://circ.ahajournals.org/cgi/content/full/118/8/887.

Richter SS, Heilmann KP, Dohrn CL, Riahi F, Beekmann SE, Doern GV. Changing epidemiology of antimicrobial-resistant Streptococcus pneumoniae in the United States, 2004-2005. *Clin Infect Dis.* 2009;48(3):e23–e33.

Wilson W, Taubert KA, Gewitz M, et al. Prevention of infective endocarditis: guidelines from the American Heart Association. A guideline from the American Heart Association Rheumatic Fever, Endocarditis, and Kawasaki Disease Committee; Council on Cardiovascular Disease in the Young; and the Council on Clinical Cardiology; Council on Cardiovascular Surgery and Anesthesia; and the Quality of Care and Outcomes Research Interdisciplinary

Table 1-1 SBE Prophylaxis Regimens for Dental and Incisional Nasolacrimal Procedures

Situation	Agent	Regimen: Single Dose 30 to 60 min Before Procedure	
		Adults	Children
Oral	Amoxicillin	2 g	50 mg/kg
Unable to take oral medication	Ampicillin	2 g IM or IV	50 mg/kg IM or IV
	OR Cefazolin or ceftriaxone	1 g IM or IV	50 mg/kg IM or IV
Allergic to penicillins or ampicillin—oral	Cephalexin*†	2 g	50 mg/kg
	OR Clindamycin	600 mg	20 mg/kg
	OR Azithromycin or clarithromycin	500 mg	15 mg/kg
Allergic to penicillins or ampicillin and unable to take oral medication	Cefazolin or ceftriaxone†	1 g IM or IV	50 mg/kg IM or IV
	OR Clindamycin	600 mg IM or IV	20 mg/kg IM or IV

IM = intramuscular, IV = intravenous, SBE = subacute bacterial endocarditis.

*Or other first- or second-generation oral cephalosporin in equivalent adult or pediatric dosage.

†Cephalosporins should not be used in an individual with a history of anaphylaxis, angioedema, or urticaria with penicillins or ampicillin.

Adapted from Wilson W, Taubert KA, Gewitz M, et al. Prevention of infective endocarditis: guidelines from the American Heart Association. A guideline from the American Heart Association Rheumatic Fever, Endocarditis, and Kawasaki Disease Committee; Council on Cardiovascular Disease in the Young; and the Council on Clinical Cardiology; Council on Cardiovascular Surgery and Anesthesia; and the Quality of Care and Outcomes Research Interdisciplinary Working Group. *Circulation.* 2007;116(15): 1736–1754, Table 5. Full online text available at: http://circ.ahajournals.org/cgi/content/full/116/15/1736.

Working Group. *Circulation.* 2007;116(15):1736–1754. Full online text available at: http://circ.ahajournals.org/cgi/content/full/116/15/1736.

Clostridium difficile

Clostridium difficile is an endemic anaerobic gram-positive bacillus that is part of the normal gastrointestinal flora. It has acquired importance because of its role in the development of pseudomembranous enterocolitis following the use of antibiotics. Typically, within 1–14 days of starting antibiotic therapy, patients develop fever and diarrhea. The diarrhea occasionally becomes bloody and typically contains a cytopathic toxin that is elaborated by *C difficile*.

In the past, a tissue-culture assay for the toxin has been the best diagnostic test. Newer enzyme immunoassay and PCR tests allow more rapid detection. The most frequently implicated antibiotics include clindamycin, ampicillin, chloramphenicol, tetracycline, erythromycin, and the cephalosporins. Recently, new hypervirulent strains of *C difficile* infection have emerged in the United States, Europe, and Japan. Initial treatment includes discontinuing the causative antibiotic and administering metronidazole for 10 days. Vancomycin is also effective, but its use should be limited to decrease the development of vancomycin-resistant organisms such as enterococci and staphylococci. It is also much more expensive than metronidazole. Vancomycin should be limited to those who cannot tolerate or have not responded to metronidazole, or to situations in which metronidazole use is contraindicated, such as during the first trimester of pregnancy. Rifampin, fusidic acid, nitazoxanide, ramoplanin, rifaximin, intravenous immunoglobulin, and a new toxin-binding polymer have been evaluated as potential alternative therapies, and trials are in progress with a new toxoid vaccine. Corticosteroids have been proven to reduce the diarrhea associated with *C difficile* infection.

DuPont HL, Garey K, Caeiro JP, Jiang ZD. New advances in Clostridium difficile infection: changing epidemiology, diagnosis, treatment and control. *Curr Opin Infect Dis.* 2008;21(5): 500–507.

Guiles J, Critchley I, Sun X. New agents for Clostridium difficile-associated disease. *Expert Opin Investig Drugs.* 2008;17(11):1671–1683.

Persson S, Torpdahl M, Olsen KE. New multiplex PCR method for the detection of Clostridium difficile toxin (tcdA) and toxin B (tcdB) and the binary toxin (cdtA/cdtB) genes applied to a Danish strain collection. *Clin Microbiol Infect.* 2008;14(11):1057–1064.

Haemophilus influenzae

Haemophilus influenzae is a common inhabitant of the upper respiratory tract in 20%–50% of healthy adults and 80% of children. *H influenzae* is divided into 6 serotypes, based on differing capsular polysaccharide antigens. Both encapsulated and unencapsulated species cause disease, but systemic spread is typical of the encapsulated strain, whose capsule protects it against phagocytosis. Infants are usually protected for a few months by passively acquired maternal antibodies; thereafter, active antibody levels increase with age, being inversely related to the risk of infection. Of the patients with meningitis, roughly 14% develop significant neurologic damage. Other infections include epiglottitis, orbital cellulitis, arthritis, otitis media, bronchitis, pericarditis, sinusitis, and pneumonia. DNA PCR probe assay is available for rapid diagnosis of *H influenzae* type B infections.

Treatment of acute infections has been complicated by the emergence of ampicillin-resistant strains, with an incidence approaching 50% in some geographic areas. Current recommendations are to start empirical therapy with amoxicillin-clavulanate (Augmentin), trimethoprim-sulfamethoxazole (Bactrim), a quinolone such as ciprofloxacin, or a third-generation cephalosporin, pending susceptibility testing of the organism. Nearly all isolates of *H influenzae* are now resistant to macrolides. Serious or life-threatening infections should be treated with an intravenous third-generation cephalosporin with known activity against *H influenzae,* such as ceftriaxone or cefotaxime, while results of sensitivity testing are pending. Recent reports note an increase in the number of isolates with reduced sensitivity to cephalosporins and quinolones, especially in patients with chronic pulmonary disease.

H influenzae type B conjugate vaccines are available for use in infants and have demonstrated their effectiveness in protecting infants and older children against meningitis and other invasive diseases caused by *H influenzae* type B. In studies of fully immunized populations, *H influenzae* infection has been nearly eradicated since these vaccines were introduced. Also, the incidence of meningitis, orbital cellulitis, and other infections caused by *H influenzae* has been reduced significantly since *H influenzae* type B conjugate vaccines became available. It is important to remember that immunized patients are still susceptible to infections caused by strains of *H influenzae* other than type B.

Ambati BK, Ambati J, Azar N, Stratton L, Schmidt EV. Periorbital and orbital cellulitis be-fore and after the advent of Haemophilus influenzae type B vaccination. *Ophthalmology.* 2000;107(8):1450–1453.

Marty A, Greiner O, Day PJ, Gunziger S, Mühlemann K, Nadal D. Detection of Haemophilus influenzae type b by real-time PCR. *J Clin Microbiol.* 2004;42(8):3813–3815.

Schmitt HJ, Maechler G, Habermehl P, et al. Immunogenicity, reactogenicity, and immune memory after primary vaccination with a novel Haemophilus influenzae-Neisseria menin-gitidis serogroup C conjugate vaccine. *Clin Vaccine Immunol.* 2007;14(4):426–434.

Neisseria

Most *Neisseria* organisms are normal inhabitants of the upper respiratory and alimen-tary tracts; the commonly recognized pathogenic species are the meningococci and the gonococci.

Meningococci can be cultured in up to 15% of healthy persons in nonepidemic pe-riods. Virulence is determined by the polysaccharide capsule and the potent endotoxic activity of the cell wall, which can cause cardiovascular collapse, shock, and disseminated intravascular coagulation. Complement-deficient or asplenic persons are at risk for seri-ous clinical infections. Diagnostic testing may include Gram stain, blood and cerebrospi-nal fluid cultures, *enzyme-linked immunosorbent assay (ELISA),* and PCR. An automated fluorescent multiplex PCR assay that can simultaneously detect *N meningitidis, H influen-zae,* and *S pneumoniae* can be used for evaluating patients with suspected meningitis. This test provides extremely high sensitivity and a specificity of 100% for each organism.

The range of meningococcal infections includes meningitis; mild to severe upper res-piratory tract infections; and, less often, endocarditis, arthritis, pericarditis, pneumonia, endophthalmitis, and purpura fulminans. *N meningitidis* serogroup B is the most common cause of bacterial meningitis in children and young adults. Meningitis with a petechial or pupuric exanthem is the classic presentation, although each may occur in isolation.

Historically, the treatment of choice for meningococcal meningitis has been high-dose penicillin or, in the case of allergy, chloramphenicol or a third-generation cephalosporin. However, in one European study, 39% of asymptomatic carriers and about 55% of infected patients had isolates with decreased susceptibility to penicillin. Rifampin or minocycline is used as chemoprophylaxis for family members or intimate personal contacts of the in-fected individual. Polysaccharide vaccines are most effective in older children and adults. The routine administration of meningococcal vaccines is not recommended, except in patients who have undergone splenectomy, complement-deficient persons, military per-sonnel, travelers to endemic regions, and close contacts of infected patients.

Gonococci are not normal inhabitants of the respiratory or genital flora, and their major reservoir is the asymptomatic patient. Among infected women, 50% are asymptom-atic, whereas 95% of infected men have symptoms. Asymptomatic patients are infectious for several months, with a transmissibility rate of 20%–50%. Nonsexual transmission is rare. The key to prevention is identification and treatment of asymptomatic carriers and their sexual contacts.

Chlamydia trachomatis coexists with gonorrhea in 25%–50% of women with endocervical gonorrhea and 20%–33% of men with gonococcal urethritis. Diagnosis of gonococcal infections, as well as infections caused by many other bacteria, mycobacteria, viruses, and mycoplasma, has been enhanced with the development of highly sensitive DNA probes that use PCR techniques.

The range of gonococcal infections includes cervicitis, urethritis, pelvic inflammatory disease, pharyngitis, conjunctivitis, ophthalmia neonatorum, and disseminated gonococcal disease with fever, polyarthralgias, and rash.

Because penicillin-resistant and tetracycline-resistant gonococcal strains have become common in many areas of the United States, treatment should be tailored to their local prevalence. Tetracycline is effective for susceptible strains, penicillin-allergic persons, or concurrent chlamydial infections. Ceftriaxone (via intramuscular injection) is the drug of choice for penicillinase-resistant strains; thus far, reduced susceptibility to this antibiotic is extremely rare. Other alternatives include oral cefixime; cefuroxime; azithromycin; and the fluoroquinolones. The macrolides and fluoroquinolones have the added benefit of excellent activity against concomitant *C trachomatis* infection. However, gonococcal isolates with reduced sensitivity to macrolides and fluoroquinolones have been reported with increasing frequency, and the CDC recently recommended that clinicians no longer use fluoroquinolones as a first-line treatment for gonorrhea in one high-risk group, homosexual men.

Matsumoto T. Trends of sexually transmitted diseases and antimicrobial resistance in Neisseria gonorrhoeae. *Int J Antimicrob Agents.* 2008;31(Suppl 1):S35–S39.

Wang SA, Harvey AB, Conner SM, et al.Antimicrobial resistance for Neisseria gonorrhoeae in the United States, 1988 to 2003: the spread of fluoroquinolone resistance. *Ann Intern Med.* 2007;147(2):81–88.

Workowski KA, Berman SM, Douglas JM Jr. Emerging antimicrobial resistance in Neisseria gonorrhoeae: urgent need to strengthen prevention strategies. *Ann Intern Med.* 2008;148(8): 606–613.

Pseudomonas aeruginosa

Pseudomonas aeruginosa is a gram-negative bacillus found free living in moist environments. Together with *Serratia marcescens, P aeruginosa* is 1 of the 2 most consistently antimicrobial-resistant pathogenic bacteria. Infection usually requires either a break in the first-line defenses or altered immunity resulting in a local pyogenic response. The virulence of this organism is related to extracellular toxins, endotoxin, and a polysaccharide protection from phagocytosis. Systemic spread can result in disseminated intravascular coagulation, shock, and death.

Usual sites of infection include the respiratory system, skin, eye, urinary tract, bone, and wounds. Systemic infections caused by a resistant organism carry a high mortality rate and are usually associated with depressed immunity, often in a hospital setting.

Over half of *P aeruginosa* isolates are now resistant to aminoglycosides. Therefore, treatment of serious infections relies on combined antimicrobial coverage with either a semisynthetic penicillin or a third-generation cephalosporin with an aminoglycoside. Ceftazidime has been the most effective cephalosporin for treatment of pseudomonal infections. Piperacillin/tazobactam, imipenem, and meropenem also remain highly effective against most isolates, but resistance to the carbapenems and fluoroquinolones has been rising gradually. The initial choice of antimicrobials depends on local susceptibility prevalence and should be guided by susceptibility testing. Multidrug-resistant *P aeruginosa* arises in a stepwise manner following prolonged exposure to antipseudomonal antibiotics and results in adverse outcomes, with high mortality.

The use of vaccines incorporating multiple *P aeruginosa* serotypes is under investigation for the treatment of patients with severe burns, cystic fibrosis, or immunosuppression. Oral fluoroquinolones as well as newer macrolides such as azithromycin have been useful as prophylactic agents in patients with cystic fibrosis.

Hocquet D, Berthelot P, Roussel-Delvallez M, et al. Pseudomonas aeruginosa may accumulate drug resistance mechanisms without losing its ability to cause bloodstream infections. *Antimicrob Agents Chemother.* 2007;51(10):3531–3536.

Mesaros N, Nordmann P, Plésiat P, et al. Pseudomonas aeruginosa: resistance and therapeutic options at the turn of the new millennium. *Clin Microbiol Infect.* 2007;13(6):560–578.

Tam VH, Chang KT, LaRocco MT, et al. Prevalence, mechanisms, and risk factors of carbapenem resistance in bloodstream isolates of Pseudomonas aeruginosa. *Diagn Microbiol Infect Dis.* 2007;58(3):309–314.

Treponema pallidum

The spirochete *Treponema pallidum* (syphilis) is exclusively a human pathogen. Infection usually follows direct sexual contact. Transplacental transmission from an untreated pregnant woman to her fetus before 16 weeks' gestation results in *congenital syphilis.*

Stages

The course of the disease is divided into 4 stages: primary, secondary, latent, and tertiary (late). Initial inoculation occurs through intact mucous membranes or abraded skin and, within 6 weeks, results in a broad, ulcerated, painless papule called a *chancre.* The spirochetes readily enter the lymphatic system and bloodstream. The ulcer heals spontaneously, and signs of dissemination appear after a variable quiescent period of several weeks to months.

The secondary stage is heralded by fever, malaise, adenopathy, and patchy loss of hair. Meningitis, uveitis, optic neuritis, and hepatitis are less common. Maculopapular lesions may develop into wartlike condylomata in moist areas, and oral mucosal patches sometimes appear, all of which are highly infectious. The secondary lesions usually resolve in 2–6 weeks, although up to 25% of patients may experience relapse in the first 2–4 years. Without treatment, these persons enter the latent stage of disease.

Latent syphilis, characterized by positive serologic results without clinical signs, is divided into 2 stages. The *early latent stage* is within 1 year of infection. During this time, the disease is potentially transmissible, because relapses associated with spirochetemia are possible. The *late latent stage* is associated with immunity to relapse and resistance to infectious lesions.

Tertiary manifestations can occur from 2 to 20 years after infection, and one third of untreated cases of latent disease progress to this stage. The remaining two thirds of cases either are subclinical or resolve spontaneously. *Tertiary disease* is characterized by destructive granulomatous lesions with a typical endarteritis that can affect the skin, bone, joints, oral and nasal cavities, parenchymal organs, cardiovascular system, eyes, meninges, and CNS. Few spirochetes are found in lesions outside the CNS.

Pathologically, obliterative endarteritis with a perivascular infiltrate of lymphocytes, monocytes, and plasma cells is a feature of all active stages of syphilis. Gummata of tertiary syphilis are evidenced by a central area of caseating necrosis with a surrounding granulomatous response.

Diagnosis

Most cases of syphilis are diagnosed serologically. *Nontreponemal tests,* such as the VDRL (Venereal Disease Research Laboratory) test or RPR (rapid plasma reagin) test, are usually positive during the early stages of the primary lesion, uniformly positive during the secondary stage, and progressively nonreactive in the later stages. In neurosyphilis, the serum VDRL test result may be negative and the cerebrospinal fluid VDRL result may be positive. These patients require careful evaluation and aggressive treatment with close follow-up. Nontreponemal test results become predictably negative after successful therapy and can be used to assess the efficacy of treatment; however, they can be falsely positive in a variety of autoimmune diseases, especially systemic lupus erythematosus and the antiphospholipid antibody syndrome. In this disorder, the autoantibodies, anticardiolipin, and the lupus anticoagulant may result in vasculopathy and a hypercoagulable state, with arterial and venous thrombosis (including retinal vascular occlusion), preeclampsia, and spontaneous abortions. Less than 50% of patients with the antiphospholipid antibody syndrome have lupus. False-positive VDRL results can also occur in liver disease, diseases with a substantial amount of tissue destruction, pregnancy, or infections caused by other treponemae.

The *fluorescent treponemal antibody absorption test (FTA-ABS)* involves specific detection of antibody to *T pallidum* after the patient's serum is treated with nonpathogenic treponemal antigens to avoid nonspecific reactions. Hemagglutination tests specific for treponemal antibodies also have high sensitivity and specificity for detecting syphilis. These tests include the hemagglutination treponemal test for syphilis (HATTS), the *T pallidum* hemagglutination assay (TPHA), and the microhemagglutination test for *T pallidum* (MHA-TP). Treponemal antibody detection tests are more specific than nontreponemal tests, but the titers do not decrease with successful treatment; thus, such tests should be considered as confirmatory tests, especially in later stages of disease.

Results of treponemal tests can be falsely positive in 15% of patients with systemic lupus erythematosus, in patients with other treponemal infections or Lyme disease, and, in rare instances, in patients who have lymphosarcoma or who are pregnant, although the fluorescent staining is typically weak.

Table 1-2 Treatment of Syphilis

Syphilis	Drug of Choice and Dosage
Early <1 yr	Penicillin G 2.4 million U IM × 1
Late >1 yr, no CNS	Penicillin G 2.4 million U IM weekly × 3 wk
Neurosyphilis	Penicillin G 2–4 million U IV q 4 hr × 10 days

Newer, more sensitive diagnostic tests for syphilis are ELISA, Western blot, and DNA PCR techniques. These methods may also improve our ability to diagnose congenital syphilis and neurosyphilis.

Management

Treatment of syphilis is determined by stage and by CNS involvement. *Treponema pallidum* is exquisitely sensitive to penicillin, which remains the antimicrobial of choice (Table 1-2). Erythromycin, azithromycin, chloramphenicol, tetracycline, doxycycline, and the cephalosporins are acceptable alternatives to penicillin. Lumbar puncture should be performed to determine cerebrospinal fluid involvement in a number of circumstances. They are as follows: latent syphilis of more than 1 year's duration; suspected neurosyphilis; treatment failure; HIV coinfection; high RPR titers (>1:32); evidence of other late manifestations (cardiac involvement, gummata). Either penicillin G or a single oral dose of azithromycin has been recommended for treatment of patients recently exposed to a sexual partner with infectious syphilis. There have been reports of syphilis treatment failures with use of azithromycin, but the cure rate is still higher than that of penicillin G.

Many reports have described an accelerated clinical course of syphilis in patients infected with HIV; furthermore, such patients may experience an incomplete response to standard therapy. An HIV-infected patient with syphilis often requires a longer and more intensive treatment regimen, ongoing follow-up to assess for recurrence, and complete neurologic workup with an aggressive cerebrospinal fluid investigation for evidence of neurosyphilis. Ceftriaxone compares favorably with intravenous penicillin for the treatment of neurosyphilis in HIV-infected patients. Patients with any stage of clinical syphilis should also be tested for HIV status.

Bai ZG, Yang KH, Liu YL, et al. Azithromycin vs. benzathine penicillin G for early syphilis: a meta-analysis of randomized clinical trials. *Int J STD AIDS.* 2008;19(4):217–221.

Gottlieb SL, Pope V, Sternberg MR, et al. Prevalence of syphilis seroreactivity in the United States: data from the National Health and Nutrition Examination Surveys (NHANES) 2001-2004. *Sex Transm Dis.* 2008;35(5):507–511.

McMillan A, Young H. Qualitative and quantitative aspects of the serological diagnosis of early syphilis. *Int J STD AIDS.* 2008;19(9):620–624.

Pialoux G, Vimont S, Moulignier A, Buteux M, Abraham B, Bonnard P. Effect of HIV infection on the course of syphilis. *AIDS Rev.* 2008;10(2):85–92.

Borrelia burgdorferi

Borrelia burgdorferi is a large, microaerophilic, plasmid-containing spirochete. When transmitted to humans and domestic animals through the bite of the *Ixodes* genus of ticks, this organism can cause both acute and chronic illness, now known as *Lyme disease*. First recognized in 1975, Lyme disease is the most common vectorborne infection in the United States. Although cases have been reported in nearly all states, clusters are apparent in the northeast Atlantic, the upper Midwest, and the Pacific southwest areas, corresponding to the distribution of the *Ixodes* tick population. The range of the disease extends throughout Europe and Asia.

The life cycle of the spirochete depends on its horizontal transmission through a mouse. Early in the summer, an infected *Ixodes* tick nymph (juvenile) bites a mouse, which becomes infected; then, in late summer, the infection is transmitted to an immature uninfected larva after it bites the infected mouse. This immature larva then molts to become a nymph, and the cycle is repeated. Once a nymph matures to an adult, its favorite host is the white-tailed deer, although it can survive with other hosts. Recently, it has been discovered that 2 other tickborne zoonoses (babesiosis and human granulocytic ehrlichiosis) can be cotransmitted with Lyme disease.

Stages

Lyme disease usually occurs in 3 stages following a tick bite: *localized (stage 1), disseminated (stage 2),* and *persistent (stage 3).* Localized disease (stage 1), present in 86% of infected patients, is characterized by skin involvement, initially as a red macule or papule, which later expands in a circular manner, usually with a bright red border and a central clear indurated area, known as *erythema chronicum migrans.* Hematogenous dissemination (stage 2) can then occur within days to weeks and is manifested as a flulike illness with headaches, fatigue, and musculoskeletal aching.

More profound symptoms occur as the infection localizes to the nervous, cardiovascular, and musculoskeletal systems (stage 3). Neurologic complications such as meningitis, encephalitis, cranial neuritis (including Bell palsy), radiculopathy, and neuropathy occur in 10%–15% of patients. A recent study from Boston revealed that Lyme disease was responsible for 34% of pediatric cases of acute facial nerve palsy. Cardiac manifestations include myopericarditis and variable heart block in 5% of patients. Unilateral asymmetric arthritis occurs in up to 80% of untreated patients.

Late persistent manifestations are usually confined to the nervous system, skin, and joints. Late neurologic signs include encephalomyelitis as well as demyelinating and psychiatric syndromes. Joint involvement includes asymmetric pauciarticular arthritis; skin involvement is characterized by localized scleroderma-type lesions or acrodermatitis chronica atrophicans.

Other systemic manifestations during the initial dissemination or the late persistent state include lymphadenopathy, conjunctivitis, keratitis, neuritis, uveitis, orbital myositis, hematuria, and orchitis. In some studies, serologic testing of patients with chronic fatigue syndrome has shown an increased incidence of positive *B burgdorferi* antibodies.

Diagnosis

During the early stages of infection, the immune response is minimal, with little cellular reactivity to *B burgdorferi* antigens and nonspecific elevation of IgM. During the disseminated phase, cellular antigenic response is markedly increased and specific IgM is followed by a polyclonal B-lymphocyte activation, with development of specific IgG antibody within weeks of the initial infection. Histopathology shows lymphocytic tissue infiltration, often in a perivascular distribution. Late manifestations may be either HLA-mediated autoimmune damage or prolonged latency followed by persistent infection.

Laboratory diagnosis of *B burgdorferi* infection depends on serodiagnosis. However, there is a poor recovery rate of positive serology from blood, cerebrospinal fluid, and synovial fluid during the early stages of infection. Skin-biopsy specimens with monoclonal antibody staining have demonstrated good sensitivity in identifying the organism. Although serodiagnosis remains the practical solution for establishing the diagnosis, laboratory methodology is not standardized.

The most commonly used serologic tests are the immunofluorescence antibody assay or the more sensitive *ELISA*. The ELISA is 50% sensitive during the early stages of the disease, and almost all symptomatic patients are seropositive during the later disseminated and persistent phases of the infection. These tests should be used only to support a clinical diagnosis of Lyme disease, not as the primary basis for making diagnostic or treatment decisions. Positive IgG and IgM ELISA results are usually confirmed with Western immunoblot testing. Serologic testing is not useful early in the course of Lyme disease because of the low sensitivity of tests in early disease. Serologic testing is more helpful in later disease, when the sensitivity and specificity are greater. False-positive results can occur in patients with syphilis, Rocky Mountain spotted fever, yaws, pinta, *B recurrentis,* and various rheumatologic disorders. PCR has been used to detect *B burgdorferi* DNA in serum and cerebrospinal fluid, but its sensitivity in neuroborreliosis is no better than that of the ELISA methods. Although the FTA-ABS test result for syphilis may be positive in patients with Lyme disease, the VDRL test result should be nonreactive.

Management

Treatment of *B burgdorferi* infection depends on the stage and the severity of the infection. Early Lyme disease is typically treated with oral doxycycline, amoxicillin, cefuroxime, or erythromycin. Mild disseminated disease is treated with oral doxycycline or amoxicillin. Serious disease (with cardiac or neurologic manifestations) is typically treated with ceftriaxone or high-dose penicillin G intravenously for up to 6 weeks. Patients who do not respond to the initial regimen may require alternate or combination therapy. Up to 15% of patients may develop a *Jarisch-Herxheimer reaction,* in which symptoms worsen during the first day of treatment.

Bacon RM, Kugeler KJ, Mead PS; Centers for Disease Control and Prevention (CDC). Surveillance for Lyme disease—United States, 1992-2006. *MMWR Surveill Summ.* 2008;57(10):1–9.

Bratton RL, Whiteside JW, Hovan MJ, Engle RL, Edwards FD. Diagnosis and treatment of Lyme disease. *Mayo Clin Proc.* 2008;83(5):566–571.

Halperin JJ. Nervous system Lyme disease. *Infect Dis Clin North Am.* 2008;22(2):261–274.

Marques A. Chronic Lyme disease: a review. *Infect Dis Clin North Am.* 2008;22(2):341–360.

Chlamydia trachomatis

Members of *Chlamydia trachomatis* are small, obligate, intracellular parasites that contain DNA and RNA and have a unique biphasic life cycle. These prokaryotes use the host cell's energy-generating capacity for their own reproduction. *C trachomatis* can survive only briefly outside the body. Transmitted by close contact, it is the most common sexually transmitted infection, with 4 million new cases per year. More than 15% of infected pregnant women and 10% of infected men are asymptomatic.

Infection is initiated by local inoculation and ingestion of the organism by phagocytes, followed by intracellular reproduction and eventual spread to other cells. The mechanism for immunologic eradication of *Chlamydia* is uncertain but appears to involve cell-mediated immunity. Infections in humans include trachoma, inclusion conjunctivitis, nongonococcal urethritis, epididymitis, mucopurulent cervicitis, proctitis, salpingitis, infant pneumonia syndrome, and lymphogranuloma venereum. Genital *C trachomatis* infection can result in pelvic inflammatory disease, tubal infertility, and ectopic pregnancy. In one study, 80% of ocular adnexal lymphoma samples carried DNA of a related organism, *Chlamydia psittaci,* suggesting an etiologic role of the organism in some cases of lymphoma.

Another recent study revealed a 12-fold increase in the risk of progression of age-related macular degeneration (AMD) in patients with the Y4203H variant of the complement factor H (*CFH)* gene, along with an elevated titer of antibodies to *C pneumoniae.* Smoking was a significant risk factor for AMD progression in this study as well.

Diagnostic techniques include culture, direct immunofluorescent antibody testing of exudates, enzyme immunoassay, and DNA probes using PCR.

Chlamydial infections are readily treated with tetracycline, erythromycin, or one of the quinolones or newer macrolides. Although single-dose azithromycin or sparfloxacin therapy for urethritis and cervicitis has proven effective in some studies, it is usually recommended that patients continue treatment for at least 7 days to ensure complete eradication. Sexual partners of patients with *Chlamydia* infections, as well as other sexually transmitted diseases, should be examined and counseled for consideration of antibiotic treatment as well.

Ferreri AJ, Guidoboni M, Ponzoni M, et al. Evidence for an association between Chlamydia psittaci and ocular adnexal lymphomas. *J Natl Cancer Inst.* 2004;96(8):586–594.

Gaydos CA, Ferrero DV, Papp J. Laboratory aspects of screening men for Chlamydia trachomatis in the new millennium. *Sex Transm Dis.* 2008;35(11 Suppl):S45–S50.

Karunakaran KP, Rey-Ladino J, Stoynov N, et al. Immunoproteomic discovery of novel T cell antigens from the obligate intracellular pathogen Chlamydia. *J Immunol.* 2008;180(4):2459–2465.

Mycoplasma pneumoniae

Mycoplasma pneumoniae is a unique bacterium that may cause multiple disorders—including pharyngitis, otitis media, tracheobronchitis, pneumonia, endocarditis, nephritis, encephalitis, meningitis, optic neuritis, and facial nerve palsy—and has been implicated in some cases of chronic fatigue and fibromyalgia syndromes. Recent serologic studies indicate that *M pneumoniae,* varicella-zoster, and *B burgdorferi* cause the majority of cases of Bell palsy.

Serious *M pneumoniae* infections requiring hospitalization occur in both adults and children and may involve multiple organ systems. Extrapulmonary complications involving all the major organ systems can occur in association with *M pneumoniae* infection as a result of direct invasion or autoimmune response. Recent evidence suggests that *M pneumoniae* may play a contributory role in chronic lung disorders such as asthma.

PCR assays have been adapted for the direct detection of *M pneumoniae* organisms, but in clinical practice, sensitive serologic tests are usually used initially to detect antibodies. Initial treatment of *M pneumoniae* infections usually involves use of a macrolide, tetracycline, or fluoroquinolone.

Atkinson TP, Balish MF, Waites KB. Epidemiology, clinical manifestations, pathogenesis and laboratory detection of Mycoplasma pneumoniae infections. *FEMS Microbiol Rev.* 2008; 32(6):956–973.

Defilippi A, Silvestri M, Tacchella A, et al. Epidemiology and clinical features of Mycoplasma pneumoniae infection in children. *Respir Med.* 2008;102(12):1762–1768.

Martínez MA, Ruiz M, Zunino E, Luchsinger V, Avendaño LF. Detection of Mycoplasma pneumoniae in adult community-acquired pneumonia by PCR and serology. *J Med Microbiol.* 2008;57(Pt 12):1491–1495.

Nilsson AC, Björkman P, Persson K. Polymerase chain reaction is superior to serology for the diagnosis of acute Mycoplasma pneumoniae infection and reveals a high rate of persistent infection. *BMC Microbiol.* 2008;8:93.

Mycobacteria

Mycobacteria include a range of pathogenic and nonpathogenic species distributed widely in the environment. *Mycobacterium tuberculosis* is the most significant human pathogenic species. *M tuberculosis* infects an estimated 1.8 billion persons worldwide (32% global prevalence) and causes approximately 2 million deaths each year. There are at least 8 million new cases of tuberculosis each year, most of these occurring in Africa and Southeast Asia. *Nontuberculous mycobacteria* may be responsible for up to 5% of all clinical mycobacterial infections. Atypical mycobacterial infections are more prevalent in immunosuppressed patients, including those with AIDS. Infections caused by nontuberculous mycobacteria include lymphadenitis, pulmonary infections, skin granulomas, prosthetic valve infections, and bacteremia. Despite their low virulence, atypical mycobacterial infections are difficult to treat because of resistance to standard antituberculous regimens.

Tuberculosis

Tuberculosis (TB) infection usually occurs through inhalation of infective droplets and, in rare cases, by way of the skin or gastrointestinal tract. Cell-mediated hypersensitivity to tuberculoprotein develops 3–9 weeks after infection, with a typical granulomatous response that slows or contains bacterial multiplication. Most organisms die during the fibrotic phase of the response. Reactivation is usually associated with depressed immunity and aging. Systemic spread occurs with reactivation and results in a granulomatous response to the infected foci. Acquired immunity is cell-mediated but incomplete, and the role of delayed hypersensitivity is complex: high degrees of sensitivity to tuberculoprotein can cause caseous necrosis, which leads to spread of the disease. Infections include pulmonary involvement, which can lead to systemic spread with involvement of any organ system.

Laboratory diagnosis involves culture of infective material on Lowenstein-Jensen medium for 6–8 weeks and use of the acid-fast type of Ziehl-Neelsen stain or fluorescent antibody staining of infected material. In addition, DNA probes using PCR techniques for *M tuberculosis* and other mycobacteria are available. Newer PCR assays can identify resistant strains of TB by detecting isoniazid and rifampin resistance mutations in organisms from cultures or from smear-positive specimens.

The tuberculin skin test measures delayed hypersensitivity to tuberculoprotein. Purified protein derivative (PPD) produced from a culture filtrate of *M tuberculosis* is standardized and its activity expressed as tuberculin units (TU). A positive PPD reaction is defined as an area of induration 10 mm or greater in the area of intradermal injection of 0.1 mL of PPD read 48–72 hours later. For children, the tine test is an easily administered alternative to the PPD. In 2005, the QuantiFERON-TB Gold test received final approval from the FDA as an alternative to the PPD skin test. This test detects the release of interferon-γ from sensitized patients. Its specificity is higher, but the sensitivity is similar to that of the PPD skin test. It also appears to be less affected by previous BCG (bacille Calmette-Guérin) vaccination.

The BCG vaccine causes false-positive reactions to the PPD skin test and thus interferes with the efficacy of the test as a diagnostic and epidemiologic tool. The false-positive effect of BCG decreases over time, so PPD may still be useful in patients with previous BCG administration.

Among patients in whom skin testing yields positive results, the overall risk of reactivation of the disease is 3%–5%. A positive PPD test result should be considered in light of the individual patient's radiologic and clinical data as well as age to determine the need for prophylactic treatment. Administration of isoniazid daily for 1 year reduces the risk of reactivation by 80%; however, the risk of isoniazid hepatotoxicity increases with age and alcohol use. Nevertheless, patients with a positive tuberculin skin test result who require long-term high-dose corticosteroids or other immunosuppressive agents should be treated prophylactically with isoniazid for the duration of their immunosuppressive therapy in order to prevent reactivation.

Treatment of active infection involves use of 2 or 3 drugs because of the emergence of resistance and of delay in culture susceptibility studies. Standard regimens employ multiple drugs for 18–24 months, but with the addition of newer agents, treatment for 6–9 months has been found equally effective. Drugs currently used include isoniazid, rifampin, rifabutin, ethambutol, streptomycin, pyrazinamide, aminosalicylic acid, ethionamide, and cycloserine. All of the agents currently used have toxic side effects, especially hepatic and neurologic, which should be carefully monitored during the course of therapy. Isoniazid and ethambutol can cause optic neuritis in a small percentage of patients, and rifampin may cause pink-tinged tears and blepharoconjunctivitis.

Outbreaks of nosocomial and community-acquired multidrug-resistant TB (MDRTB) have increased, particularly in the presence of concurrent HIV infection. MDRTB in patients infected with HIV is associated with widely disseminated disease, poor treatment response, and substantial mortality. Infection has also been documented in health care workers exposed to these patients. MDRTB represents a serious public health threat that will require an aggressive governmental and medical response to limit its spread. Newer fluoroquinolones and some of the newer classes of broad-spectrum antibiotics, such as linezolid, are effective against many isolates of MDRTB, as well as against atypical mycobacteria, and have been recommended as potential therapeutic alternatives.

Dover LG, Bhatt A, Bhowruth V, Willcox BE, Besra GS. New drugs and vaccines for drug-resistant Mycobacterium tuberculosis infections. *Expert Rev Vaccines.* 2008;7(5):481–497.

Ly LH, McMurray DN. Tuberculosis: vaccines in the pipeline. *Expert Rev Vaccines.* 2008;7(5): 635–650.

Takahashi T, Tamura M, Asami Y, et al. Novel wide-range quantitative nested real-time PCR assay for Mycobacterium tuberculosis DNA: development and methodology. *J Clin Microbiol.* 2008;46(5):1708–1715.

van Doorn HR, An DD, de Jong MD, et al. Fluoroquinolone resistance detection in Mycobacterium tuberculosis with locked nucleic acid probe real-time PCR. *Int J Tuberc Lung Dis.* 2008;12(7):736–742.

Fungal Infections

Candida albicans is a yeast that is normally present in the oral cavity, lower gastrointestinal tract, and female genital tract. Under conditions of disrupted local defenses or depressed immunity, overgrowth and parenchymal invasion occur, with the potential for systemic spread. Increased virulence of *Candida* is related to its mycelial phase, when it is more resistant to the host's cellular immune system, which acts as the primary modulator of infection. Infections include oral lesions (thrush) and vaginal, skin, esophageal, and urinary tract involvement. Chronic mucocutaneous lesions may occur in persons with specific T-lymphocyte defects. Disseminated disease can involve any organ system, most commonly the kidneys, brain, heart, and eyes, and is more common in immune-compromised patients and those with indwelling vascular catheters.

Other important invasive fungal infections are cryptococcosis, histoplasmosis, blastomycosis, aspergillosis, and coccidioidomycosis. Invasive fungal infections have become a major problem in immunocompromised patients. Fungal PCR assays provide more rapid diagnosis of serious fungal infections than do fungal cultures, while offering increased sensitivity.

Treatment of serious systemic infections has traditionally involved the use of intravenous amphotericin B, sometimes in combined therapy with flucytosine or an imidazole. Lipid complex and liposome-encapsulated formulations of amphotericin B (AmBisome, Amphotec) were developed to reduce the drug's nephrotoxicity and myelosuppression. A controlled study revealed that intravenous amphotericin B prophylaxis reduced the incidence of systemic fungal infections in immunocompromised patients with leukemia. Newer imidazoles, such as fluconazole, itraconazole, and voriconazole, are less toxic and better-tolerated alternatives. In fact, itraconazole has replaced ketoconazole as the treatment of choice for nonmeningeal, non–life-threatening cases of histoplasmosis, blastomycosis, and paracoccidioidomycosis. Itraconazole is also effective in treating patients with cryptococcosis and coccidioidomycosis, including those with meningitis. A new monoclonal antifungal antibody (Mycograb) is an experimental therapy for refractory invasive fungal infections.

Lehmann LE, Hunfeld KP, Emrich T, et al. A multiplex real-time PCR assay for rapid detection and differentiation of 25 bacterial and fungal pathogens from whole blood samples. *Med Microbiol Immunol.* 2008;197(3):313–324.

Prasad PA, Coffin SE, Leckerman KH, Walsh TJ, Zaoutis TE. Pediatric antifungal utilization: new drugs, new trends. *Pediatr Infect Dis J.* 2008;27(12):1083–1088.

Scheinfeld N. Ketoconazole: a review of a workhorse antifungal molecule with a focus on new foam and gel formulations. *Drugs Today.* 2008;44(5):369–380.

Subirà M, Martino R, Gómez L, Martí JM, Estany C, Sierra J. Low-dose amphotericin B lipid complex vs. conventional amphotericin B for empirical antifungal therapy of neutropenic fever in patients with hematologic malignancies—a randomized, controlled trial. *Eur J Haematol.* 2004;72(5):342–347.

Toxoplasma

Toxoplasmosis is caused by infection with the protozoan parasite *Toxoplasma gondii,* which infects up to a third of the world's population. Acute infections may be asymptomatic in pregnant women, but they can be transmitted to the fetus and cause severe complications, including mental retardation, blindness, and epilepsy. As many as 4000 new cases of congenital toxoplasmosis occur each year in the United States. Of the nearly 750 US deaths attributed to toxoplasmosis each year, approximately half are believed to be caused by eating contaminated undercooked or raw meat. Toxoplasma can also be transmitted to humans by ingestion of oocysts, an environmentally resistant form of the organism, through exposure to cat feces, water, or soil containing the parasite or from eating unwashed contaminated fruits or vegetables.

Toxoplasma infection can be prevented in large part by cooking meat to a safe temperature, peeling or thoroughly washing fruits and vegetables before eating, and cleaning cooking surfaces and utensils after they have contacted raw meat. Pregnant women should avoid changing cat litter and handling raw or undercooked meat. Also, they should keep cats indoors, where cats are less likely to eat infected prey and subsequently acquire toxoplasma.

Primary infection is usually subclinical, but in some patients cervical lymphadenopathy or ocular disease can be present. The ocular manifestations include uveitis and chorioretinitis with macular scarring. The clinical picture and histopathology of toxoplasmosis are a reflection of the immune response, which includes an early humoral response, followed by the cellular response, which varies from low-grade mononuclear infiltrate to total tissue destruction. In immunocompromised patients, reactivation of latent disease can cause life-threatening encephalitis.

Diagnosis of toxoplasmosis can be established by direct detection of the parasite or by serologic techniques. Real-time PCR is a very sensitive technique for diagnosing infection caused by *T gondii* and for determining the precise genotype of the organism. The most commonly used therapeutic regimen, and probably the most effective, comprises a combination of pyrimethamine with sulfadiazine and folinic acid. Recently, sulfadiazine has been replaced by sulfadoxine, which has a longer half-life and provides a dosing schedule resulting in improved compliance. Newer drugs with activity against *T gondii* include azithromycin, atovaquone, and clindamycin.

Alfonso Y, Fraga J, Cox R, et al. Comparison of four DNA extraction methods from cerebrospinal fluid for the detection of Toxoplasma gondii by polymerase chain reaction in AIDS patients. *Med Sci Monit.* 2008;14(3):MT1–MT6.

Fricker-Hidalgo H, Bulabois CE, Brenier-Pinchart MP, et al. Diagnosis of toxoplasmosis after allogeneic stem cell transplantation: results of DNA detection and serological techniques. *Clin Infect Dis.* 2009;48(2):e9–e15.

Montoya JG, Liesenfeld O. Toxoplasmosis. *Lancet.* 2004;363(9425):1965–1976.

Rothova A. Ocular manifestations of toxoplasmosis. *Curr Opin Ophthalmol.* 2003;14(6): 384–388.

Herpesvirus

As a class, viruses are strictly intracellular parasites, relying on the host cell for their replication. Herpesviruses, which are large-enveloped, double-stranded DNA viruses, are one of the most common human infectious agents, responsible for a wide spectrum of acute and chronic diseases. The major members of the group are herpes simplex viruses (HSV-1 and HSV-2), varicella-zoster virus (VZV), cytomegalovirus (CMV), and Epstein-Barr virus (EBV). There are now 8 recognized types of human herpesviruses: herpesvirus 1 is HSV-1; type 2 is HSV-2; type 3 is VZV; type 4 is EBV; type 5 is CMV; types 6 and 7, Roseolovirus, cause roseola infantum and encephalitis; and type 8 is associated with Kaposi sarcoma and HIV-related lymphomas.

Herpes Simplex

Herpes simplex virus has 2 antigenic types, each with numerous antigenic strains. Each type has different epidemiologic patterns of infection. Seroepidemiologic studies show a high prevalence of HSV-1 antibodies with a lower prevalence of HSV-2 antibodies. Many people with HSV antibodies are asymptomatic. Infection is modulated by a predominantly cellular response. The presence of high titers of neutralizing antibodies to HSV does not seem to retard the cell-to-cell transmission of the virus, which can spread within nerves and cause a latent infection of sensory and autonomic ganglia. Reactivation of HSV from the trigeminal ganglia may be associated with asymptomatic excretion or with the development of mucosal herpetic ulceration. Serologic testing, DNA PCR testing, and viral culture can help diagnose difficult cases, particularly CNS infections.

Herpes simplex type 1 is associated with mucocutaneous superficial infections of the pharynx, skin, oral cavity, vagina, eye, and brain. Ophthalmic infection most often manifests as corneal dendritic or stromal disease but may present as acute retinal necrosis. (The ocular manifestations of HSV infection are discussed in more detail in BCSC Section 8, *External Disease and Cornea,* Section 9, *Intraocular Inflammation and Uveitis,* and Section 12, *Retina and Vitreous.*) Herpes encephalitis carries a 15% mortality rate. *Herpes simplex type 2* is an important sexually transmitted disease that is associated with genital infections, aseptic meningitis, and congenital infection. *Neonatal herpes infection* involves multiple systems and, if untreated, has a mortality rate as high as 80%.

The drug of choice for treating acute systemic infections is acyclovir. Localized disease can be treated with oral acyclovir. Topical treatment of skin or mucocutaneous lesions with acyclovir ointment decreases the healing time. Oral acyclovir can also be used pro- phylactically for severe and recurrent genital herpes. Long-term suppressive oral acyclovir (400 mg twice a day) also reduces the recurrence of herpes simplex epithelial keratitis and stromal keratitis. Intravenous acyclovir is used in the treatment of herpes encephalitis.

Two newer antiviral agents, famciclovir and valacyclovir, are approved for the treat- ment of herpes zoster and herpes simplex. Compared with acyclovir, these agents have better bioavailability and achieve higher blood levels. HSV is also sensitive to vidarabine. Cidofovir, an antiviral drug used for treating CMV infections, is also very effective against acyclovir-resistant herpes simplex.

Varicella-Zoster

Varicella-zoster virus, also sometimes referred to as *herpes zoster*, produces infection in a manner similar to that of herpes simplex. After a primary infection, the virus remains latent in dorsal root ganglia, with host cellular immune interaction inhibiting reactivation. Primary infection usually occurs in childhood in the form of chickenpox (varicella), a gen- eralized vesicular rash accompanied by mild constitutional symptoms. Reactivation may be heralded by pain in a sensory nerve distribution, followed by a unilateral vesicular erup- tion occurring over 1 to 3 dermatomic areas. New crops of lesions appear in the same area within 7 days. Resolution of the lesions may be followed by postherpetic neuralgia. Other neurologic sequelae following VZV reactivation include segmental myelitis, Guillain- Barré syndrome, and Ramsay Hunt syndrome. The incidence of VZV is 2 to 3 times higher in patients older than age 60. Postherpetic neuralgia occurs after VZV infection in ap- proximately 50% of patients older than 50 years. The pain of postherpetic neuralgia can be severe and debilitating and may persist for months or even years. Immunosuppressed persons experience recurrent lesions and an increased incidence of disseminated disease.

Recommended 7-day treatment regimens of immunocompetent adults with cutane- ous VZV infection include famciclovir (Famvir) 500 mg 2 times daily, valacyclovir (Val- trex) 100 mg 3 times a day, or acyclovir 800 mg 5 times daily.

Treatment of acute infection in immunocompromised patients or those with vis- ceral involvement may include acyclovir, famciclovir, or valacyclovir. Newer drugs being evaluated for resistant VZV strains or concomitant HIV infection include sorivudine, brivudine, fialuridine, fiacitabine, netivudine, lobucavir, foscarnet, and cidofovir. A live attenuated varicella vaccine (Varivax), available for prevention of primary disease, also reduces the incidence of recurrent VZV infection and neuralgia. This vaccine is recom- mended for children, patients with chronic diseases or leukemia, and patients receiving immunosuppressive therapy. In some patients, tricyclic antidepressants, carbamazepine, gabapentin (Neurontin), and topical capsaicin cream reduce the pain of postherpetic neu- ralgia. For refractory cases, transcutaneous electronic nerve stimulation or nerve blocks are sometimes helpful.

Engelmann I, Petzold DR, Kosinska A, Hepkema BG, Schulz TF, Heim A. Rapid quantitative PCR assays for the simultaneous detection of herpes simplex virus, varicella zoster virus, cytomegalovirus, Epstein-Barr virus, and human herpesvirus 6 DNA in blood and other clinical specimens. *J Med Virol.* 2008;80(3):467–477.

Hjalmarsson A, Blomqvist P, Sköldenberg B. Herpes simplex encephalitis in Sweden, 1990-2001: incidence, morbidity, and mortality. *Clin Infect Dis.* 2007;45(7):875–880.

Plentz A, Jilg W, Kochanowski B, Ibach B, Knöll A. Detection of herpesvirus DNA in cerebrospinal fluid and correlation with clinical symptoms. *Infection.* 2008;36(2):158–162.

Shafran SD, Tyring SK, Ashton R, et al. Once, twice, or three times daily famciclovir compared with acyclovir for the oral treatment of herpes zoster in immunocompetent adults: a randomized, multicenter, double-blind clinical trial. *J Clin Virol.* 2004;29(4):248–253.

Cytomegalovirus

Cytomegalovirus is a ubiquitous human virus: 50% of adults in developed countries harbor antibodies, which are usually acquired during the first 5 years of life. The virus can be isolated from all body fluids, even in the presence of circulating neutralizing antibody, for up to several years after infection. Serologic and PCR testing are available to assist in the diagnosis of CMV infection. Presence of the pp65 antigen, as detected by PCR, indicates the need for preemptive therapy against CMV.

Congenital CMV disease carries a 20% incidence of hearing loss or mental retardation and a 0.1% incidence of various other severe congenital disorders, including jaundice, hepatosplenomegaly, anemia, microcephaly, and chorioretinitis. Infections in adults include heterophile-negative mononucleosis, pneumonia, hepatitis, and Guillain-Barré syndrome. In immunocompromised patients, CMV interstitial pneumonia carries a 90% mortality rate. Disseminated spread to the gastrointestinal tract, CNS, and eyes is common in patients with AIDS. Latent infection within leukocytes accounts for transfusion-associated disease. Recent cases of CMV retinitis have been reported following intravitreous corticosteroid injections. CMV replication itself can further suppress cell-mediated immunity, with resultant depressed lymphocyte response and development of severe opportunistic infections.

CMV retinitis is initially treated with ganciclovir, which is administered via intravenous, oral, or intravitreal routes. A slow-release intraocular ganciclovir insert is also available for the treatment of CMV retinitis. Intravenous foscarnet (Foscavir), cidofovir (Vistide), fomivirsen (Vitravene), and leflunomide are also effective in the treatment of CMV retinitis. One study showed that intravitreal cidofovir given at 6-week intervals was highly effective for treating CMV retinitis. Valganciclovir (Valcyte) is a well-tolerated, newer oral agent that is highly effective in the treatment of CMV infection, including retinitis.

Allice T, Cerutti F, Pittaluga F, et al. Evaluation of a novel real-time PCR system for cytomegalovirus DNA quantitation on whole blood and correlation with pp65-antigen test in guiding pre-emptive antiviral treatment. *J Virol Methods.* 2008;148(1-2):9–16.

Lazzarotto T, Guerra B, Lanari M, Gabrielli L, Landini MP. New advances in the diagnosis of congenital cytomegalovirus infection. *J Clin Virol.* 2008;41(3):192–197.

Razonable RR, Paya CV. Valganciclovir for the prevention and treatment of cytomegalovirus disease in immunocompromised hosts. *Expert Rev Anti Infect Ther.* 2004;2(1):27–41.

Epstein-Barr Virus

Epstein-Barr virus antibodies are found in 90%–95% of all adults. Childhood infections are usually asymptomatic, with symptomatic disease occurring in young adults. Infectious mononucleosis is the usual clinical disease in most symptomatic adults. Transplant recipients on cyclosporine or patients with AIDS may develop lymphoproliferative disorders. EBV is epidemiologically associated with Burkitt lymphoma and nasopharyngeal carcinoma and has been reported in EBV-associated hemophagocytic lymphohistiocytosis (EBV-HLH), also known as *EBV-associated hemophagocytic syndrome,* which develops mostly in children and young adults and may be fatal. EBV also has been reported as a cause of pediatric acute renal failure. A highly sensitive PCR assay is available for detecting primary EBV infection and infectious mononucleosis.

Treatment of acute disease is largely supportive, although the EBV DNA polymerase is sensitive to acyclovir and ganciclovir, which decrease viral replication in tissue culture. No vaccine is currently available against EBV, but research is ongoing toward developing a cytotoxic T-lymphocyte–based vaccine.

Imashuku S, Kuriyama K, Sakai R, et al. Treatment of Epstein-Barr virus-associated hemo-phagocytic lymphohistiocytosis (EBV-HLH) in young adults: a report from the HLH study center. *Med Pediatr Oncol.* 2003;41(2):103–109.

Paramita DK, Fachiroh J, Haryana SM, Middledorp JM. Evaluation of commercial EBV Recomb-Line assay for diagnosis of nasopharyngeal carcinoma. *J Clin Virol.* 2008;42(4):343–352.

Rey J, Xerri L, Bouabdallah R, Keuppens M, Brousset P, Meggetto F. Detection of different clonal EBV strains in Hodgkin lymphoma and nasopharyngeal carcinoma tissues from the same patient. *Br J Haematol.* 2008;142(1):79–81.

Influenza

See Chapter 13 for a discussion of influenza and immunization.

Hepatitis

Hepatitis A

Hepatitis A is usually transmitted by the oral route and may be acquired from contaminated water supplies and unwashed or poorly cooked foods. Patients at high risk (travelers to endemic areas, military personnel, drug abusers, family contacts of infected patients, and laboratory workers exposed to the virus) should be given the hepatitis A vaccine (Havrix). Many adults in the United States are already immune, so antibody testing can be performed first, followed by vaccination if antibodies are not present.

Hepatitis B

See Chapter 13 for a discussion of hepatitis B and immunization.

Hepatitis C and Other Forms of Hepatitis

Approximately 20%–40% of acute viral hepatitis cases reported in the United States are of the non-A, non-B type; of this group, the majority of cases are caused by the hepatitis C virus (HCV). Worldwide prevalence is approximately 1%. Current estimates suggest that 170,000 new cases of HCV occur annually in the United States; 50%–80% of these patients develop evidence of chronic hepatitis, and 20% of these patients develop cirrhosis. Only 6% of reported cases of hepatitis C are transfusion-related. Other recognized risk factors for hepatitis C transmission include parenteral drug use, hemodialysis, and occupational exposure to blood. Although the role of sexual activity in the transmission of HCV remains to be fully elucidated, this mode is clearly not a predominant source of transmission. Of all the hepatitis viruses, HCV causes the most damage in immunocompetent hosts because of direct hepatocyte cytotoxicity and may result in cirrhosis, fulminant hepatitis, and hepatocellular carcinoma. At present, cirrhosis from HCV infection is the most common indication for liver transplantation in the United States.

A sensitive enzyme immunoassay has been developed for detecting and quantifying total HCV core antigen in anti-HCV-positive or anti-HCV-negative sera. Also, a 1-step PCR assay is available to detect HCV RNA and provide HCV genotyping.

Treatment of acute hepatitis C infection with interferon-α_{2a} reduces the rate of acute infections converting to chronic hepatitis C infections. The current treatment of choice for chronic active hepatitis C is combination therapy with peginterferon-α_{2a} and the antiviral agent ribavirin. This combination can achieve up to 80% response rates for hepatitis C genotypes 2 and 3 and approximately a 50% response rate for patients with genotype 1, cirrhosis, or nonresponse to previous treatments. Management of chronic persistent hepatitis C is largely supportive, but some studies advocate prolonged therapy with peginterferon. No vaccine is currently available against HCV, but researchers are hopeful that a vaccine will soon be developed.

Chronic delta hepatitis is a severe form of chronic liver disease caused by hepatitis delta virus (hepatitis D virus) infection superimposed on chronic hepatitis B. Both interferon-α_{2a} and lamivudine have been found to be beneficial in treating chronic hepatitis D infection.

Hepatitis E virus is a small, nonenveloped RNA virus that is transmitted enterically and causes sporadic as well as epidemic acute viral hepatitis in many developing countries. As a superinfection in patients with preexisting chronic liver disease, hepatitis E may cause severe liver decompensation, often complicated by hepatic encephalopathy and renal failure. Acute hepatitis E in these patients has a protracted course, with high morbidity and mortality.

Hepatitis G virus may cause coinfection with HBV or HCV but usually does not increase their pathogenicity. GB virus C and the hepatitis G virus (GBV-C/HGV) are variants of the same RNA flavivirus, which has been found to be a lymphotropic virus that replicates primarily in the spleen and bone marrow.

Transfusion-transmitted virus (TTV) is a virus identified in a small percentage of patients with non-A, G posttransfusion hepatitis. In some patients, the virus causes coinfection with hepatitis C. TTV DNA is common in high-risk populations, such as patients with hemophilia, those on hemodialysis, and intravenous drug abusers. TTV has recently been implicated alone, as well as in coinfection with EBV, as a potential cause of 30%–50% of cases of lymphoma and Hodgkin disease.

Aitken CK, Lewis J, Tracy SL, et al. High incidence of hepatitis C virus reinfection in a cohort of injecting drug users. *Hepatology.* 2008;48(6):1746–1752.

Brant LJ, Ramsay ME, Balogun MA, et al. Diagnosis of acute hepatitis C virus infection and estimated incidence in low- and high-risk English populations. *J Viral Hepat.* 2008;15(12): 871–877.

Farci P, Roskams T, Chessa L, et al. Long-term benefit of interferon alpha therapy of chronic hepatitis D: regression of advanced hepatic fibrosis. *Gastroenterology.* 2004;126(7):1740–1749.

Fried MW, Hadziyannis SJ. Treatment of chronic hepatitis C infection with peginterferons plus ribavirin. *Semin Liver Dis.* 2004;24(suppl 2):47–54.

Tang YW, Li H, Roberto A, Warner D, Yen-Lieberman B. Detection of hepatitis C virus by a user-developed reverse transcriptase-PCR and use of amplification products for subsequent genotyping. *J Clin Virol.* 2004;31(2):148–152.

Human Papillomavirus

Human papillomavirus (HPV) infection is highly prevalent and is closely associated with condylomata (genital warts), cervical intraepithelial neoplasia, cervical cancer (95% of cervical cancers contain HPV DNA), conjunctival intraepithelial neoplasia, and some cases of head and neck squamous cell carcinoma. A recent review suggests that HPV has a possible etiologic role in some cases of lung adenocarcinoma as well. More than 50% of all persons are infected with HPV during their lifetimes, via either intrauterine or sexually transmitted infection. HPV can be detected with PCR assay techniques, and women at high risk for HPV should receive HPV testing at the time of the Papanicolaou (Pap) test. Vaccines to prevent HPV infection and its sequelae have recently become available. HPV in association with cervical cancer is discussed further in Chapter 13.

Cuzick J, Arbyn M, Sankaranarayanan R, et al. Overview of human papillomavirus-based and other novel options for cervical cancer screening in developed and developing countries. *Vaccine.* 2008;26(Suppl 10):K29–K41.

Fisher R, Darrow DH, Tranter M, Williams JV. Human papillomavirus vaccine: recommendations, issues and controversies. *Curr Opin Pediatr.* 2008;20(4):441–445.

Gillison ML. Human papillomavirus-associated head and neck cancer is a distinct epidemiologic, clinical, and molecular entity. *Semin Oncol.* 2004;31(6):744–754.

Heymann WR. The human papillomavirus vaccine. *J Am Acad Dermatol.* 2008;58(6): 1047–1048.

Acquired Immunodeficiency Syndrome

During the 1980s, AIDS emerged as a major public health problem. AIDS was originally described in 1981, when *Pneumocystis carinii* pneumonia (PCP) and Kaposi sarcoma were noted to occur in homosexual men and intravenous drug abusers. Since then, the number of cases has increased exponentially. In 1983, it was discovered that AIDS was caused by the retrovirus HIV (human immunodeficiency virus). Subsequently, it became evident that HIV caused a spectrum of disease, including an asymptomatic carrier state, the AIDS-related complex (ARC), and AIDS itself.

As of the end of 2006, an estimated 982,498 cases of AIDS in the United States have been reported to the CDC. The total cumulative number of deaths of persons reported with AIDS was 545,805. It is estimated that over 1.1 million Americans are currently infected with HIV, with more than 25% of these persons unaware that they are infected. In 2006, an estimated 56,300 new cases of HIV infection occurred in the United States. Over 70% of these new cases are males, and half of them are younger than 25 years. On the positive side, improved antiretroviral therapy in recent years has resulted in a significant decline in the number of AIDS cases in the United States and a 70% reduction in deaths due to AIDS since 1995. Further, AIDS is no longer the leading cause of death in young adults in the United States.

Worldwide, AIDS continues to take a devastating toll, particularly in countries of sub-Saharan Africa and in Asian nations with large, impoverished populations. However, the number of cases per year has actually decreased in recent years, due to increasing awareness and funding of HIV prevention and treatment programs.

According to the Joint United Nations Program on HIV/AIDS, as of the end of 2007, 33 million people were estimated to be living with HIV/AIDS, and 2.7 million more people became infected during that year. Approximately two thirds of those infected live in sub-Saharan Africa and 20% live in Asia and the Pacific. An estimated 28 million people have died from AIDS since the epidemic began, including 13 million women and 6 million children younger than age 15. In 2007 alone, AIDS caused the deaths of an estimated 2 million people, including nearly 500,000 children younger than age 15. Women are increasingly affected by HIV: approximately 50% of the estimated 33 million adults now living with HIV or AIDS worldwide are women. The overwhelming majority of people with HIV, approximately 95% of the global total, are in developing countries. In Africa and Asia, HIV causes more loss of productivity than any other disease. It is estimated that 16,000 new infections occur worldwide each day. More than 50% of the infections are in young adults between the ages of 15 and 25. Only 10% of the world's HIV-infected people know that they are infected. More than 15 million children have been orphaned because of HIV infection of 1 or both of their parents.

Etiology and Pathogenesis

AIDS is caused by infection with HIV (HIV-1), previously known as the human T-lymphotropic virus type 3 (HTLV-3), lymphadenopathy-associated virus, and AIDS-related virus. Thus far, there are 9 known serotypes of HIV-1 group M, and 1 each of HIV-1 groups O and N. In the United States, HIV-1 group M, serotype B is the most common form of HIV. Another human T-lymphotropic virus, HIV-2, has been isolated from West Africans and is associated with AIDS as well. HIV-2 is closely related to simian immunodeficiency virus.

HIV belongs to a family of viruses known as *retroviruses*. A retrovirus encodes its genetic information in RNA and uses a unique viral enzyme called *reverse transcriptase* to copy its genome into DNA. Other members of this retrovirus family include the human

T-lymphotropic retrovirus type 1 (HTLV-1), which can cause adult T-lymphocyte leukemia and chronic progressive myelopathy with atrophy of the spinal cord. HTLV-2 is associated with hairy cell leukemia.

HIV preferentially infects T lymphocytes, especially helper T (CD4$^+$) lymphocytes. The virus infects mature T lymphocytes in vitro, although other cells can serve as targets. CD4 is the phenotypic marker for this subset and is identified by monoclonal antibodies OKT4 and Leu3.

The hallmark of the immunodeficiency in AIDS is a depletion of the CD4$^+$ helper-inducer T lymphocytes. HIV selectively infects these lymphocytes as well as macrophages; with HIV replication, the helper T lymphocyte is killed. Because of the central role of the helper T lymphocyte in the immune response, loss of this subset results in a profound immune deficiency, leading to the life-threatening opportunistic infections indicative of AIDS. This selective depletion of CD4$^+$ helper T lymphocytes leads to the characteristic inverted CD4$^+$/CD8$^+$ ratio (also known as the *T4/T8 ratio*). Years may pass between the initial HIV infection and the development of these immune abnormalities.

In addition to the cellular immune deficiency, patients with AIDS have abnormalities of B-lymphocyte function. These patients fail to mount an antibody response to novel T lymphocyte–dependent B-lymphocyte challenges, although they have B-lymphocyte hyperfunction with polyclonal B-lymphocyte activation, hypergammaglobulinemia, and circulating immune complexes. This B-lymphocyte hyperfunction may be a direct consequence of HIV infection: studies have demonstrated that polyclonal activation can be induced in vitro by adding HIV to B lymphocytes.

HIV has also been documented to infect the brains of patients with AIDS. It is thought that HIV infection of the brain is responsible for the HIV encephalopathy syndrome. HIV-infected cells in the brain have generally been identified as macrophages.

Clinical Syndromes

The clinical syndrome of AIDS consists of recurrent severe opportunistic infections or unusual neoplasms. In 1982, the CDC published an original case definition of AIDS as the presence of a reliably diagnosed disease at least moderately indicative of an underlying cellular immune deficiency (Kaposi sarcoma in a patient younger than 60 years, PCP, or other opportunistic infection) and the absence of known causes of an underlying immune deficiency or of any other stage of resistance reported to be associated with the disease (immunosuppressive therapy, lymphoreticular malignancy). This original surveillance case definition has been modified by the CDC as new data have become available. HIV-related primary encephalopathy and HIV-associated nephropathy are also frequently encountered in HIV-infected patients. HIV-associated nephropathy, which is a glomerulosclerosis, is the most common cause of chronic renal failure in HIV patients and occurs almost exclusively in blacks. It is now clear that this disorder is caused by a direct infection of renal cells by HIV.

The CDC has classified HIV infection into the 3 stages outlined in Table 1-3. The older categories A, B, and C of HIV infection are now designated as stages 1, 2, and 3, respectively. Stage 1 HIV infection is defined by either CD4$^+$ T-lymphocyte count of more

Table 1-3 Surveillance Case Definition for Human Immunodeficiency Virus (HIV) Infection Among Adults and Adolescents (aged ≥13 Years)—United States, 2008

Stage	Laboratory Evidence*	Clinical Evidence
Stage 1	Laboratory confirmation of HIV infection *and* CD4+ T-lymphocyte count of ≥500 cells/µL *or* CD4+ T-lymphocyte percentage of ≥29	None required (but no AIDS-defining condition)
Stage 2	Laboratory confirmation of HIV infection *and* CD4+ T-lymphocyte count of 200–499 cells/µL *or* CD4+ T-lymphocyte percentage of 14–28	None required (but no AIDS-defining condition)
Stage 3 (AIDS)	Laboratory confirmation of HIV infection *and* CD4+ T-lymphocyte count of <200 cells/µL *or* CD4+ T-lymphocyte percentage of <14†	*or* documentation of an AIDS-defining condition (with laboratory confirmation of HIV infection)†
Stage unknown§	Laboratory confirmation of HIV infection *and* no information on CD4+ T-lymphocyte count or percentage	*and* no information on presence of AIDS-defining conditions

*The CD4+ T-lymphocyte percentage is the percentage of total lymphocytes. If the CD4+ T-lymphocyte count and percentage do not correspond to the same HIV infection stage, select the more severe stage.
†Documentation of an AIDS-defining condition supersedes a CD4+ T-lymphocyte count of ≥200 cells/µL and a CD4+ T-lymphocyte percentage of total lymphocytes of ≥14. Definitive diagnostic methods for these conditions are available in Appendix C of the 1993 revised HIV classification system and the expanded AIDS case definition (CDC. 1993 Revised classification system for HIV infection and expanded surveillance case definition for AIDS among adolescents and adults. *MMWR Recomm Rep.* 1992; 41(RR-17):1–19 and from the National Notifiable Diseases Surveillance System (available at cdc.gov/epo).
§Although cases with no information on CD4+ T-lymphocyte count or percentage or on the presence of AIDS-defining conditions can be classified as stage unknown, every effort should be made to report CD4+ T-lymphocyte counts or percentages and the presence of AIDS-defining conditions at the time of diagnosis. Additional CD4+ T-lymphocyte counts or percentages and any identified AIDS-defining conditions can be reported as recommended. (Council of State and Territorial Epidemiologists. Laboratory reporting of clinical test results indicative of HIV infection: new standards for a new era of surveillance and prevention [Position Statement 04-ID-07]: 2004. Available at http://www.cste.org/ps/2004pdf/04-ID-07-final.pdf.)

From Schneider E, Whitmore S, Glynn KM, Dominguez K, Mitsch A, McKenna MT; CDC. Revised surveillance case definitions for HIV infection among adults, adolescents, and children aged <18 months and for HIV infection and AIDS among children aged 18 months to <13 years, United States, 2008. *MMWR Recomm Rep.* 2008;57(RR–10):1–12.

than 500 cells/µL or CD4+ T-lymphocyte percentage of total lymphocytes of greater than 29, and the presence of no AIDS-defining conditions. Stage 2 HIV infection is defined by either CD4+ T-lymphocyte count of 200–499 cells/µL or CD4+ T-lymphocyte percentage of total lymphocytes of 14–28, and the presence of no AIDS-defining conditions. Stage 3 HIV infection (AIDS) is designated by CD4+ T-lymphocyte count of less than 200 cells/µL or CD4+ T-lymphocyte percentage of total lymphocytes of less than 14 or documentation of one or more of the past or present AIDS-defining conditions listed in Table 1-4.

Acute infection with HIV often manifests as a transient mononucleosis-like syndrome. This syndrome has been called *primary HIV infection,* the typical symptoms of which are fever, fatigue, weight loss, myalgias, headache, pharyngitis, and nausea. Primary

Table 1-4 AIDS-Defining Conditions

- Bacterial infections, multiple or recurrent*
- Candidiasis of bronchi, trachea, or lungs
- Candidiasis of esophagus†
- Cervical cancer, invasive§
- Coccidioidomycosis, disseminated or extrapulmonary
- Cryptococcosis, extrapulmonary
- Cryptosporidiosis, chronic intestinal (>1 month's duration)
- Cytomegalovirus disease (other than liver, spleen, or nodes), onset at age >1 month
- Cytomegalovirus retinitis (with loss of vision)†
- Encephalopathy, HIV related
- Herpes simplex: chronic ulcers (>1 month's duration) or bronchitis, pneumonitis, or esophagitis (onset at age >1 month)
- Histoplasmosis, disseminated or extrapulmonary
- Isosporiasis, chronic intestinal (>1 month's duration)
- Kaposi sarcoma†
- Lymphoid interstitial pneumonia or pulmonary lymphoid hyperplasia complex*†
- Lymphoma, burkitt (or equivalent term)
- Lymphoma, immunoblastic (or equivalent term)
- Lymphoma, primary, of brain
- *Mycobacterium avium* complex or *mycobacterium kansasii,* disseminated or extrapulmonary†
- *Mycobacterium tuberculosis* of any site, pulmonary,†§ disseminated,† or extrapulmonary†
- *Mycobacterium,* other species or unidentified species, disseminated† or extrapulmonary†
- *Pneumocystis carinii* pneumonia†
- Pneumonia, recurrent†§
- Progressive multifocal leukoencephalopathy
- *Salmonella* septicemia, recurrent
- Toxoplasmosis of brain, onset at age >1 month†
- Wasting syndrome attributed to HIV

*Only among children aged <13 years.
†Condition that might be diagnosed presumptively.
§Only among adults and adolescents aged ≥13 years.

HIV infection is diagnosed when a positive result on the plasma HIV RNA test and a negative result on the Western blot assay are obtained on the same day. To confirm seroconversion, patients should have a repeat HIV antibody test 2–3 weeks after resolution of symptoms.

Patients may then enter a prolonged asymptomatic carrier state (the majority of HIV-infected patients in the United States are in this condition). There is also a syndrome of persistent generalized lymphadenopathy, which is associated with depleted helper T lymphocytes and HIV infection. Constitutional symptoms include fever, weight loss, chronic diarrhea, oral thrush, and lymphadenopathy.

Seroepidemiology

Antibodies to HIV can be detected in HIV-infected persons. Such screening is now performed with commercially available kits, based on an ELISA using whole, disrupted HIV antigens. The ELISA test for HIV antibodies is sensitive (99%) and specific (99%). However, false-negative results can occur, especially in the first weeks after HIV infection. False-positive ELISA results are also possible; thus, the ELISA must yield positive results twice and be confirmed by Western blot analysis or immunofluorescence assay before a patient is said to have antibodies to HIV. Persons with antibodies to HIV should be considered infectious for HIV. Currently, HIV p24 antigen testing or HIV-1 RNA analysis can be performed. These tests yield positive results earlier than anti-HIV antibody tests do.

Current screening recommendations for HIV testing include routine testing of all high-risk adults and adolescents and all pregnant women. Some even advocate routine testing of all patients in all clinical settings. Persons at high risk for HIV should be screened for HIV at least annually. Specific signed consent for HIV testing should not be required. General informed consent for medical care should be considered sufficient to include informed consent for HIV testing. However, patients must not be tested without their knowledge. Perinatal transmission rates can be reduced to less than 2% with universal screening of pregnant women, prophylactic antiretroviral drugs, scheduled cesarean delivery when appropriate, and avoidance of breast feeding.

Seroepidemiologic studies conducted in high-risk populations revealed an increasing prevalence of HIV infection, from almost none before 1979 to as high as 70% by 1988. The rate of increase of HIV infection slowed during the 1990s in the United States but accelerated in Africa and other developing regions. In the past, 100% of patients with HIV infection ultimately developed AIDS, but this percentage has gradually fallen as many patients have responded to HAART, resulting in a corresponding decrease in the incidence of opportunistic infections. The median incubation period between acquisition of HIV infection and the development of AIDS is more than 10 years.

Modes of Transmission

Modes of transmission of HIV infection are

- sexual contact
- intravenous drug use
- transfusion
- perinatal transmission from an infected mother to her child

There have been no documented cases of transmission by casual contact. Furthermore, although HIV infection may be transmitted by blood or blood products, the risk of transmission by accidental needle-stick appears quite low (<0.5%). Studies of nonsexual household contacts of patients with AIDS have revealed that these people are at minimal or possibly no risk of infection with HIV.

At the beginning of the AIDS epidemic, almost all the cases were confined to gay men in the United States, but that proportion has been steadily decreasing, with corresponding increases in the number of cases in intravenous drug users and in patients infected through heterosexual contact. Furthermore, in Africa the male/female ratio is 1:1, and epidemiologic data have suggested that the disease is transmitted predominantly by heterosexual activity, perinatal exposure from infected mothers to their newborns, and parenteral exposure to blood transfusion and unsterilized needles.

Prognosis and Treatment

AIDS is still considered an incurable and potentially fatal disease. Nevertheless, infected patients are living much longer and have had better quality of life than infected patients in previous years because of significant improvements in antiviral therapy. For that reason, AIDS is now managed more as a chronic illness rather than as a terminal disease. The risk factors that are most closely associated with decreased survival in patients with AIDS are reduced CD4 levels, length of time since diagnosis, previous opportunistic infections, high viral load, and new "clinical progression" events. CD4 counts are good predictors of risk of opportunistic infection. Plasma HIV RNA levels are even better predictors of disease progression and are the best single predictors of response to therapy.

It is now well established that superinfection with a second strain, or clade, of HIV-1 virus occurs in humans, often following a period of immunologic stability. Detection of increasing viral DNA, which results from infection of a cell by 2 or more HIV clades, suggests that superinfection occurs more frequently than previously thought. The second virus (usually from a different clade) can superinfect cells well after the initial infection, and this is associated with rapid viral rebound and immunologic decline. Primary infection with a specific HIV clade appears to provide inadequate immune protection against superinfection with a different clade.

Recommended laboratory studies with a newly diagnosed case of HIV infection include complete blood count with differential; CD4 count; HIV viral load (RNA level); electrolytes; renal and liver function tests; urinalysis; PPD (TB test); and serologic tests for syphilis, hepatitis B virus and HCV, toxoplasma, CMV, and VZV. Female patients should undergo a Papanicolaou test because of the high risk of invasive cervical cancer in HIV-infected persons. The recommended vaccinations in HIV-positive patients are *Pneumococcus* (every 5 years), hepatitis B virus, hepatitis A virus (especially if the patient is HCV-positive), influenza virus (yearly), diphtheria/tetanus (every 10 years), and measles (contraindicated in severe immunosuppression). Immunizations that are contraindicated and should not be administered in HIV-infected patients include live attenuated influenza, varicella-zoster, oral polio, smallpox, typhoid, and yellow fever vaccines.

In 1986, the drug *zidovudine* (also known as azidothymidine [AZT]; Retrovir), a synthetic analogue of thymidine, became available for the treatment of AIDS. Zidovudine is incorporated into DNA by the DNA polymerase (reverse transcriptase) of HIV and prevents further viral DNA synthesis. In the early AIDS treatment trials, zidovudine decreased mortality among patients with AIDS and decreased the number of episodes of opportunistic infections. The major limiting side effect of this therapy was bone marrow suppression. Currently, zidovudine and other nucleoside analogues are used only in combination therapy, because of the rapid emergence of HIV resistance in patients treated with a nucleoside analogue alone.

Some of the other nucleoside analogue reverse transcriptase inhibitors approved as combined therapy for HIV infection are *didanosine* (or ddI; Videx), *lamivudine* (or 3TC; Epivir), and *stavudine* (or d4T; Zerit). These drugs have in vitro activity against HIV similar to that of zidovudine. The primary benefit of these drugs over zidovudine is reduced bone marrow toxicity. However, didanosine has been associated with peripheral retinal toxicity. Lamivudine is available as a combination drug with zidovudine (Combivir). *Abacavir* (Ziagen) was the first clinically available guanosine analogue reverse transcriptase inhibitor. *Trizivir* is a combination drug containing abacavir, lamivudine, and zidovudine. *Tenofovir* (PMPA; Viread) is a *nucleotide* reverse transcriptase inhibitor (NRTI) that allows for once-daily dosing and has been well tolerated in clinical trials to date, without evidence of long-term toxicity. *Truvada* is a combination drug containing emtricitabine and tenofovir. *Apricitabine* (ATC) is a novel deoxycytidine analogue reverse transcriptase inhibitor that is well tolerated and has good clinical efficacy against drug-resistant HIV.

Nonnucleoside reverse transcriptase inhibitors (NNRTIs), such as *nevirapine* (Viramune), also share the disadvantage of rapid emergence of viral resistance. Therefore, they are currently used in combination therapy. A newer NNRTI, *efavirenz* (Sustiva), is taken once daily, has excellent activity against HIV, and has fewer side effects than other NNRTIs. This agent has become a cornerstone of antiretroviral therapy, and its efficacy over other antiretrovirals has been established in many clinical trials. *Etravirine* (or TMC-125; Intelence,) is a new NNRTI and was granted accelerated approval in the United States and Europe in 2008. Etravirine has been evaluated in multiple controlled trials, and in one study, it possessed such initial antiviral potency, that it was equivalent to a 5-drug, triple-class antiretroviral regimen.

The protease inhibitors are a class of antiretroviral drugs that prevent the cleavage of precursor proteins into the viral elements needed for viral assembly, thereby resulting in the production of nonfunctional, noninfectious virions. These agents are used primarily in multidrug therapy along with one or more nucleoside analogues. The protease inhibitors currently approved for the treatment of HIV infection include *saquinavir* (Invirase), *indinavir* (Crixivan), *ritonavir* (Norvir), *nelfinavir* (Viracept), *atazanavir* (Reyataz), and a *lopinavir/ritonavir combination* (Kaletra). *Fosamprenavir* (Lexiva, Telzir) is well-tolerated and is indicated as initial combination therapy. *Tipranivir* (Aptivus), *rupintrivir, raltegravir* (Isentress), and *darunavir* (Prezista) are newer protease inhibitors that are highly selective for the HIV protease enzyme and demonstrate potent in vitro activity against wild-type strains of HIV-1 and HIV-2. In combination therapy with low-dose ritonavir and efavirenz (Sustiva, Stocrin), tipranivir is highly effective against HIV isolates resistant to other protease inhibitors.

Fusion inhibitors are a new class of investigational antiviral agents that block fusion of HIV with the human cell by blocking the function of the gp120 envelope glycoprotein. *Enfuvirtide* (T-20; Fuzeon) provides clinically relevant improvements in CD4 cell counts and reductions in HIV viral load across all subgroups of the treatment-experienced patients studied.

A small percentage of the population appears to be naturally immune to HIV infection. These persons have defective genes for CCR5, a surface receptor that HIV requires to attach to T lymphocytes. Also, approximately 50% of long-term survivors of HIV are heterozygous for the CCR5 defect. This has led to some speculation concerning the possibilities for genetic therapy, in which anti-HIV genes could be "injected" into a patient's chromosomes with a harmless viral vector. In one recent study, recombinant lentiviral vectors were used to deliver the *CCR5-delta32* gene into human cell lines, and resistance to HIV was transmitted to most of these cells. This may become useful for stem cell–based or T-lymphocyte–based gene therapy for HIV-1 infection. Several small-molecule CCR5 receptor inhibitors are now being evaluated in clinical trials. Two new agents, vicriviroc and maraviroc (Selzentry), received accelerated FDA approval in 2007 and are currently being used in combined therapy regimens and phase 3 controlled trials.

Other new experimental classes of antiretroviral drugs currently under investigation include the entry, coreceptor, integrase, and p7 nucleocapsid zinc finger inhibitors; and the coreceptor CXCR4 and CCR5 antagonists, as well as potential inhibitors of genome transport to the nucleus, HIV interaction with nuclear pores, and virus budding.

In response to the extremely high prices of many AIDS drugs, several states have established AIDS drug assistance programs. Also, many AIDS drug manufacturers now offer patient assistance programs to help patients locate sources for reimbursement or provide drugs free to patients who have no means of obtaining them.

Multidrug therapy, or HAART, has been the standard of care since 1998 and usually involves drug regimens with 3 or more agents. To prevent early drug resistance, patients should be given all drugs simultaneously rather than sequentially. Most of the clinical trials recommend a drug regimen that includes a potent protease inhibitor in combination with 2 nucleoside analogue reverse transcriptase inhibitors or 2 protease inhibitors combined with 1 or 2 nucleoside analogue reverse transcriptase inhibitors. Recently, alternative treatment regimens have omitted protease inhibitors *(protease-sparing regimen)*. Protease-sparing regimens such as abacavir/AZT/3TC (Trizivir) and drug combinations that include efavirenz appear to be as effective as regimens that contain protease inhibitors.

HAART has been shown to result in a dramatic reduction of the HIV viral load, increased CD4 cell counts, delay of disease progression, reduction in the number of opportunistic infections, decreased number of hospitalizations, and prolonged survival. Some statistics show up to an 82% decline in the number of opportunistic infections in patients on HAART. These advantages are translating into improved survival and enhanced quality of life for HIV-infected patients. It is interesting to note that the number of AIDS cases in the United States peaked in 1993 and has been gradually decreasing since then. The HIV mortality rate has declined more than 70% since 1995, mostly because of HAART. In just the 2-year period from 1995 to 1997, the AIDS mortality rate decreased from 29.4 to 8.8 per 100 person-years. Despite the high cost of antiretroviral medications, it is still less expensive to treat HIV-infected patients with HAART and prevent them from developing AIDS than it is to provide the extensive care required once they develop AIDS.

Over the past few years, HIV prevention and drug treatment programs have slowly but consistently improved throughout much of the developing world and the number of AIDS cases and the AIDS-related mortality rate have leveled off, and in some areas have actually begun to decline.

At present, the most common treatment end point or goal of HAART is reduction of HIV RNA levels, preferably to undetectable levels (<500 copies/mL). In some studies, HAART reduced HIV RNA to undetectable levels in up to 78% of patients. Baseline levels should be checked before the initiation of or change in antiretroviral therapy, again at 1 month after treatment begins to show efficacy, and then every 3 or 4 months. For consistency, all HIV RNA testing in a single patient should be obtained via the same assay. Assays are now available for monitoring drug levels of most of the antiretroviral agents. Also, detection of specific mutations for drug resistance helps guide therapy for multidrug-resistant HIV infections.

Discontinuation of HAART after 1 year of successful treatment is usually followed by a rapid rebound of viral load. However, viral antigen quickly returns to undetectable levels following reintroduction of HAART. For patients in whom HAART fails because of drug resistance, some studies have offered alternative aggressive salvage therapy regimens that use 5 or more agents. HIV drug sensitivity testing is now available for most of the approved antiretroviral agents and should be performed in patients with suspected drug-resistant infections. In some patients, HAART is interrupted because of drug toxicity.

In recent years, drug resistance has emerged as a significant problem in treating HIV infection. HAART does not result in long-term suppression of HIV replication in 20%–50% of treatment-naive patients and in up to 50%–70% of treatment-experienced patients. In the majority of patients with viral rebound, mutations of drug resistance are detected. New HIV infections through transmission of drug-resistant strains to patients who have never been exposed to antiretroviral therapy are increasingly reported. Also, recent reports correlate new infections by drug-resistant HIV with suboptimal treatment response.

The immunomodulators are a diverse group of drugs and immunologic adjuvants that have been evaluated for their efficacy in enhancing the host immune response to HIV and related opportunistic infections. They employ multiple novel mechanisms of action to suppress HIV replication by targeting host cellular proteins that are not susceptible to mutation. Drug resistance, therefore, may be less of a problem with these agents. Actual clinical results, however, have been disappointing. The immunomodulators have been used primarily as a supplement to antiretroviral agents in combined therapy study protocols and have been discussed much less in the literature since the availability of HAART. *Hematopoietic agents,* such as erythropoietin and interleukin-3, enhance the proliferation of blood cells and are useful in treating cytopenias. Thalidomide has been beneficial in some patients for treating HIV wasting syndrome, HIV-associated colitis, hypertrophic genital herpes, and recurrent aphthous ulcerations in HIV-infected patients.

Although no highly successful HIV vaccines have been developed, clinical trials of several vaccines are in progress. Viral components, such as gp120 and gp160 envelope glycoproteins, and p17 and p24 viral antigens have been incorporated into vaccines that generate limited immune protection. The potential applications for an effective HIV vaccine would include the prevention of infection in high-risk populations, as well as enhanced viral clearance in chronically infected patients. One study demonstrated improved CD4 levels in patients with AIDS given recombinant envelope glycoprotein gp160 vaccine. Two DNA vaccines are currently being investigated. HIV-1 delta4 is a vaccine in development that uses a mutated form of the virus. However, there is reluctance to use vaccines made up of whole inactivated virions or live attenuated HIV because of the perceived possible risk of transmitting the infection through the vaccine. Another obstacle to vaccine development is the need to provide protection for the 10 or so known subtypes of HIV now in existence around the world, as well as the new mutations that continue to arise.

In September 2007, phase 2b trials for Merck's much-anticipated MRKAd5 trivalent vaccine showed no protection from HIV-1 infection in the vaccinated group compared with a control group, and the vaccine trial was terminated. This vaccine was expected to stimulate HIV-specific T-lymphocyte immune response and thus prevent infection or significantly reduce levels of HIV viral load, but it failed on all counts. This disappointing outcome has led to a critical review of all current vaccine studies and a call for a renewed effort toward developing novel immunogens to be tested in large primate trials.

Following occupational exposure to HIV by accidental needle-stick or mucous membrane contact, postexposure prophylactic therapy is strongly advised. Current recommendations by the CDC categorize combination therapy into basic, alternate, and expanded multidrug regimens.

Panlilio AL, Cardo DM, Grohskopf LA, Heneine W, Ross CS; US Public Health Service. Updated U.S. Public Health Service guidelines for the management of occupational exposures to HIV and recommendations for postexposure prophylaxis. *MMWR Recomm Rep.* 2005;54(RR-9):1–17. Full text available online at: cdc.gov/mmwr/preview/mmwrhtml/rr5409a1.htm.

Opportunistic Infections

Treatment of Pneumocystis carinii *pneumonia*

Pneumocystis carinii pneumonia (PCP) continues to affect a significant percentage of patients with AIDS and is a major cause of mortality in these patients. (The organism was recently renamed *P jiroveci,* but all previous medical literature and textbooks refer to it as *P carinii.*) However, recent advances in diagnosis and management, appropriately targeting chemoprophylaxis to HIV-infected patients at high clinical risk for PCP, and the introduction of HAART have contributed to a dramatic reduction in the incidence of PCP. Nevertheless, PCP remains the most common opportunistic pneumonia and the most common life-threatening infectious complication in HIV-infected patients.

PCP is generally treated with IV trimethoprim-sulfamethoxazole (TMP-SMX; Bactrim, Septra). Inhaled pentamidine (NebuPent) prevents the recurrence of PCP (secondary prophylaxis) and appears to be efficacious for primary prophylaxis when used in patients with HIV infection and CD4 counts less than $200/mm^3$. The regimen for inhaled pentamidine is generally 300 mg every 4 weeks using a nebulizer. This form of therapy avoids the toxicity of systemically administered pentamidine.

Several studies show that oral TMP-SMX prophylaxis is more effective than aerosolized pentamidine for PCP prophylaxis in those patients who can tolerate it. This regimen may also provide systemic prophylaxis against toxoplasmosis infection. However, adverse reactions are frequent in HIV-infected patients. Dapsone, alone or in combination with pyrimethamine, is effective for primary and secondary prophylaxis against PCP and is tolerated by most patients who develop rashes with use of TMP-SMX. Primaquine, clindamycin, and atovaquone (Mepron) have been used successfully in treating PCP, but these drugs are reserved for use in patients intolerant of TMP-SMX or pentamidine, or for those with resistant infections. Judicious use of corticosteroids may help reduce morbidity in patients with severe pulmonary inflammation caused by PCP.

Treatment of CMV infections

Ganciclovir is still used in treating CMV retinitis and colitis in immunocompromised patients. Studies of the drug suggest a response in 80%–100% of patients treated for CMV retinitis and remissions in 60%–80% of these patients. Intravitreal ganciclovir injections have been effective in treating the disease, and a slow-release ganciclovir implant (Vitrasert) has been approved. The implants are surgically inserted within the vitreal cavity and attached at the pars plana. Combination therapy with oral ganciclovir and the ganciclovir implant is more effective than the implant alone. Usually recommended for maintenance therapy after intravenous induction, oral ganciclovir is effective and has fewer side effects than the intravenous form. Ganciclovir's major toxicity is reversible bone marrow suppression. One third of patients using ganciclovir develop significant granulocytopenia, requiring them to discontinue the drug. The treatment of CMV retinitis is discussed in further detail in BCSC Section 9, *Intraocular Inflammation and Uveitis,* and Section 12, *Retina and Vitreous.*

Foscarnet (Foscavir) is also effective in treating CMV infections. Foscarnet inhibits the DNA polymerase of herpesvirus and HIV and demonstrates in vitro activity against CMV, herpes simplex, varicella-zoster, and HIV at concentrations readily achieved with intravenous therapy. Because oral bioavailability is poor, intravenous therapy is required for suppression of CMV retinitis in HIV disease. Foscarnet's primary value is that it is not generally myelosuppressive and therefore may be used without discontinuing zidovudine therapy.

Cidofovir (Vistide) is a potent antiviral agent with activity against herpes simplex, herpes zoster, CMV, adenovirus, EBV, and HIV. Cidofovir blocks DNA synthesis by viral DNA polymerase. It provides a prolonged antiviral activity that lasts up to several weeks, thereby allowing infrequent dosing. In one study, intravitreal cidofovir led to healing of CMV retinitis in all 53 participating patients. Anterior uveitis occurs in up to 37% of patients receiving cidofovir therapy for the disease, but it responds well to topical corticosteroid treatment and does not require cessation of cidofovir in most cases.

Fomivirsen (Vitravene), an antisense drug that targets CMV mRNA, has been shown to be effective in controlling early or advanced CMV retinitis. Valganciclovir (Valcyte), a prodrug of ganciclovir, is an oral agent that is as effective as IV ganciclovir in treating the disease.

The incidence and recurrence rate of CMV retinitis, as well as the frequency of drug resistance, have all decreased since 1995, largely because of enhanced immune system function resulting from HAART. Maintenance CMV therapy can often be discontinued in patients with immune recovery following HAART.

Treatment of spore-forming intestinal protozoa

Spore-forming intestinal protozoa are a frequent cause of gastrointestinal tract infections in patients with AIDS. This group of infections includes cryptosporidiosis (caused by *Cryptosporidium parvum*), microsporidiosis (Microsporida), isosporiasis *(Isospora belli),* and cyclosporiasis *(Cyclospora cayetanensis).*

Cryptosporidiosis can be treated with clarithromycin, azithromycin, rifabutin, albendazole, metronidazole, or a newer, more effective agent, nitazoxanide. HIV-infected patients on HAART have a dramatically lower incidence of cryptosporidiosis, which is attributable to the effects of intestinal immune reconstitution.

Isosporiasis and cyclosporiasis have been treated successfully with TMP-SMX. There are no curative drugs for invasive microsporidiosis, but recent studies have revealed that albendazole or fumagillin may control disease symptoms.

It is important to realize that chronic diarrhea in HIV-infected patients also may be caused by many nonprotozoan pathogens, particularly *Salmonella, Shigella, Campylobacter, C difficile, Vibrio parahaemolyticus, Escherichia coli, M avium,* and CMV.

Treatment of tuberculosis and atypical mycobacteria

The incidence of TB is increasing in HIV-infected patients in Africa and Asia. HIV-induced immunosuppression alters the typical clinical presentation of TB, causing atypical signs and symptoms and more frequent extrapulmonary disease dissemination. Also, the treatment of TB is more difficult to manage in HIV-infected patients, because of drug interactions between protease inhibitors and rifampicin or rifabutin. In addition, increased use of HAART in developed countries may be responsible for a paradoxical worsening of TB clinical manifestations, due to immune restoration and the subsequent inflammatory responses against TB.

Multidrug resistance has become an increasing problem—particularly in Africa and Asia—in patients with AIDS who have TB or atypical mycobacterial (*M avium, M kansasii*) infections. Delay in diagnosis and multidrug resistance are strong risk factors for mortality.

Standard drugs used in treating mycobacterial infections include isoniazid, rifampin, ethambutol, streptomycin, para-aminosalicylic acid, ethionamide, pyrazinamide, cycloserine, kanamycin, and amikacin. Some of the newer drugs found to be effective in treating these refractory infections are clofazimine (also used in treating leprosy), capreomycin, rifabutin, azithromycin, clarithromycin, and the quinolones (ciprofloxacin, ofloxacin, and sparfloxacin). The quinolones are promising because they possess a high level of antimycobacterial activity with few adverse effects. Combined therapy with rifampin or rifabutin, ethambutol, clofazimine, and clarithromycin or ciprofloxacin has been successful in treating atypical mycobacterial infections in patients with AIDS. Rifabutin may cause uveitis and hypotony in some patients. Isoniazid prophylaxis has been recommended in HIV-positive patients at high risk for TB.

Prophylactic therapy with azithromycin, clarithromycin, rifabutin, or combined therapy may help prevent disseminated *M avium* complex (MAC) in patients with AIDS. However, a significant reduction in the incidence of disseminated atypical mycobacterial infections in the HAART era has been documented. Also, the clinical picture of atypical mycobacterial infections in patients treated with HAART has shifted from one of primarily disseminated disease with bacteremia to one of localized infections. Data from several controlled trials led to the current practice of discontinuing prophylaxis against disseminated MAC infections when the CD4+ cell counts remain stable at over 100 cells/μL. Furthermore, because of the potential drug interactions and adverse effects of antimycobacterial therapy, some authors suggest that routine prophylaxis should not be recommended, even in patients with low CD4+ counts, unless these patients do not respond to HAART.

Treatment of other opportunistic infections

Other opportunistic infections encountered in patients with AIDS include CNS toxoplasmosis, disseminated fungal infections, and coinfection with viral hepatitis, herpes simplex, or herpes zoster infections. Although toxoplasmosis has traditionally been treated with sulfadiazine, pyrimethamine, or clindamycin, more recent data suggest that TMP-SMX may be equally effective, with far fewer side effects. Also, TMP-SMX has been used as prophylactic therapy against PCP as well as toxoplasmosis.

Hepatitis B or C coinfection has been encountered more frequently in HIV-infected patients. Recent guidelines for screening and prevention of opportunistic infections suggest testing all HIV-infected patients for hepatitis B and C. HIV coinfection accelerates HCV-related liver disease, causing more rapid progression to cirrhosis, end-stage liver disease, and hepatocellular carcinoma. Although some antiretroviral agents, such as protease inhibitors, have significant anti-HBV activity, they have little direct impact on HCV infection.

The new antiviral agents valacyclovir and famciclovir, as well as other antiviral agents such as cidofovir, offer alternatives to acyclovir in treating AIDS in patients with refractory or disseminated herpes simplex or herpes zoster infections.

Treatment of disseminated fungal infections is evolving with the availability of the newer imidazoles, fluconazole and itraconazole. Amphotericin B continues to be important in treating advanced invasive fungal disease, and new formulations of the drug in lipid complexes or liposomes reduce systemic toxicity. In addition to the commonly recognized benefits of HAART for opportunistic infections (such as reestablishing immune competency), a recent study has proven that the protease inhibitor indinavir (Crixivan) directly inhibits the growth rate of the opportunistic fungal pathogen *Cryptococcus neoformans.*

In the past few years, recommendations have been made to discontinue prophylaxis in treating opportunistic infections in patients whose CD4+ T-lymphocyte counts have increased in response to HAART.

Treatment of AIDS-related malignancies

Kaposi sarcoma is usually a localized disease that can be treated with radiotherapy, but metastatic or disseminated disease may require combined chemotherapy. In addition, immunotherapy with β-interferon has been used in some patients with Kaposi sarcoma. B-lymphocyte lymphomas in patients with AIDS often involve the lymph nodes, CNS, and lungs and may require treatment with multidrug chemotherapy and sometimes with regional radiotherapy. Since the advent of HAART, the incidence of Kaposi sarcoma in HIV-infected patients has declined dramatically—as much as 87%, according to one review.

Hodgkin lymphoma is the most common non–AIDS-defining tumor in HIV-infected patients. Although the introduction of HAART led to a decreased incidence of several malignancies among HIV-infected patients, the incidence of HIV-associated Hodgkin lymphoma has been persistent. This disease's highly aggressive behavior is related to an increased frequency of unfavorable histologic types, higher tumor stages, and extranodal involvement by the time of presentation, as well as poorer therapeutic outcome, when compared with Hodgkin lymphoma in non–HIV-infected patients. Treatment of HIV-associated Hodgkin lymphoma is challenging, because of the underlying immunodeficiency caused by HIV itself, and may increase the risk of opportunistic infections by inducing further immunosuppression. Consequently, less aggressive treatment regimens have been developed to achieve tumor control in HIV-infected patients with Hodgkin lymphoma.

Other malignancies that appear to be associated with HIV infection are cervical carcinoma in situ, anogenital neoplasms, leiomyosarcoma, and conjunctival squamous cell carcinoma.

Immune reconstitution syndromes

Some patients starting HAART develop new or worsening opportunistic infections or malignancies despite improvements in the clinical markers of HIV infection. These examples of paradoxical clinical worsening, also called *immune reconstitution syndromes (IRSs),* are increased in patients with previous opportunistic infections or low CD4+ T-lymphocyte levels. IRSs are thought to result from an inflammatory response to reemergence of the immune system's ability to recognize pathogens or tumor antigens that were previously present but asymptomatic. With the increased availability of HAART, more cases and more new forms of IRS are likely to be recognized. Immune recovery uveitis (IRU) occurs in nearly 10% of HIV patients with immune recovery and a history of CMV retinitis. Of these IRU patients, 46% develop significant cystoid macular edema and 49% develop epiretinal membrane.

⊚ **Ophthalmic considerations** The ocular manifestations of AIDS are discussed in BCSC Section 9, *Intraocular Inflammation and Uveitis.*

HIV has been found in tears, conjunctival epithelial cells, corneal epithelial cells, aqueous, retinal vascular endothelium, and retina. Although transmission of AIDS or HIV infection by ophthalmic examinations or ophthalmic equipment has not been documented, the following precautions are recommended.

Health care professionals performing eye examinations or other procedures involving contact with tears should wash their hands immediately after the procedure and between patients. Hand washing alone should be sufficient, but when practical and convenient, disposable gloves may be worn. The use of gloves is advisable when the hands have cuts, scratches, or dermatologic lesions.

Instruments that come into direct contact with external surfaces of the eyes should be wiped clean and disinfected by a 5- to 10-minute exposure to one of the following: (1) a fresh solution of 3% hydrogen peroxide; (2) a fresh solution containing 5000 parts per million (ppm) free available chlorine—a one-tenth dilution of common household bleach (sodium hypochlorite); (3) 70% ethanol; or (4) 70% isopropanol. The device should be thoroughly rinsed in tap water and dried before use.

Contact lenses used in trial fittings should be disinfected between fittings with a commercially available hydrogen peroxide contact lens disinfecting system or with the standard heat disinfection regimen (78°–80°C for 10 minutes).

The demonstration of HIV in corneal epithelium has led to the recommendation that all corneal donors be screened for antibodies to HIV and that all potential donor corneas from HIV antibody–positive persons be discarded.

For more specific recommendations, see the AAO Information Statement titled "Infection Prevention in Eye Care Services and Operating Areas," available at one.aao.org/CE/PracticeGuidelines/ClinicalStatements.aspx.

Aaron L, Saadoun D, Calatroni I, et al. Tuberculosis in HIV-infected patients: a comprehensive review. *Clin Microbiol Infect.* 2004;10(15):388–398.

Barouch DH. Challenges in the development of an HIV-1 vaccine. *Nature.* 2008;455(7213):613–619.

Binford SL, Weady PT, Maldonado F, Brothers MA, Matthews DA, Patick AK. In vitro resistance study of rupintrivir, a novel inhibitor of human rhinovirus 3C protease. *Antimicrob Agents Chemother*. 2007;51(12):4366–4373.

Branson BM, Handsfield HH, Lampe MA, et al. Revised recommendations for HIV testing of adults, adolescents, and pregnant women in health-care settings. *MMWR: Recomm Rep*. 2006;55(RR14):1–17. Full text available online at http://www.cdc.gov/mmwr/preview/mmwrhtml/rr5514a1.htm.

Cahn P, Rolon M, Cassetti I, Shiveley L, Holdich T, Sawyer J. Multiple-dose pharmacokinetics of apricitabine, a novel nucleoside reverse transcriptase inhibitor, in patients with HIV-1 infection. *Clin Drug Investig*. 2008;28(2):129–138.

Centers for Disease Control and Prevention (CDC). Epidemiology of HIV/AIDS—United States, 1981-2005. *MMWR Morb Mortal Wkly Rep*. 2006;55(21):589–592.

Centers for Disease Control and Prevention (CDC). HIV prevalence estimates—United States, 2006. *MMWR Morb Mortal Wkly Rep*. 2008;57(39):1073–1076.

Centers for Disease Control and Prevention (CDC). Twenty-five years of HIV/AIDS—United States, 1981-2006. *MMWR Morb Mortal Wkly Rep*. 2006;55(21):585–589.

Chapman TM, Plosker GL, Perry CM. Fosamprenavir: a review of its use in the management of antiretroviral therapy–naive patients with HIV infection. *Drugs*. 2004;64(18):2101–2124.

Clotet B, Raffi F, Cooper D, et al. Clinical management of treatment-experienced, HIV-infected patients with the fusion inhibitor enfuvirtide: consensus recommendations. *AIDS*. 2004; 18(8):1137–1146.

Cooper DA, Steigbigel RT, Gatell JM, et al; BENCHMRK Study Teams. Subgroup and resistance analyses of raltegravir for resistant HIV-1 infection. *N Engl J Med*. 2008;359(4):355–365.

De Clercq E. HIV-chemotherapy and -prophylaxis: new drugs, leads and approaches. *Int J Biochem Cell Biol*. 2004;36(9):1800–1822.

Delyfer MN, Rougier MB, Hubschman JP, Aouizérate F, Korobelnik JF. Cytomegalovirus retinitis following intravitreal injection of triamcinolone: report of two cases. *Acta Ophthalmol Scand*. 2007;85(6):681–683.

de Mendoza C, Morelló J, Garcia-Gascó P, Rodríguez-Novoa S, Soriano V. Tipranavir: a new protease inhibitor for the treatment of antiretroviral-experienced HIV-infected patients. *Expert Opin Pharmacother*. 2007;8(6):839–850.

Esté JA, Telenti A. HIV entry inhibitors. *Lancet*. 2007;370(9581):81–88.

Fätkenheuer G, Nelson M, Lazzarin A, et al; MOTIVATE 1 and MOTIVATE 2 Study Teams. Subgroup analyses of maraviroc in previously treated R5 HIV-1 infection. *N Engl J Med*. 2008; 359(14):1442–1455.

Fortin C, Joly V. Efavirenz for HIV-1 infection in adults: an overview. *Expert Rev Anti Infect Ther*. 2004;2(5):671–684.

Gardner EM, Connick E. Illness of immune reconstitution: recognition and management. *Curr Infect Dis Rep*. 2004;6(6):483–493.

Gewurz BE, Jacobs M, Proper JA, Dahl TA, Fujiwara T, Dezube BJ. Capravirine, a nonnucleoside reverse-transcriptase inhibitor in patients infected with HIV-1: a phase 1 study. *J Infect Dis*. 2004;190(11):1957–1961.

Glynn MK, Lee LM, McKenna MT. The status of national HIV case surveillance, United States 2006. *Public Health Rep*. 2007;122(Suppl 1):63–71.

Hall HI, Song R, Rhodes P, et al. Estimation of HIV incidence in the United States. *JAMA*. 2008;300(5):520–529.

Hammer SM, Eron JJ Jr, Reiss P, et al; International AIDS Society-USA. Antiretroviral treatment of adult HIV infection: 2008 recommendations of the International AIDS Society-USA panel. *JAMA*. 2008;300(5):555–570.

Holland GN. AIDS and ophthalmology: the first quarter century. *Am J Ophthalmol.* 2008; 145(3):397–408.

Hulgan T, Shepherd BE, Raffanti SP, et al. Absolute count and percentage of CD4+ lymphocytes are independent predictors of disease progression in HIV-infected persons initiating highly active antiretroviral therapy. *J Infect Dis.* 2007;195(3):425–431.

Hutchinson AB, Farnham PG, Dean HD, et al. The economic burden of HIV in the United States in the era of highly active antiretroviral therapy: evidence of continuing racial and ethnic differences. *J Acquir Immune Defic Syndr.* 2006;43(4):451–457.

Iaccino E, Schiavone M, Fiume G, Quinto I, Scala G. The aftermath of the Merck's HIV vaccine trial. *Retrovirology.* 2008;5:56.

Jin Q, Marsh J, Cornetta K, Alkhatib G. Resistance to human immunodeficiency virus type 1 (HIV-1) generated by lentivirus vector-mediated delivery of the CCR5{Delta}32 gene despite detectable expression of the HIV-1 co-receptors. *J Gen Virol.* 2008;89(Pt 10):2611–2621.

Jlizi A, Edouard J, Fadhlaoui-Zid K, et al. Identification of the CCR5-Delta32 HIV resistance allele and new mutations of the CCR5 gene in different Tunisian populations. *Hum Immunol.* 2007;68(12):993–1000.

Kempen JH, Min YI, Freeman WR, et al; Studies of Ocular Complications of AIDS Research Group. Risk of immune recovery uveitis in patients with AIDS and cytomegalovirus retinitis. *Ophthalmology.* 2006;113(4):684–694.

Kimberlin DW, Acosta EP, Sánchez PJ, et al; National Institute of Allergy and Infectious Diseases Collaborative Antiviral Study Group. Pharmacokinetic and pharmacodynamic assessment of oral valganciclovir in the treatment of symptomatic congenital cytomegalovirus disease. *J Infect Dis.* 2008;197(6):836–845.

Knoll BM, Vento S, Temesgen Z. Etravirine. *Drugs Today (Barc).* 2008;44(1):23–33.

Lalezari J, Yadavalli GK, Para M, et al. Safety, pharmacokinetics, and antiviral activity of HGS004, a novel fully human IgG4 monoclonal antibody against CCR5, in HIV-1-infected patients. *J Infect Dis.* 2008;197(5):721–727.

Lange CG, Woolley IJ, Brodt RH. Disseminated Mycobacterium avium-intracellulare complex (MAC) infection in the era of effective antiretroviral therapy: is prophylaxis still indicated? *Drugs.* 2004;64(7):679–692.

Lima VD, Johnston K, Hogg RS, et al. Expanded access to highly active antiretroviral therapy: a potentially powerful strategy to curb the growth of the HIV epidemic. *J Infect Dis.* 2008;198(1):59–67.

Miedema F. A brief history of HIV vaccine research: stepping back to the drawing board? *AIDS.* 2008;22(14):1699–1703.

Onyebujoh PC, Ribeiro I, Whalen CC. Treatment options for HIV-associated tuberculosis. *J Infect Dis.* 2007;196(Suppl 1):S35–S45.

Panlilio AL, Cardo DM, Grohskopf LA, Heneine W, Ross CS; US Public Health Service. Updated U.S. Public Health Service guidelines for the management of occupational exposures to HIV and recommendations for postexposure prophylaxis. *MMWR Recomm Rep.* 2005;54(RR-9):1–17.

Patel N, Koziel H. Pneumocystis jiroveci pneumonia in adult patients with AIDS: treatment strategies and emerging challenges to antimicrobial therapy. *Treat Respir Med.* 2004;3(6): 381–397.

Schneider E, Whitmore S, Glynn KM, Dominguez K, Mitsch A, McKenna MT; Centers for Disease Control and Prevention (CDC). Revised surveillance case definitions for HIV infection among adults, adolescents, and children aged <18 months and for HIV infection and AIDS among children aged 18 months to <13 years—United States, 2008. *MMWR Recomm Rep.* 2008;57(RR-10):1–12.

Spach DH. Immunizations for HIV-infected adults: indications, timing, and response. *Top HIV Med.* 2006;14(5):154–158.

UNAIDS: Joint United Nations Programme on HIV/AIDS. 2008 report on the global AIDS epidemic. Full text online available at: http://www.unaids.org/en/knowledgecentre/hivdata/globalreport/2008.

Weng FL, Patel AM, Wanchoo R, et al. Oral ganciclovir versus low-dose valganciclovir for prevention of cytomegalovirus disease in recipients of kidney and pancreas transplants. *Transplantation.* 2007;83(3):290–296.

Update on Antibiotics

For over 60 years, the main trend in infectious disease management has been the evolution and refinement of antibiotic therapy. Factors that have stimulated the development of new antibiotics include the continuous emergence of resistant bacteria, economics, and the desire to eliminate undesirable side effects. During the last couple of decades, emphasis has gradually shifted from aminoglycosides to β-lactams and the development of new classes of antibiotics such as carbapenems and monobactams. In addition, vancomycin, TMP-SMX, erythromycin, and rifampin have enjoyed a popular resurgence and new applications. Quinolones offer the possibility of treating serious infections on an outpatient basis.

For the characteristics of selected antibiotics, see Table 1-5. Antiretroviral agents are discussed in detail earlier in this chapter.

Antibacterial Agents

Antibacterial agents can be separated into groups according to their specific targets on or within bacteria:

- β-Lactams and glycopeptides inhibit cell wall synthesis.
- Polymyxins distort cytoplasmic membrane function.
- Quinolones and rifampicins inhibit nucleic acid synthesis.
- Macrolides, aminoglycosides, and tetracyclines inhibit ribosome function.
- Trimethoprim and sulfonamides inhibit folate metabolism.

All antibiotics facilitate the growth of resistant bacteria consequent to the destruction of susceptible bacteria. Although the wide use of antimicrobial agents for veterinary and agricultural purposes has contributed to the emergence of multiresistant microorganisms, the excessive use of antibiotics, especially in hospitals, has been the most significant catalyst for resistance. Bacteria resist antibiotics by inactivation of the antibiotic, decreased accumulation of the antibiotic within the microorganism, or alteration of the target site on the microbe. For example, resistance to penicillins and cephalosporins is initiated by β-lactamase enzymes that hydrolyze the β-lactam ring, thus destroying the antibiotic's effectiveness. Resistance can be mediated by chromosomal mutations or the presence of extrachromosomal DNA, also known as *plasmid resistance*. Plasmid resistance is more important from an epidemiologic point of view because it is transmissible and usually highly stable; also, it confers resistance to many different classes of antibiotics simultaneously and is often associated with other characteristics that enable a microorganism to colonize and invade a susceptible host.

Table 1-5 Characteristics of Selected Antibiotics

Antibiotic	Spectrum	Route	Side Effects/Special Uses
	Antibacterial Agents		
Sulfonamides (bacteriostatic)			
Sulfisoxazole (Gantrisin)	Urinary tract infections, +, −, *Nocardia*, lymphogranuloma venereum, trachoma	PO	Crystalluria, allergic reactions (rashes, photosensitivity, and drug fever), kernicterus in newborns, renal damage, Stevens-Johnson syndrome (more likely with long-acting sulfonamides), blood dyscrasia (agranulocytosis), disseminated vasculitis.
Trimethoprim-sulfamethoxazole, TMP-SMX (Bactrim, Septra)	Urinary tract infections, +, −, shigellosis, *Nocardia*, *Pneumocystis* pneumonia	PO, IV	Same as above, plus nausea and vomiting, diarrhea, rashes, CNS irritability, bone marrow toxicity. Liver damage and Stevens-Johnson syndrome may be fatal.
Penicillin G (bactericidal)			
Aqueous (many brands)	+, *Neisseria*, spirochetes, actinomycosis	IV only	Penicillin allergy.* CNS toxicity with high blood levels, Coombs-positive hemolytic anemia, rare nephritis.
Procaine (many brands)	Same as above	IM only	Same as above, plus -*caine* reactions.
Benzathine (Bicillin)	Spirochetes, *Streptococcus* prophylaxis	IM only	Prolonged penicillin allergy.*
Semisynthetic penicillins (bactericidal)			
Penicillin V (Pen-Vee K)	+, *Neisseria*, spirochetes, actinomycosis	PO	Much better absorption than penicillin G when given orally in the fasting state.
Nafcillin (Unipen)	Penicillinase-producing *Staph*	IV	Penicillin allergy,* phlebitis, interstitial nephritis, diarrhea; rare bone marrow toxicity.
Cloxacillin (Tegopen)	+, especially *Staph*	PO	Penicillin allergy,* GI symptoms. Better absorbed and better tolerated than nafcillin and oxacillin given orally in the fasting state.
Dicloxacillin (Dynapen)	+, especially *Staph*	PO	Same as above.

+ = gram-positive, − = gram-negative, *Staph* = penicillinase-producers.
*Penicillin allergy includes spectrum from anaphylaxis to serum sickness.

(Continued)

Table 1-5 Characteristics of Selected Antibiotics (continued)

Antibiotic	Spectrum	Route	Side Effects/Special Uses
Ampicillin (Polycillin)	+, especially Enterococcus (except Staph) and some −, especially Haemophilus influenzae, Proteus mirabilis, Salmonella sp, Escherichia coli	IV, PO	Penicillin allergy,* GI symptoms (from PO administration). Rash common in viral illnesses (maculopapular eruption that is not necessarily allergy).
Ampicillin-sulbactam (Unasyn)	Same as ampicillin plus β-lactamase producers and some anaerobes	IV	Penicillin allergy,* diarrhea, elevated liver enzymes.
Amoxicillin (Amoxil)	Same as above, except Shigella	PO	Same as above. Better absorbed than oral ampicillin. Should replace oral ampicillin for everything except bacillary dysentery.
Amoxicillin–potassium clavulanate (Augmentin)	Same as amoxicillin plus β-lactamase producers (Haemophilus influenzae, Branhamella sp, and Staph sp)	PO	Same as amoxicillin plus more diarrhea.
Ticarcillin (Ticar)	−, especially Pseudomonas aeruginosa and Proteus sp, abdominal anaerobes, and some +, except Staph	IV	Penicillin allergy,* rare bleeding diathesis, hypokalemia (4.0 mEq Na$^+$/gm), abnormal liver function tests, Candida overgrowth.
Ticarcillin–potassium clavulanate (Timentin)	Same as ticarcillin plus β-lactamase producers (Klebsiella sp, Bacteroides fragilis, and Serratia sp)	IV	Same as ticarcillin plus more diarrhea and nausea. Candida overgrowth frequent.
Mezlocillin (Mezlin)	Same as ticarcillin	IV	Same as ticarcillin.
Piperacillin (Pipracil)	−, most active of all semisynthetic penicillins against Pseudomonas and many other aerobic gram-negative rods, including Klebsiella; abdominal anaerobes	IV	One half as much Na$^+$ as ticarcillin. Similar to ticarcillin, but approximately 25% of patients develop a hypersensitivity reaction and/or diarrhea. Must be used with an aminoglycoside. Rare bleeding diathesis.

+ = gram-positive, − = gram-negative, Staph = penicillinase-producers.
*Penicillin allergy includes spectrum from anaphylaxis to serum sickness.

Antibiotic	Spectrum	Route	Side Effects/Special Uses
Piperacillin-tazobactam (Zosyn)	Same as piperacillin with increased coverage of β-lactamase producers and anaerobes	IV	Same as piperacillin.
Cephalosporins (bactericidal)			
First-generation cephalosporins			
Cefazolin (Kefzol, Ancef)	+ and some –; not a good *Staph* treatment	IM, IV	Thrombophlebitis or pain at injection site, rash, urticaria, eosinophilia, neutropenia.
Cephalexin (Keflex)	+, *Staph*, and some –	PO	Same as above plus GI symptoms.
Cephradine (Anspor, Velosef)	+, *Staph*, and some –	PO	Same as above.
Cefadroxil monohydrate (Duracef)	+, *Staph*, and some –	PO	Rash, urticaria, GI symptoms.
Second-generation (extended-spectrum) cephalosporins			
Cefamandole (Mandol)	+, especially *Staph*, and some –	IV	Less thrombophlebitis than above, rash, drug fever, eosinophilia, hypoprothrombinemia ± bleeding. Extremely effective prophylaxis for *Staph*, including MRSE.
Cefoxitin (Mefoxin)	+, –, abdominal anaerobes (the best of all cephalosporins)	IV	Thrombophlebitis, fever, rash, eosinophilia, nausea, vomiting, diarrhea, bone marrow and liver toxicity.
Cefonicid (Monocid)	– and some anaerobes	IV	Often used for prophylaxis with colorectal or gynecologic surgeries; may cause pain at injection site, eosinophilia, GI symptoms, rash.
Cefaclor (Ceclor, Distaclor)	+ and some –, *Haemophilus* sp	PO	Toxicity similar to other cephalosporins. Major uses are treating ENT infections in children and respiratory tract infections in adults with COPD.

+ = gram-positive, – = gram-negative, Staph = penicillinase-producers.

(Continued)

Table 1-5 Characteristics of Selected Antibiotics (*continued*)

Antibiotic	Spectrum	Route	Side Effects/Special Uses
Cefuroxime sodium (IV: Zinacef, Kefurox); cefuroxime axetil (PO: Ceftin)	+ and some –, *Haemophilus* sp	IV, PO	Rash, GI symptoms.
Cefotetan (Cefotan)	–, anaerobes	IM or IV	A long half-life cefoxitin. Hypoprothrombinemia, hemolytic anemia, and disulfiram-like reaction.
Third-generation (ultrabroad-spectrum) cephalosporins			
Cefotaxime (Claforan)	–, including many multidrug-resistant organisms	IV	Cephalosporin hypersensitivity reaction, thrombophlebitis. Good penetration into CSF in meningitis.
Cefoperazone (Cefobid)	–, including *Pseudomonas* sp and many multidrug-resistant organisms, some anaerobes	IM or IV	Cephalosporin hypersensitivity, hypoprothrombinemia, diarrhea. Can be given q 8–12 hr.
Ceftriaxone (Rocephin)	Like cefotaxime; gonorrhea, *Borrelia burgdorferi*	IM or IV	Very long half-life makes it attractive for outpatient therapy. Treatment of choice for gonorrhea. Effective for all forms of Lyme disease. Good CNS penetration for meningitis.
Ceftazidime (Fortaz, Tazidime, Tazicef)	–, especially *Pseudomonas* sp	IM, IV	Good anti-pseudomonal cephalosporin, long half-life: q 8–12 hr administration. The best all-purpose third-generation cephalosporin.
Ceftizoxime (Cefizox)	Many – and anaerobes	IV	Rash, GI symptoms, elevated liver enzymes.
Cefixime (Suprax)	+, some – (*Haemophilus influenzae*, *Branhamella catarrhalis*)	PO	Diarrhea, nausea, abdominal pain, flatulence. First oral third-generation cephalosporin.
Cefpodoxime proxetil (Vantin)	+, –, *Enterobacter*, *Pseudomonas*, *Serratia*, *Morganella*, *Enterococcus*, generally resistant infections	PO	Twice daily for ENT, respiratory and urinary tract, and soft tissue infections. Single dose for uncomplicated gonorrhea.
Cefprozil (Cefzil)	+, –, including *Haemophilus*	PO	Rash, GI symptoms.

+ = gram-positive, – = gram-negative, *Staph* = penicillinase-producers.

Antibiotic	Spectrum	Route	Side Effects/Special Uses
Ceftibuten (Cedax)	+, −, including *Haemophilus, Moraxella*	PO	No real advantages.
Cefdinir (Omnicef)	+, −, including *Haemophilus*	PO	Rash, GI symptoms.
Cefditoren (Spectracef)	+, −, including *Haemophilus*	PO	Very broad spectrum but not active against *Pseudomonas*.
Fourth-generation (*very broad spectrum*) cephalosporins			
Cefepime (Maxipime)	+, −, some anaerobes	IV, IM	Expensive; slightly better gram-negative coverage than ceftazidime.
Cefpirome	+, −, some anaerobes	IV, IM	Effective for sepsis.
Carbacephems (bactericidal)			
Loracarbef (Lorabid)	+, −, including *Haemophilus*	PO	Rash, GI symptoms.
Cephamycins (bactericidal)			
Cefmetazole (Zefazone)	Similar to that of second-generation cephalosporins	IV	GI symptoms, rash, seizures in patients with renal insufficiency, more side effects than second-generation cephalosporins.
Monobactams (bactericidal)			
Aztreonam (Azactam)	Most −; no activity for + or anaerobes	IM, IV	First of this class of monocyclic β-lactams. The spectrum of an aminoglycoside without oto- or nephrotoxicity. No cross-reaction in penicillin–allergic patients.
Carbapenems (bactericidal)			
Imipenem-cilastatin (Primaxin)	+, −, including *Pseudomonas* sp and multidrug-resistant strains, anaerobes	IV	Nausea, diarrhea, phlebitis, elevated serum glutamic-oxaloacetic transaminase (SGOT), elevated serum glutamic-pyruvic transaminase (SGPT), seizures. Prototype of carbapenems. *Candida* superinfection frequent. Extremely broad spectrum.

+ = gram-positive, − = gram-negative, *Staph* = penicillinase-producers.

(Continued)

Table 1-5 Characteristics of Selected Antibiotics (continued)

Antibiotic	Spectrum	Route	Side Effects/Special Uses
Meropenem (Merrem)	Similar to imipenem, but less active against +, more active against −	IV	Does not require cilastatin component because more resistant to enzyme degradation; less problem with seizures.
Ertapenem	Similar to meropenem	IM, IV	Similar to meropenem; once-daily dosing.
Faropenem	Similar to meropenem	PO	Similar to meropenem.
Macrolides (bacteriostatic)			
Erythromycin	+, spirochetes, *Mycoplasma*, *Legionella*, *Campylobacter*	PO, IV	GI upset, altered liver function test, hepatic damage, stomatitis, thrombophlebitis (with IV administration). Take with meals or a snack when given orally.
Clindamycin (Cleocin)	+, anaerobes, actinomycosis	PO, IV	GI toxicity can be severe and even lethal.
Azalides			
Clarithromycin (Biaxin) Azithromycin (Zithromax) Dirithromycin (Dynabac) Roxithromycin Spiramycin Josamycin	+, *Mycoplasma*, *Chlamydia*, *Legionella*	PO	Reversible dose-related hearing loss in high doses. Less GI than erythromycin.
Ketolides			
Telithromycin (Ketek)	+, *Mycoplasma*, *Chlamydia*, *Legionella*. Good for multidrug-resistant +	PO	Associated with hepatotoxicity, exacerbation of Myasthenia gravis, and blurred vision.
Glycopeptides (bactericidal)			
Vancomycin (Vancocin)	+, especially *Staph* and *Enterococcus*, *Clostridia*, and other β-lactam-resistant +	IV, PO	Thrombophlebitis, leukopenia. Resistant enterococci and reduced-sensitivity *Staph* strains are increasing.

+ = gram-positive, − = gram-negative, *Staph* = penicillinase-producers.

Antibiotic	Spectrum	Route	Side Effects/Special Uses
Teicoplanin (Targocid)	Similar to vancomycin with better activity against *Streptococcus* and *Enterococcus*. Effective for some vancomycin-resistant strains of *Enterococcus*.	IV, IM	Longer half-life (allows daily dosing), lower toxicity, less nephrotoxicity, better tissue penetration than vancomycin.
Tetracyclines* (bacteriostatic) *In order of bacterial activity:*			
Minocycline (Minocin)	+ and −, spirochetes, *Mycoplasma*, lymphogranuloma venereum, psittacosis, *Rickettsia*	PO, IV	Most active. Useful as an alternative to vancomycin for treatment of methicillin-resistant staphylococci, particularly MRSE, and for meningococcal prophylaxis. Vertigo. May cause a drug-induced lupus syndrome.
Doxycycline (Vibramycin)	Same as above	PO, IV	Hepatic excretion, so may be best in renal failure. Do not use in urinary tract infections. Phototoxic reactions. Useful for the treatment of blepharitis.
Tetracycline	Same as above	PO, IV	Probably best choice for routine use. *Candida* overgrowth.
Aminoglycosides (bactericidal)			
Streptomycin	Tuberculosis, −, *Pasteurella* sp, *Franciscella* sp	IM only	Vestibular damage, drug fever, peripheral neuropathy.
Gentamicin (Garamycin)	Community-acquired −; not effective for + or anaerobes	IM or IV slowly	Vestibular damage, renal damage, curare-like effect.
Tobramycin (Nebcin)	−, especially *Pseudomonas* and *Aeromonas*	IM or IV slowly	Less nephrotoxic than gentamicin. Most active against *Pseudomonas*.
Netilmicin (Netromycin)	−, including some gentamicin/ tobramycin-resistant organisms	IM or IV slowly	May be less toxic than gentamicin or tobramycin.

+ = gram-positive, − = gram-negative, *Staph* = penicillinase-producers.

* *Side effects of tetracyclines:* GI disturbance; bone lesions; staining and deformity of teeth in children up to 8 years old and in newborns when given to pregnant women after the fourth month; malabsorption; enterocolitis; photosensitivity reaction (most frequent with demethylchlortetracycline). Parenteral doses may cause serious liver damage, especially in pregnant women and patients with renal disease; allergic reactions, blood dyscrasia, interference with protein metabolism, increased intracranial pressure in infants, Fanconi-like syndrome from deteriorated tetracyclines. Take with meals or a snack, but avoid milk and milk products.

(Continued)

Table 1-5 Characteristics of Selected Antibiotics *(continued)*

Antibiotic	Spectrum	Route	Side Effects/Special Uses
Amikacin (Amikin)	−, active against many gentamicin/tobramycin-resistant gram-negatives. Ideal for nosocomial gram-negative infection.	IM or IV slowly	Nephrotoxic and ototoxic (more deafness than vestibular effects). Curare-like effect.
Quinolones (bactericidal)	+, most −, including multidrug-resistant isolates, and MRSA and MRSE. Not good for *Enterococcus*.		Expensive, *Candida* overgrowth, photosensitivity reactions, hypoglycemia, hyperglycemia.
Norfloxacin (Noroxin)	Same as above	PO	Very broad treatment for complicated urinary tract infections.
Ciprofloxacin (Cipro)	Same as above	PO, IV	Very broad spectrum makes this a useful oral agent for mixed infections, infectious diarrhea, and multidrug-resistant organisms at any body site except CNS.
New quinolones Ofloxacin (Floxin) Sparfloxacin (Zagam) Enoxacin (Penetrex) Temafloxacin (Omniflox) Lomefloxacin (Maxaquin) Levofloxacin (Levaquin) Trovafloxacin (Trovan) Moxifloxacin (Avelox) Gatifloxacin (Tequin) Gemifloxacin (Factive) Clinafloxacin	Increased activity for + and −	PO	Same as above.
Miscellaneous agents Chloramphenicol (Chloromycetin)	+, −, anaerobes, *Rickettsia*; bacteriostatic	PO, IV	"Gray baby" syndrome in newborns, bone marrow toxicity, optic atrophy, and peripheral neuropathy.
Metronidazole (Flagyl, Flagyl IV)	Anaerobes, *Campylobacter*, amebae, *Trichomonas*, *C difficile*; bacteriostatic	PO, IV	GI upset, vertigo, ataxia, peripheral neuropathy, phlebitis, carcinogenic (?), Antabuse-like reaction.

+ = gram-positive, − = gram-negative, *Staph* = penicillinase-producers.

Antibiotic	Spectrum	Route	Side Effects/Special Uses
Rifampin (Rifadin)	TB, *Staph* (synergy), meningococcal prophylaxis; bactericidal	PO	Hepatotoxicity, flulike syndrome, discoloration of body secretions, drug interactions.
Pentamidine (Pentam 300)	*Pneumocystis* pneumonia	IV, aerosol	Hypotension, hypoglycemia, abnormal liver function tests, azotemia, bone marrow toxicity.
New Antibiotic Classes			
Streptogramins (bactericidal) Quinupristin/dalfopristin (Synercid)	Active against multidrug-resistant + organisms, even those with reduced sensitivity to vancomycin	IV	Bactericidal as a combined drug. No cross-resistance with other antibiotics. GI side effects, rash, myalgias.
Oxazolidinones (bactericidal) Linezolid (Zyvox) Eperezolid (investigational)	Similar to quinupristin/dalfopristin	IV, PO	Has monoamine oxidase (MAO) inhibitor effects, so drug interactions are possible.
Everninomicins (bactericidal) Evernimicin (Ziracin)	Similar to quinupristin/dalfopristin	IV	Effective for methicillin-resistant and vancomycin-intermediate-sensitivity organisms.
Avilamycin	Similar to quinupristin/dalfopristin	IV	Similar to above.
Lipopeptides (bactericidal) Daptomycin (investigational)	Similar to quinupristin/dalfopristin	IV, PO	Most bactericidal of all in a study of new antibiotics for drug-resistant + strain.

+ = gram-positive, – = gram-negative, *Staph* = penicillinase-producers.

(Continued)

Table 1-5 Characteristics of Selected Antibiotics *(continued)*

Antibiotic	Spectrum	Route	Side Effects/Special Uses
Antifungal Agents (Fungistatic)			
Nystatin (Mycostatin)	*Candida*	PO tabs or suspension; topical cream, ointment, powder; GU irrigant, vaginal suppository	Useful for prevention of *Candida* overgrowth or for topical treatment of GI, mucosal, or skin candidiasis.
5-fluorocytosine (Ancobon, Ancotil)	*Candida, Cryptococcus*	PO	GI distress, leukopenia, hepatotoxicity. Particularly toxic in patients with compromised renal function.
Amphotericin B (Fungizone, Amphotec)	Most invasive fungi, oral candidiasis	IV for systemic use; PO only for oral candidiasis	Chills, fever, nausea, vomiting, thrombophlebitis, nephrotoxicity, hypokalemia, bone marrow suppression, shock, cardiotoxicity.
Miconazole (Micatin, Monistat)	*Candida*, dermatophytes	Topical or vaginal cream; IV	Topical treatment of *Candida* and dermatophytes. When used IV thrombophlebitis, thrombocytosis, anemia.
Clotrimazole (Lotrimin, Gyne-Lotrimin, Mycelex)	*Candida*, dermatophytes	Topical solution, vaginal suppository; PO	Same as above.
Ketoconazole (Nizoral)	Many fungi	PO	Rash, pruritus, nausea, gynecomastia, liver toxicity, impaired fertility.
Newer imidazoles			
Fluconazole (Diflucan) Itraconazole (Sporanox) Voriconazole (Vfend) Croconazole	*Candida, Cryptococcus*	PO, IV	Less toxicity than amphotericin and flucytosine. Better tolerated than ketoconazole.
Allylamines			
Terbinafine (Lamisil)	Dermatophytes causing onychomycosis	PO	Headache, GI symptoms, rash.

+ = gram-positive, − = gram-negative, *Staph* = penicillinase-producers.

Antibiotic	Spectrum	Route	Side Effects/Special Uses
Benzylamines			
Butenafine (Mentax)	Dermatophyte skin and nail infections	Topical	Rash.
Antiviral Agents*			
Acyclovir (Zovirax)	HSV, varicella-zoster	IV, PO, topical	Nephrotoxicity, CNS toxicity, nausea, vomiting.
Famciclovir (Famvir)	HSV, varicella-zoster	PO	Less frequent dosing (q 8 hr) than acyclovir.
Valacyclovir (Valtrex)	HSV, varicella-zoster	PO	Pro-drug for acyclovir. Less frequent dosing (q 8 hr).
Ganciclovir (Cytovene)	CMV, EBV, HSV	IV, PO, intraocular	Bone-marrow toxicity, phlebitis, headache, disorientation, nausea, anorexia, myalgia, rash.
Foscarnet (Foscavir)	CMV, EBV, HSV	IV	Nephrotoxicity.
Cidofovir (Vistide)	CMV, EBV, HSV	IV, intraocular	Effective for CMV and acyclovir-resistant HSV; prolonged duration of action allows infrequent dosing (every other week for IV).
Valganciclovir (Valcyte)	CMV	PO	Active against CMV strains that are resistant to other agents.
Amantadine (Symmetrel, Symadine)	Influenza A	PO	CNS toxicity, anticholinergic reactions.
Rimantadine (Flumadine)	Influenza A	PO	Fewer side effects than amantadine.
Zanamivir (Relenza)	Influenza A and B	Inhaled	An inhaled neuraminidase inhibitor. Approved for treatment and prophylaxis of contacts.
Oseltamivir (Tamiflu)	Influenza A and B	PO	Oral neuraminidase inhibitor. Fewer side effects and less resistance than with others. Approved for treatment and prophylaxis of contacts.
Ribavirin (Virazole)	Respiratory syncytial virus (RSV), hepatitis C; being studied for use with hantavirus	Inhaled, IV, PO	Synergistic with interferon-α for hepatitis C.

+ = gram-positive, − = gram-negative, *Staph* = penicillinase-producers.

*Antiretroviral agents for HIV infection are covered in the AIDS discussion in this chapter.

Resistance-conferring plasmids have been identified in virtually all bacteria. Moreover, many bacteria contain transposons that can enter plasmids or chromosomes. Plasmids can therefore pick up chromosomal genes for resistance and transfer them to species not currently resistant.

Bacteria that have acquired chromosomal and plasmid-mediated resistance can neutralize or destroy antibiotics in 3 different ways (they can use one or more of these mechanisms simultaneously):

1. by preventing the antibacterial agent from reaching its receptor site
2. by modifying or duplicating the target enzyme so that it is insensitive to the antibacterial agent
3. by synthesizing enzymes that destroy the antibacterial agent or modify the agent to alter its entry or receptor binding

Antimicrobial susceptibility testing permits a rational choice of antibiotics, although correlation of in vivo and in vitro susceptibility is not always precise. Disk-diffusion susceptibility testing has provided qualitative data about the inhibitory activity of commonly used antimicrobials against an isolated pathogen, and these data are usually sufficient. In serious infections, such as infective endocarditis, it is useful to quantify the drug concentrations that inhibit and kill the pathogen. The lowest drug concentration that prevents the growth of a defined inoculum of the isolated pathogen is the *minimal inhibitory concentration (MIC)*; the lowest concentration that kills 99.9% of an inoculum is the *minimal lethal concentration (MLC)*. For bactericidal drugs, the MIC and MLC are usually similar.

The antimicrobial activity of a treated patient's serum can be estimated via measurement of serum bactericidal titers. Clinical experience suggests that intravascular infections usually are controlled when the peak serum bactericidal titer is 1.8 or greater. Bactericidal therapy is preferred for patients with immunologic compromise or life-threatening infection. Other patients may be treated effectively with either bactericidal or bacteriostatic drugs. Although synergistic combinations are useful in certain clinical situations (eg, enterococcal endocarditis, gram-negative septicemia in granulocytopenic patients), combined antimicrobial therapy should be used judiciously so that potential antagonism and toxicity can be minimized.

β-Lactam antibiotics

The β-lactam group includes the penicillins, cephalosporins, and monobactams, all of which possess a β-lactam ring that binds to specific microbial binding sites and interferes with cell wall synthesis. The carbapenems and carbacephems are often grouped with β-lactams but have a slightly different ring structure. The majority of new agents have been created by side-chain manipulation of the β-lactam ring, which has improved resistance to enzymatic degradation. However, some of the newer antibiotics (such as third-generation cephalosporins) show diminished potency against gram-positive cocci, especially staphylococci.

Penicillins The first *natural penicillins,* types G and V, were degraded by the enzyme penicillinase. The *penicillinase-resistant penicillins,* such as methicillin, nafcillin, oxacillin, and cloxacillin, were developed for treating resistant *Staphylococcus* species, and except for a strain of methicillin-resistant *S epidermidis*, they were effective. The next generation of penicillins included the *aminopenicillins*, ampicillin and amoxicillin, created by placing an amino group on the acyl side chain of the penicillin nucleus. This change broadened their effectiveness to include *H influenzae*, *E coli*, and *Proteus mirabilis*. The next advance was the *carboxypenicillins*, carbenicillin and ticarcillin, active against aerobic gram-negative rods such as *P aeruginosa*, *Enterobacter* species, and indole-positive strains of *Proteus*. Therefore, carboxypenicillins are particularly effective for intra-abdominal conditions such as cholangitis, diverticular rupture, and gynecologic infections. The fourth-generation penicillins, known as *acylureidopenicillins*, included azlocillin, mezlocillin, and piperacillin. Currently, their usefulness is in treating Enterobacteriaceae, *P aeruginosa*, and febrile neutropenic patients, as well as for infections secondary to a combination of flora found in skin, soft tissue, intra-abdominal, and pelvic infections. However, because of the possibility of emergence of resistance, the newer penicillins are usually administered with an aminoglycoside.

Allergic reactions are the chief adverse effects encountered in using the penicillins; among antimicrobial agents, the penicillins are the leading cause of allergy. This allergy may be present in 3%–5% of the general population and in as many as 10% of those who have previously received a penicillin. Furthermore, the reported mortality rate with penicillin-induced anaphylaxis is approximately 10%. Large doses or prolonged administration seems to be associated with a high frequency of untoward reaction. Allergic reactions to penicillin are less frequent when the drug is administered orally. Reactions are somewhat higher in frequency when aqueous crystalline penicillin G is given by injection and distinctly higher when procaine penicillin G is given intramuscularly. Cross-allergenicity among the semisynthetic and natural penicillins apparently reflects their common 6-aminopenicillanic acid nucleus and sensitizing derivatives. Cross-allergenicity to cephalosporins may occur in 3%–5% of patients and should be of particular concern when the allergic reaction to either group of antimicrobial agents has been of the immediate type, such as anaphylaxis, angioneurotic edema, or hives.

Cephalosporins   The first-generation cephalosporins are active against β-lactamase–producing gram-positive cocci and gram-negative bacilli, which are responsible for most community-acquired infections. *Bacillus fragilis*, *P aeruginosa*, and *Enterobacter* species are typically resistant, as are methicillin-resistant staphylococci. None of the first-generation cephalosporins cross the meninges in concentrations sufficient for treating meningitis.

The second-generation extended-spectrum cephalosporins have expanded coverage against gram-negative bacilli.

Third-generation cephalosporins have greater activity against gram-negative bacilli than the earlier cephalosporins, specifically inhibiting the majority of Enterobacteriaceae. Unfortunately, none of the third-generation cephalosporins is effective against enterococci. In general, third-generation cephalosporins are less active than their predecessors against gram-positive organisms, especially *S aureus*. Activity against *B fragilis* varies. Third-generation cephalosporins penetrate the cerebrospinal fluid and have been used successfully to treat meningitis caused by susceptible microorganisms. It is advisable to limit these expensive antibiotics to situations in which they offer a clear advantage, such as in gram-negative bacillary infections or in place of more toxic agents. With the possible exception of ceftazidime, none of these agents is effective enough to be used by itself against *P aeruginosa* or in a febrile neutropenic patient. Likewise, these agents are not to be used for surgical prophylaxis because of their limited activity against gram-positive organisms. Although several oral third-generation cephalosporins are now available, their antimicrobial spectrum is not as broad as that of the parenteral third-generation cephalosporins.

The fourth-generation cephalosporins, cefepime and cefpirome, have a very broad spectrum of activity and are active against most gram-positive bacteria, as well as against *Pseudomonas* and other gram-negative organisms that are resistant to other β-lactam antibiotics. The fourth-generation cephalosporins also provide good coverage for most anaerobic infections. A new investigational cephalosporin, cefozopran, has similar activity and antibacterial spectrum. Two others, S-3578 and BAL9141, are active against methicillin-resistant staphylococci and penicillin-resistant *S pneumoniae*. Ceftobiprole (Zeftera) is being called a fifth-generation cephalosporin and is very effective in treating MRSA, as well as other serious gram-positive and gram-negative infections. It is approved in Canada and, as of 2009, is in the final stages of FDA approval in the United States.

In recent years, the benefits of continuous intravenous infusion of β-lactam antibiotics, such as nafcillin and ceftazidime, have been demonstrated. This method of dosing provides continuous and stable therapeutic blood and tissue levels of an antibiotic.

Parenteral cephalosporins have a direct effect on prothrombin production and on suppression of vitamin K–producing intestinal flora. The risk of hemorrhagic complications is increased in patients who are taking parenteral cephalosporins in conjunction with heparin, possibly the result of an additive or synergistic pharmacologic effect. The hypoprothrombinemic effects of oral anticoagulants may be increased by such cephalosporins as cefoxitin, leading to a coagulopathy. Acute intolerance to alcohol may occur in persons receiving cephalosporins that have an N-methylthiotetrazole side chain, such as cefamandole or cefoperazone. Patients should avoid alcohol during therapy and for 2–3 days after completion.

Monobactams   *Monobactams* are a monocyclic class of antibiotics that use only the β-lactam ring as their core structure. This group possesses excellent activity against aerobic gram-negative bacilli but is ineffective against both gram-positive cocci and anaerobes. The monobactams are similar in antimicrobial spectrum to the aminoglycosides and are generally better tolerated. However, the use of monobactams is limited by their narrow spectrum: many nosocomial infections are polymicrobial, involving gram-positive bacteria or anaerobes in addition to gram-negative aerobic bacilli. *Aztreonam* (Azactam), the first approved monobactam antibiotic, has an excellent safety profile and good success rate in the treatment of infections caused by aerobic gram-negative bacilli. Aztreonam is usually combined with a semisynthetic antistaphylococcal penicillin or clindamycin in presumptive therapy of known mixed infections.

Carbapenems   Carbapenems are a class of antibiotics with a basic ring structure similar to that of penicillins, except that a carbon atom replaces sulfur at the number 1 position.

The antibacterial spectrum of the carbapenems is broader than that of any other existing antibiotic and includes *S aureus*, *Enterobacter* species, and *P aeruginosa*. However, carbapenem-resistant strains of *Staphylococcus*, *Pseudomonas*, *Klebsiella*, *Acinetobacter*, and *Bacteroides* have been reported recently. Carbapenems also have excellent activity against anaerobic bacteria, including *B fragilis*. Cross-resistance between the carbapenems and between carbapenems and piperacillin/tazobactam has been reported recently in *Pseudomonas* isolates. Carbapenems produce a postantibiotic killing effect against some organisms, with a delay in regrowth of damaged organisms similar to that seen with aminoglycosides but not with cephalosporins or acylureidopenicillins. This quality can be particularly important for settings in which host defenses are compromised, such as granulocytopenia or sequestered foci of infection.

Imipenem-cilastatin (Primaxin) combines imipenem, a carbapenem, with cilastatin, an inhibitor of renal dehydropeptidase. Cilastatin has no antimicrobial activity and is present solely to prevent degradation of imipenem by dehydropeptidase. As monotherapy for mixed infections, imipenem-cilastatin is an appropriate compound. Up to 50% of penicillin-allergic patients are also allergic to imipenem.

Meropenem (Merrem), *biapenem*, *panipenem*, *ertapenem*, *faropenem*, *tomopenem*, and *ritipenem* are newer penems that have increased stability against degradation by dehydropeptidases. *Doripenem* is a new agent that appears to be most effective in treating carbapenem-resistant gram-negative bacilli and penicillin-resistant streptococci.

Loracarbef (Lorabid) is an oral carbacephem, a class of antibiotic that is structurally similar to cephalosporins but that possesses a broader spectrum due to higher stability against both plasmid and chromosomally mediated β-lactamases. Loracarbef provides good coverage for most gram-positive and gram-negative aerobic bacteria.

Clavulanic acid, sulbactam, and *tazobactam* are β-lactam molecules that possess little intrinsic antibacterial activity, but they are potent inhibitors of many plasmid-mediated class A β-lactamases. Currently, 4 combinations of β-lactam antibiotics plus β-lactamase inhibitors are available in the United States: *Augmentin* (oral amoxicillin and clavulanic acid), *Timentin* (intravenous ticarcillin and clavulanic acid), *Unasyn* (intravenous ampicillin and sulbactam), and *Zosyn* (intravenous piperacillin and tazobactam). These drugs have excellent activity against β-lactamase–producing gram-positive and gram-negative bacteria as well as many anaerobes. Recent research has illuminated new broad-spectrum inhibitors that are capable of simultaneously inactivating several classes of β-lactamases (including classes A, C, and D) and has explored potential new cephalosporin-derived β-lactamase inactivators.

Glycopeptides

Vancomycin regained popularity because of the emergence of methicillin-resistant staphylococci and the recognition that *C difficile* is a cause of pseudomembranous colitis. It has excellent activity against *Clostridium* and against most gram-positive bacteria, including methicillin-resistant staphylococci, *Corynebacterium* species, and other diphtheroids. Vancomycin has been used alone to treat serious infections caused by methicillin-resistant staphylococci. In cases of prosthetic-valve endocarditis caused by methicillin-resistant *S epidermidis*, a combination of vancomycin, rifampin, and gentamicin has proven effective.

In recent years, several cases of vancomycin-resistant enterococcal infection have been reported. In one study of hospitalized patients, approximately 1% carried vancomycin-resistant enterococci in their gastrointestinal tract. These infections are very difficult or impossible to treat because of multidrug resistance. In vitro studies have shown that plasmid-mediated vancomycin resistance can be easily transferred to staphylococci; indeed, since July 2002, there have been several confirmed isolated reports of *S aureus* and *S epidermidis* infections resistant to vancomycin.

The CDC has issued recommendations regarding appropriate use of vancomycin to help counteract the emergence of bacterial drug resistance. These guidelines include discouraging the use of vancomycin for routine surgical prophylaxis, avoiding its empirical use in febrile neutropenic patients unless there is strong evidence of a β-lactam–resistant gram-positive infection, and avoiding prophylactic therapy for patients with intravascular catheters or vascular grafts. The rationale for these recommendations is that inappropriate use of this drug will only hasten the emergence of new resistant bacterial strains. Similarly, many authors think that prophylactic use of vancomycin in routine ophthalmic surgery is not advisable from an infectious disease and public health standpoint.

Teicoplanin (Targocid), a newer glycopeptide, has several advantages over vancomycin, including longer half-life, lower nephrotoxicity, and no requirement for monitoring drug levels. Teicoplanin is effective for treatment of staphylococcal infections, including endocarditis, bacteremia, osteomyelitis, and septic arthritis. The once-daily or alternate-day dosage allows home administration of treatment of serious infections caused by MRSA and enterococci, with significant savings in hospital costs and enhanced quality of life. Teicoplanin may be preferable to vancomycin for surgical prophylaxis because of its excellent tissue penetration, lower toxicity, and long half-life, allowing single-dose administration in several surgical procedures. The antibacterial activity of teicoplanin is similar to that of vancomycin but with increased potency, particularly against *Streptococcus* and *Enterococcus*. Teicoplanin is active against vancomycin-resistant organisms such as VanB-resistant and VanC-resistant strains. An investigational drug, it is available from the manufacturer for compassionate use. The new investigational glycopeptides oritavancin, telavancin, and dalbavancin and the glycolipodepsipeptide ramoplanin are highly active against vancomycin-resistant infections.

Quinolones

In 1962, *nalidixic acid* was discovered as an accidental by-product of research on quinolones as antimalarial agents. Nalidixic acid has relatively good activity against aerobic gram-negative bacteria but only limited activity against gram-positive species. It can provide adequate therapy for urinary tract infections, but if taken orally, it does not produce tissue concentrations sufficient to treat systemic infections. When administered intravenously, it produces CNS and cardiac toxicity. Consequently, for years the quinolones were not considered an important class of drugs.

The introduction of a fluorine into the basic quinolone nucleus has produced compounds known as *fluoroquinolones,* which have excellent gram-positive activity. The subsequent addition of piperazine produced compounds such as *norfloxacin* (Noroxin) and *ciprofloxacin* (Cipro), which have a broad spectrum of activity, encompassing staphylococci and most of the significant gram-negative bacilli, including *Pseudomonas.* Cipro-floxacin is available in both oral and parenteral forms and can be used to treat urinary tract infections, gonorrhea, and diarrheal diseases, as well as respiratory, skin, and, par-ticularly, bone infections. Fluoroquinolones introduced more recently into the US market include *ofloxacin* (Floxin), *temafloxacin* (Omniflox), *lomefloxacin* (Maxaquin), *enoxacin* (Penetrex), *sparfloxacin* (Zagam), *levofloxacin* (Levaquin), *moxifloxacin* (Avelox), *gati-floxacin* (Tequin), *trovafloxacin* (Trovan), and *gemifloxacin* (Factive). *Besifloxacin,* devel-oped by Bausch and Lomb for ocular surface infections, was approved by the FDA in December 2008. So far, more than 10,000 fluoroquinolone agents have been synthesized and tested since the discovery of nalidixic acid. Newer drugs awaiting FDA approval in-clude *garenoxacin, nadifloxacin,* and *prulifloxacin.* The new fluoroquinolones possess even greater activity against gram-positive and gram-negative bacteria. Either moxifloxa-cin or levofloxacin appears to be a good treatment choice for pneumococcal infections that are resistant to penicillin and the macrolides. Oral quinolones are an alternative form of therapy to β-lactams and aminoglycosides and have allowed physicians to treat more patients outside the hospital setting.

Macrolides

The macrolide *erythromycin* is often employed for the initial treatment of community-acquired pneumonia. This agent is effective against infections caused by pneumococci, group A streptococci, *M pneumoniae,* and *Chlamydia.* It is also effective against *Legion-ella* species, which have been recognized as a significant cause of community-acquired pneumonia. Erythromycin is used to treat upper-respiratory tract infections and sexually transmitted diseases in penicillin-allergic patients.

Clarithromycin (Biaxin), *azithromycin* (Zithromax), and *dirithromycin* (Dynabac) are newer macrolide antibiotics chemically related to erythromycin. All are well-tolerated al-ternatives to erythromycin and may offer particular advantages in treating gonococcal and *Chlamydia* infections and in the treatment of *M avium* and other recalcitrant infections associated with AIDS. Azithromycin is subclassified as an *azalide,* and it causes far fewer drug interactions than erythromycin. Increasing cross-resistance among the macrolides has been shown. Additional new macrolide antibiotics, such as roxithromycin, spiramy-cin, and josamycin, are being evaluated and have similar antimicrobial spectra.

Telithromycin and cethromycin, newer ketolide antibiotics that belong to a new class of semisynthetic 14-membered-ring macrolides, are discussed in New Antibiotic Classes, later in this chapter.

Clindamycin has a gram-positive spectrum similar to that of erythromycin and is also active against most anaerobes, including *B fragilis.* Except for treating anaerobic infection, clindamycin is rarely the drug of choice, although it is well absorbed orally, and parenteral formulations are available. Its major adverse effect is diarrhea, which may progress to pseudomembranous enterocolitis in some patients.

Aminoglycosides

The aminoglycoside antibiotics inhibit protein synthesis by binding to bacterial ribo-somes. Gentamicin, tobramycin, amikacin, kanamycin, streptomycin, and netilmicin can be considered as a group because of their similar activity, pharmacology, and toxicity. Because of poor gastrointestinal absorption, parenteral administration is necessary to produce therapeutic levels.

Aminoglycosides are used to treat serious infections caused by gram-negative bacilli, including bacteremia in immunocompromised hosts, hospital-acquired pneumonia, and peritonitis. They may be combined with penicillin to treat enterococcal endocarditis. Aminoglycosides are not effective against meningitis because they do not cross the blood–brain barrier. Aminoglycosides are not used for most gram-positive infections because the β-lactams are less toxic.

The major adverse effects of the aminoglycosides are nephrotoxicity and ototoxicity. Baseline blood urea nitrogen and creatinine levels should be measured, and serial studies should be performed twice a week. Aminoglycoside peak and trough serum levels should be obtained in patients with known renal disease. Combined administration of a loop diuretic such as furosemide with aminoglycosides has a synergistic ototoxic effect, potentially leading to permanent loss of cochlear function. Penicillins may decrease the antimicrobial effectiveness of parenteral aminoglycosides, particularly in patients with impaired renal function.

Tetracyclines

The tetracyclines are bacteriostatic agents that reversibly inhibit ribosomal protein synthesis. Although they have a broad spectrum of activity (including *Rickettsia, Chlamydia, Nocardia,* and *Actinomyces*), resistance is widespread, especially among *S aureus* and gram-negative bacilli. The principal clinical uses of tetracyclines are in treatment of nongonococcal urethritis, Rocky Mountain spotted fever, chronic bronchitis, and sebaceous disorders such as acne rosacea. In addition, tetracyclines are an alternative for the penicillin-allergic patient with syphilis. Tetracyclines are well absorbed when taken on an empty stomach; however, their absorption is decreased when taken with milk, antacids, calcium, or iron. Tetracyclines are distributed throughout the extracellular fluid, but cerebrospinal fluid penetration is unreliable. Adverse effects include oral or vaginal candidiasis with prolonged use, gastrointestinal upset, photosensitivity, elevation of the blood urea nitrogen level, and pseudotumor cerebri. Tetracyclines should not be administered to pregnant women or to children younger than age 10 because of effects on developing bone and teeth. Lymecycline is a newer tetracycline agent available in Europe.

Miscellaneous antibacterial agents

Rifampin was originally developed as an anti-TB agent, but it is also used to treat a host of intractable bacterial infections. The drug is usually employed adjunctively because bacteria develop resistance to the drug when it is used as a single agent. Rifampin often demonstrates higher effectiveness in vivo than in vitro, perhaps because it penetrates directly into leukocytes and kills phagocytosed bacteria. It also penetrates well into bone and abscess cavities. Rifampin in combination with other agents is used successfully in treating *S aureus* and prosthetic valve endocarditis caused by *S epidermidis*. It is effective in eradicating the carrier state of nasal *S aureus*. The drug is also effective prophylactically against *N meningitidis* and may be useful for treating oropharyngeal carriers of *H influenzae* type B.

Another oral antibiotic with potential for treating deep-seated infections is TMP-SMX. After a single oral dose, the mean serum levels of trimethoprim and sulfamethoxazole are approximately 75% of the concentration that would be achieved through the intravenous route. In addition to its excellent pharmacokinetics, TMP-SMX has an extremely broad spectrum of activity (against Enterobacteriaceae, it is usually comparable to that of a third-generation cephalosporin or even an aminoglycoside). A number of unusual microorganisms that are resistant to cephalosporins are susceptible to TMP-SMX. One misconception is that TMP-SMX has limited activity against gram-positive bacteria; however, most streptococci, staphylococci, and *Listeria monocytogenes* are susceptible to it. Beyond the broad-spectrum effect of TMP-SMX, the concomitant use of *metronidazole* creates an antibiotic combination with activity against microorganisms surpassing that of a third-generation cephalosporin. In recent years,TMP-SMX has been used increasingly in the treatment and prophylaxis of *Pneumocystis* infection and toxoplasmosis.

Chloramphenicol is a bacteriostatic agent that reversibly inhibits ribosomal protein synthesis. This drug is active against a wide variety of gram-negative and gram-positive organisms, including anaerobes. The major concern with this agent is hematopoietic toxicity, including reversible bone marrow suppression and irreversible aplasia. Aplastic anemia is an idiosyncratic late reaction to the drug and is usually fatal. Reversible leukopenia, thrombocytopenia, and suppression of erythropoiesis are dose-related and can usually be avoided when peak serum levels are maintained at less than 25 mcg/mL. Other adverse effects include hemolysis, allergy, and peripheral neuritis.

New Antibiotic Classes

Pharmacologic research is providing entirely new classes of antibiotics that offer additional treatment options for emerging resistant bacterial strains. Most of the new drugs that have been recently developed are targeted against resistant strains of gram-positive bacteria.

The first approved *streptogramin* antibiotic is *quinupristin/dalfopristin* (Q/D; Synercid). Streptogramins, also called *synergistins,* represent a unique class of antibiotics notable for their outstanding antibacterial activity and their unique mechanism of action. Oral streptogramins have been available in Europe for years, but Q/D is the first parenteral drug in this class.

Streptogramins have excellent activity against multidrug-resistant gram-positive organisms in vitro and in vivo. This class of drugs is noted for rapid killing of bacteria and for its lack of cross-resistance with other antimicrobials. Q/D has excellent activity against all staphylococcal species tested regardless of the resistance pattern to other drug classes, including methicillin and macrolide-resistant strains, and was 2–4 times more active than vancomycin. Q/D is also active against mycoplasma, *N gonorrhoeae, H influenzae, Legionella,* and *Moraxella catarrhalis.* Despite a short half-life, an extended postantibiotic effect allows the drug to be administered every 8–12 hours. Adverse effects include rash, itching, diarrhea, vomiting, arthralgia, myalgias, and reversible elevation of serum alkaline phosphatase levels.

Linezolid (Zyvox) is the first approved *oxazolidinone* antibiotic and is highly active against multidrug-resistant strains of gram-positive bacteria. It is as effective as vancomycin in treating methicillin-resistant staphylococcal infections and is active against vancomycin-resistant enterococci, penicillin-resistant and multidrug-resistant pneumococci, and macrolide-resistant streptococci. In one study, linezolid was the most potent new antibiotic tested against gram-positive cocci, including multiresistant strains. Because it has monoamine oxidase inhibitor effects, drug interaction precautions are necessary. *Furazolidone* (Furoxone) and newer experimental agents *eperezolid, ranbezolid,* and *AZD2563* are other similar oxazolidinones.

Evernimicin (Ziracin) is a new *oligosaccharide* antibiotic of the everninomicin class. This drug offers outstanding activity against drug-resistant gram-positive strains. In one multicenter, multinational, in vitro study, evernimicin outperformed vancomycin and Q/D against methicillin-resistant staphylococcal infections and all other gram-positive organisms tested. *Avilamycin* is another, newer member of this antibiotic family.

Telithromycin (Ketek) is a new *ketolide* that belongs to a new class of semisynthetic 14-membered-ring macrolides, which also have expanded activity against multidrug-resistant gram-positive bacteria. In some studies, these drugs are 8–10 times more potent than other macrolides. Telithromycin was specifically designed to treat community-acquired respiratory tract infections and offers a wide spectrum of activity against common respiratory pathogens. Telithromycin is active against β-lactam–resistant and macrolide-resistant bacteria and does not appear to induce cross-resistance to other antimicrobials. The FDA issued a public health advisory in 2007 concerning reports of hepatotoxicity from telithromycin. More recently, telithromycin was also associated with exacerbation of myasthenia gravis and with blurred vision. *Cethromycin* is a new investigational ketolide that appears to possess antimicrobial activity similar to that of telithromycin but with less hepatotoxicity.

Daptomycin, a new cyclic *lipopeptide* antibiotic, is also highly active against multidrug-resistant gram-positive bacteria. In one comparative study, daptomycin demonstrated greater bactericidal activity against MRSA and *S epidermidis,* vancomycin-resistant enterococci, and vancomycin-intermediate *S aureus* than did vancomycin, linezolid, and Q/D. An added benefit of this drug is that it has been shown to reduce the nephrotoxicity of aminoglycosides, but the mechanism of this protection is unknown.

Other new antibiotics for treating multidrug-resistant infections include the glycylcycline antibiotic *tigecycline* (Tigacyl), which is related to the tetracyclines; the bacteriocins, *nisin* and *sakacin*; the temporins, *temporin A* and *temporin L*; the DNA nanobinders; the peptide deformylase inhibitors; a folic acid antagonist, *iclaprim*; nucleoside analogues; bacteriophage endolysins, which are derived from viral phage-infected bacterial cells; and antimicrobial proteins (AMPs), natural endogenous proteins able to kill bacteria, fungi, and viruses at nanomolar concentrations.

Antifungal Agents

Fluconazole (Diflucan) and *itraconazole* (Sporanox) are newer antifungal *imidazoles* for treating cryptococcal meningitis, candidiasis, and other invasive fungal infections. These drugs are more effective and better tolerated than ketoconazole in treating candidiasis and invasive fungal disease. Imidazoles function by inhibiting fungal cytochrome P-450–dependent enzymes, thereby blocking synthesis of the fungal cell membrane. The newer imidazoles offer a less toxic alternative to amphotericin B in treating cryptococcal meningitis and may play a role in chronic suppression of *Cryptococcus* after remission of acute infection in severely immunocompromised patients. Voriconazole (Vfend), the first approved second-generation triazole, is available in both intravenous and oral formulations. It offers a better treatment option for invasive aspergillosis and other serious fungal infections. In a recent randomized trial, voriconazole demonstrated superior efficacy compared with parenteral amphotericin B, which is followed by other antifungal agents. Additional new investigational imidazoles include *flutrimazole, croconazole, ravuconazole, posaconazole, sertaconazole, albaconazole, lanoconazole, bifonazole, eberconazole,* and *luliconazole*.

Treatment of serious deep-seated systemic fungal infections may require the use of intravenous amphotericin B, sometimes in combined therapy with either flucytosine or an imidazole. Lipid complex and liposome-encapsulated formulations of amphotericin B (AmBisome, Amphotec) are available to reduce the drug's toxicity. Nystatin, which is structurally similar to amphotericin B, is classified as a topical antifungal agent. However, a new intravenous liposomal formulation of nystatin is currently in clinical trials for treatment of systemic fungal infections.

Terbinafine (Lamisil) is an *allylamine* oral antifungal agent that is effective in controlling onychomycosis due to chronic dermatophyte infections. Treatment must be continued for 6–12 weeks to eradicate the nail infection. *Butenafine* (Mentax) is a benzylamine that effectively treats skin and nail infections caused by dermatophytes.

Several novel antifungal agents include echinocandins, pneumocandins, and improved imidazoles. *Caspofungin* (Cancidas), *micafungin* (Mycamine), and *anidulafungin* (Eraxis) are echinocandins that have recently been approved for treatment of invasive *Candida* and *Aspergillus* infections. Other promising new drugs in preclinical development include inhibitors of fungal protein, fatty acid, lipid, and cell wall synthesis.

Antiviral Agents

Acyclovir (Zovirax) is a nucleoside analogue that is effective against herpes simplex and varicella-zoster infections. It inhibits viral DNA replication. One phosphorylation step of acyclovir is catalyzed by the enzyme thymidine kinase. The viral-induced thymidine kinase is far more active than the host cell thymidine kinase. Therefore, acyclovir is very active against viruses within infected host cells and yet is generally well tolerated.

Acyclovir has proven effective in treating a variety of herpetic infections. A topical 5% ointment may be used to treat localized primary episodes of genital herpes. Oral acyclovir 200 mg 5 times daily is effective in treating acute severe genital herpes. Also, long-term suppressive therapy with oral acyclovir has demonstrated efficacy in immunocompetent patients with frequently recurring genital herpes. Intravenous acyclovir 30 mg/kg every 8 hours is the treatment of choice for herpes simplex encephalitis. Acyclovir 500 mg/M² every 8 hours has been used successfully in treating herpes zoster infections in immunocompromised patients. This dosage is also used in patients with acute retinal necrosis syndrome.

Oral acyclovir may be used to treat herpes zoster ophthalmicus: 800 mg 5 times daily is usually effective in reducing the incidence of ocular complications of herpes zoster ophthalmicus. However, postherpetic neuralgia is not affected by this therapy. A randomized controlled study of acyclovir and oral corticosteroids demonstrated that the latter did not help to reduce the incidence of postherpetic neuralgia when added to oral acyclovir.

Famciclovir (Famvir) and *valacyclovir* (Valtrex) are currently approved for the treatment of herpes zoster infections and have also been shown to be effective against herpes simplex in numerous studies. Both of these newer drugs allow less frequent dosing intervals (every 8–12 hours, depending on the indication). *Valganciclovir* (Valcyte) is used for the prevention and treatment of CMV infections in organ transplant patients and AIDS patients. In a few studies, it has also been found to be effective for treating acute retinal necrosis caused by varicella-zoster virus.

Adefovir (Preveon) is a nucleoside analogue and a potent inhibitor of many viruses, such as HIV, HSV, hepatitis B, HPV, and EBV. The nucleoside analogue *brivudine* appears to have a stronger antiviral effect against the varicella-zoster virus than does acyclovir or penciclovir. The efficacy of brivudine has been documented in several clinical trials in patients with herpes simplex and herpesvirus-related infections, particularly in patients with herpes zoster.

Ganciclovir (Cytovene), foscarnet (Foscavir), and cidofovir (Vistide) are antiviral agents used for treating CMV infections, including retinitis. These drugs and the antiretroviral agents are discussed in more detail under the earlier heading Acquired Immunodeficiency Syndrome.

Amantadine and rimantadine are M2 protein inhibitors effective for treating influenza A and for the prophylactic treatment of contacts of infected patients. However, the rapid onset of drug resistance, ineffectiveness against influenza B, and CNS side effects have limited wide acceptance of these agents. Oseltamivir is an oral neuraminidase inhibitor that initially exhibited excellent efficacy against influenza in humans, but reports in early 2009 showed a high incidence of viral resistance (up to 100%) to this agent in infections caused by influenza type A H1N1. Another neuraminidase inhibitor, zanamivir, appears to be effective for influenza, but resistance has recently been reported with this agent as well.

Anttila VJ, Salonen J, Ylipalosaari P, Koivula I, Riikonen P, Nikoskelainen J. A retrospective nationwide case study on the use of a new antifungal agent: patients treated with caspofungin during 2001-2004 in Finland. *Clin Microbiol Infect.* 2007;13(6):606–612.

Babic M, Hujer AM, Bonomo RA. What's new in antibiotic resistance? Focus on beta-lactamases. *Drug Resist Updat.* 2006;9(3):142–156.

Bailey J, Summers KM. Dalbavancin: a new lipoglycopeptide antibiotic. *Am J Health Syst Pharm.* 2008;65(7):599–610.

Boucher HW, Groll AH, Chiou CC, Walsh TJ. Newer systemic antifungal agents: pharmacokinetics, safety and efficacy. *Drugs.* 2004;64(18):1997–2020.

Bozdogan B, Esel D, Whitener C, Browne FA, Applebaum PC. Antibacterial susceptibility of a vancomycin-resistant Staphylococcus aureus strain isolated at the Hershey Medical Center. *J Antimicrob Chemother.* 2003;52(2):864–868.

Bridges EG, Selden JR, Luo S. Nonclinical safety profile of telbivudine, a novel potent antiviral agent for treatment of hepatitis B. *Antimicrob Agents Chemother.* 2008;52(7):2521–2528.

Burkhardt O, Derendorf H, Welte T. Ertapenem: the new carbapenem 5 years after first FDA licensing for clinical practice. *Expert Opin Pharmacother.* 2007;8(2):237–256.

Buynak JD. The discovery and development of modified penicillin- and cephalosporin-derived beta-lactamase inhibitors. *Curr Med Chem.* 2004;11(14):1951–1964.

Carpenter CF, Chambers HF. Daptomycin: another novel agent for treating infections due to drug-resistant gram-positive pathogens. *Clin Infect Dis.* 2004;38(7):994–1000.

Centers for Disease Control and Prevention (CDC). Vancomycin-resistant Staphylococcus aureus—New York, 2004. *MMWR Morb Mortal Wkly Rep.* 2004;53(15):322–323.

Chacko M, Weinberg JM. Famciclovir for cutaneous herpesvirus infections: an update and review of new single-day dosing indications. *Cutis.* 2007;80(1):77–81.

Cui L, Iwamoto A, Lian JQ, et al. Novel mechanism of antibiotic resistance originating in vancomycin-intermediate Staphylococcus aureus. *Antimicrob Agents Chemother.* 2006;50(2):428–438.

Doripenem (doribax)—a new parenteral carbapenem. *Obstet Gynecol.* 2008;111(5):1206–1207.

Dowell JA, Goldstein BP, Buckwalter M, Stogniew M, Damle B. Pharmacokinetic-pharmacodynamic modeling of dalbavancin, a novel glycopeptide antibiotic. *J Clin Pharmacol.* 2008;48(4):1063–1068.

Fritsche TR, Sader HS, Jones RN. Antimicrobial activity of ceftobiprole, a novel anti-methicillin-resistant Staphylococcus aureus cephalosporin, tested against contemporary pathogens: results from the SENTRY Antimicrobial Surveillance Program (2005-2006). *Diagn Microbiol Infect Dis.* 2008;61(1):86–95.

Giannarini G, Mogorovich A, Valent F, et al. Prulifloxacin versus levofloxacin in the treatment of chronic bacterial prostatitis: a prospective, randomized, double-blind trial. *J Chemother.* 2007;19(3):304–308.

Hammerschlag MR, Sharma R. Use of cethromycin, a new ketolide, for treatment of community-acquired respiratory infections. *Expert Opin Investig Drugs.* 2008;17(3):387–400.

Hoellman DB, Lin G, Ednie LM, Rattan A, Jacobs MR, Appelbaum PC. Antipneumococcal and antistaphylococcal activities of ranbezolid (RBX 7644), a new oxazolidinone, compared to those of other agents. *Antimicrob Agents Chemother.* 2003;47(3):1148–1150.

Johnson MD, Perfect JR. Caspofungin: first approved agent in a new class of antifungals. *Expert Opin Pharmacother.* 2003;4(5):807–823.

Jones RN, Huynh HK, Biedenbach DJ. Activities of doripenem (S-4661) against drug-resistant clinical pathogens. *Antimicrob Agents Chemother.* 2004;48(8):3136–3140.

Joseph JM, Jain R, Danziger LH. Micafungin: a new echinocandin antifungal. *Pharmacotherapy.* 2007;27(1):53–67.

Juang P. Update on new antifungal therapy. *AACN Adv Crit Care.* 2007;18(3):253–260.

Kwon DS, Mylonakis E. Posaconazole: a new broad-spectrum antifungal agent. *Expert Opin Pharmacother.* 2007;8(8):1167–1178.

Lee SS, Kim HS, Kang HJ, Kim JK, Chung DR. Rapid spread of methicillin-resistant Staphylococcus aureus in a new hospital in the broad-spectrum antibiotic era. *J Infect.* 2007;55(4):358–362.

Montecalvo MA. Ramoplanin: a novel antimicrobial agent with the potential to prevent vancomycin-resistant enterococcal infection in high-risk patients. *J Antimicrob Chemother.* 2003;51(Suppl 3):iii31–iii35.

Noel GJ. Clinical profile of ceftobiprole, a novel beta-lactam antibiotic. *Clin Microbiol Infect.* 2007;13(Suppl 2):25–29.

Pasqualotto AC, Denning DW. New and emerging treatments for fungal infections. *J Antimicrob Chemother.* 2008;61(Suppl 1):i19–i30.

Shanson D. New British and American guidelines for the antibiotic prophylaxis of infective endocarditis: do the changes make sense? A critical review. *Curr Opin Infect Dis.* 2008;21(2):191–199.

Spiers KM, Zervos MJ. Telithromycin. *Expert Rev Anti Infect Ther.* 2004;2(5):685–693.

Spigelman MK. New tuberculosis therapeutics: a growing pipeline. *J Infect Dis.* 2007;196(Suppl 1): S28–S34.

Stevens DL, Dotter B, Madaras-Kelly K. A review of linezolid: the first oxazolidinone antibiotic. *Expert Rev Anti Infect Ther.* 2004;2(1):51–59.

Superti F, Ammendolia MG, Marchetti M. New advances in anti-HSV chemotherapy. *Curr Med Chem.* 2008;15(9):900–911.

Takagi H, Tanaka K, Tsuda H, Kobayashi H. Clinical studies of garenoxacin. *Int J Antimicrob Agents.* 2008;32(6):468–474.

Trofe J, Pote L, Wade E, Blumberg E, Bloom RD. Maribavir: a novel antiviral agent with activity against cytomegalovirus. *Ann Pharmacother.* 2008;42(1):1447–1457.

Vazquez JA. Combination antifungal therapy: the new frontier. *Future Microbiol.* 2007;2: 115–139.

Wilcox MH. Tigecycline and the need for a new broad-spectrum antibiotic class. *Surg Infect (Larchmt).* 2006;7(1):69–80.

Zhanel GG, Karlowsky JA, Rubinstein E, Hoban DJ. Tigecycline: a novel glycylcycline antibiotic. *Expert Rev Anti Infect Ther.* 2006;4(1):9–25.

Zhang JZ, Ward KW. Besifloxacin, a novel fluoroquinolone antimicrobial agent, exhibits potent inhibition of pro-inflammatory cytokines in human THP-1 monocytes. *J Antimicrob Chemother.* 2008;61(1):111–116.

CHAPTER **2**

Hypertension

Recent Developments

- Normal blood pressure (BP) is less than 120/80 mm Hg, according to guidelines published in 2003 by the Joint National Committee on Prevention, Detection, Evaluation, and Treatment of High BP (JNC 7 report).
- Individuals with systolic BP of 120–139 mm Hg or diastolic BP of 80–89 mm Hg are considered to have prehypertension and should adopt healthy lifestyle measures to decrease BP and prevent progression to hypertension.
- The risk of cardiovascular disease, beginning at 115/75 mm Hg, doubles with each 20/10 mm Hg rise in BP.
- In persons older than age 50, systolic BP higher than 140 mm Hg is a more important cardiovascular risk factor than diastolic BP.
- Masked hypertension—that is, normal office BP but abnormal home BP readings—may occur in 10%–30% of patients and may carry a worse prognosis than white coat hypertension with regard to the development of atherosclerosis.
- A thiazide diuretic, either alone or in combination with other classes of antihypertensive drugs, can be used to treat most patients with uncomplicated hypertension.
- Antihypertensive drug classes other than diuretics (angiotensin-converting enzyme [ACE] inhibitors, angiotensin II receptor blockers, β-blockers, calcium channel blockers) are indicated in high-risk conditions such as heart disease, kidney disease, and diabetes.
- Most patients with hypertension require 2 or more antihypertensive drugs to achieve BP control (less than 140/90 mm Hg, or less than 130/80 mm Hg for patients with diabetes or kidney disease).
- Hypertension in children and adolescents is more common than previously recognized and has substantial long-term health implications.

Introduction

Hypertension affects an estimated 73 million people age 20 and older in the United States and approximately 1 billion people worldwide. Those with hypertension are at greater risk for stroke, myocardial infarction (MI), heart failure, peripheral vascular disease, kidney disease, and retinal vascular complications. The prevalence of hypertension increases with age and tends to be familial. Hypertension is more common in blacks than in whites, and the incidence of devastating complications is higher in lower socioeconomic groups because of greater prevalence, delayed detection, and poor control rates. Antihypertensive therapy is effective in reducing cardiovascular morbidity and mortality, but only 59% of patients with hypertension are treated and only 34% achieve a BP of ≤140/90 mm Hg.

Classification of Blood Pressure and Diagnosis of Hypertension

A new classification of BP for adults 18 years or older was published in 2003 by the Joint National Committee on Prevention, Detection, Evaluation, and Treatment of High BP (JNC 7). Under the guidelines outlined in Table 2-1, normal BP is less than 120/80 mm Hg. *Hypertension* is defined as systolic BP of 140 mm Hg or higher or diastolic BP of 90 mm Hg or higher. A new category, designated *prehypertension,* is systolic BP of 120–139 mm Hg or diastolic BP of 80–89 mm Hg. Stage 1 hypertension is systolic BP of 140–159 mm Hg or diastolic BP of 90–99 mm Hg. Stage 2 hypertension is systolic BP of 160 mm Hg or higher or diastolic BP of 100 mm Hg or higher. The classification is based on the average of 2 or more properly measured seated BP readings on each of 2 or more office visits.

In 10%–15% of patients, BP increases only in a physician's office; these patients are said to have "white coat" hypertension. Home BP monitoring or 24-hour ambulatory BP measurement (ABPM) is warranted in these individuals and in patients with labile hypertension, resistant hypertension, hypotensive episodes, or postural hypotension, and, more recently, in patients with masked hypertension (ie, BP that is normal in the office but elevated by home BP measurements). ABPM provides data on circadian variations of BP and readings are usually lower than measurements in the office and correlate better with target-organ injury than do office measurements. BP in most individuals decreases by 10%–20% during the night (dipping pattern); those without such a decrease (nondipping pattern) are at greater risk for cardiovascular events. Masked hypertension may occur in 10%–30% of patients and was recently shown to carry a worse prognosis than white coat hypertension with regard to the development of atherosclerosis. Thus, it is important to

Table 2-1 Classification of Blood Pressure for Adults Aged 18 Years or Older

BP Classification	Systolic, mm Hg		Diastolic, mm Hg
Normal	<120	and	<80
Prehypertension	120–139	or	80–89
Stage 1 hypertension	140–159	or	90–99
Stage 2 hypertension	≥160	or	≥100

Adapted with permission from Chobanian AV, Bakris GL, Black HR, et al; National High Blood Pressure Education Program Coordinating Committee. The Seventh Report of the Joint National Committee on Prevention, Detection, Evaluation, and Treatment of High Blood Pressure: the JNC 7 report. *JAMA.* 2003;289(19):2561. ©2003 American Medical Association.

recognize that a normal office BP does not exclude hypertension. Individuals with a mean self-measured BP of greater than 135/85 mm Hg at home are generally considered to be hypertensive.

Etiology and Pathogenesis of Hypertension

Approximately 90% of cases of hypertension are *primary (essential),* in which the etiology is unknown, and 10% are secondary to identifiable causes. Primary hypertension most likely results from a disregulation of various renal, hormonal, and cellular processes in conjunction with environmental factors such as diet and exercise. These processes include abnormal sodium transport, increased sympathetic nervous system activity, abnormal vasodilation, excess transforming growth factors β (TGF-βs), and renin-angiotensin-aldosterone system (Fig 2-1).

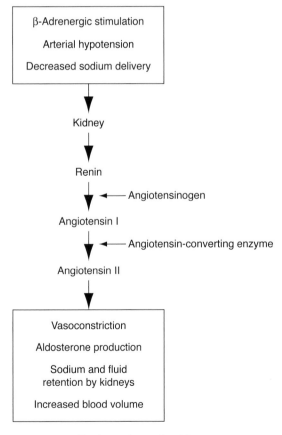

Figure 2-1   Renin-angiotensin-aldosterone system.

Causes of *secondary hypertension* are outlined in Table 2-2. Among the signs associated with secondary hypertension are

- *polycystic kidney disease:* flank mass
- *renovascular disease:* unilateral abdominal bruit in a young patient with marked hypertension; new-onset hypertension with severe end-organ disease
- *pheochromocytoma:* markedly labile BP with tachycardia and headache
- *hyperaldosteronism:* persistent hypokalemia in the absence of diuretic therapy
- *coarctation of aorta:* delayed or absent femoral pulses in a young patient
- *Cushing syndrome:* truncal obesity and abdominal striae

Secondary causes of hypertension should be suspected in persons who have accelerating hypertension or hypertension unresponsive to medication or in those who have a sudden change in previously well-controlled BP. Patients with secondary hypertension are more likely to have resistant hypertension.

Resistant hypertension is defined as a failure to achieve goal BP when a patient adheres to the maximum tolerated doses of 3 antihypertensive drugs, including a diuretic. The prevalence of resistant hypertension is currently not known, but indirect population study evidence suggests it is more common than once was thought. This is probably because of the aging population and increases in obesity, sleep apnea, and chronic kidney disease.

Most cases of resistant hypertension are due to inadequate dosing of medication and noncompliance with treatment. Other causes are listed in Table 2-2. These include NSAIDS, which have volume-retaining effects, and substances such as alcohol, oral contraceptives, licorice, cyclosporine, and antidepressants. The most common factor contributing to resistant hypertension is excess sodium intake and volume overload and failure to treat this with dietary modification or the proper diuretic usage and dosage.

Table 2-2 Causes of Secondary Hypertension

Chronic kidney disease
Obstructive uropathy
Renovascular hypertension
Genetic mutations
Primary hyperaldosteronism and other mineralocorticoid excess states
Pheochromocytoma
Cushing syndrome and corticosteroid excess
Coarctation of the aorta
Thyroid or parathyroid disease
Sleep apnea
Drugs (oral contraceptives, sympathomimetics, NSAIDS, erythropoietin calcineurin inhibitors, cyclosporine, tacrolimus, OTC medicines, ephedra, ma huang, bitter orange)
Alcohol

Adapted with permission from Chobanian AV, Bakris GL, Black HR, et al; National High Blood Pressure Education Program Coordinating Committee. The Seventh Report of the Joint National Committee on Prevention, Detection, Evaluation, and Treatment of High Blood Pressure: the JNC 7 report. *JAMA.* 2003;289(19):2563. ©2003 American Medical Association.

Evaluation of Hypertension

The evaluation of patients with hypertension should include an assessment of lifestyle and identification of other cardiovascular risk factors (Table 2-3), a search for causes of secondary hypertension, and determination of the presence or absence of target-organ damage and cardiovascular disease.

The physical examination should include measurement of BP in both arms; ophthalmoscopic examination; calculation of body mass index; measurement of waist circumference, which is considered the most important anthropometric factor associated with hypertensive risk; auscultation for carotid, abdominal, and femoral bruits; examination of the thyroid gland; examination of the heart and lungs; examination of the abdomen for masses and aortic pulsation; examination of the lower extremities for edema and pulses; and neurologic assessment.

Table 2-3 Cardiovascular Risk Factors

Major risk factors
  Hypertension*
  Cigarette smoking
  Obesity (BMI ≥30)*
  Physical inactivity
  Dyslipidemia*
  Diabetes mellitus*
  Microalbuminuria or estimated GFR <60 mL/min
  Age (>55 years for men, >65 years for women)
  Family history of premature cardiovascular disease (men <55 years of age or women <65 years
    of age)

Target-organ damage
  Heart
    Left ventricular hypertrophy
    Angina or prior myocardial infarction
    Prior coronary revascularization
    Heart failure
  Brain
    Stroke or transient ischemic attack
  Chronic kidney disease
  Peripheral arterial disease
  Retinopathy

BMI = body mass index, calculated as weight in kilograms divided by the square of height in meters, GFR = glomerular filtration rate.
*Components of the metabolic syndrome.

Adapted with permission from Chobanian AV, Bakris GL, Black HR, et al; National High Blood Pressure Education Program Coordinating Committee. The Seventh Report of the Joint National Committee on Prevention, Detection, Evaluation, and Treatment of High Blood Pressure: the JNC 7 report. *JAMA.* 2003;289(19):2563. ©2003 American Medical Association.

Laboratory tests to screen for secondary causes and exclude comorbidity (recommended before starting treatment) include an electrocardiogram, urinalysis, complete blood count, and serum chemistry studies including a lipid profile. More extensive testing for identifiable causes of hypertension usually is not indicated unless BP control is not achieved or there are other clinical findings.

Seidell JC, Han TS, Feskens EJ, Lean ME. Narrow hips and broad waist circumferences independently contribute to increased risk of non-insulin-dependent diabetes mellitus. *J Intern Med.* 1997;242(5):401–406.

Treatment of Hypertension

The primary objective of antihypertensive therapy is to reduce cardiovascular and renal morbidity and mortality. Controlling systolic BP is the major concern because, in patients older than 50 years, systolic BP greater than 140 mm Hg is a more important cardiovascular risk factor than diastolic BP. Diastolic BP usually is controlled when the systolic goal is reached. Maintaining BP at less than 140/90 mm Hg decreases cardiovascular complications. In hypertensive patients with diabetes or renal disease, the BP goal is less than 130/80 mm Hg. Effective BP control can be attained in most patients with hypertension, but the majority require 2 or more medications. It is important for patients to understand that lifelong treatment is usually necessary and that symptoms are not a reliable indicator of the severity of hypertension.

In considering the appropriate therapy for an individual patient, the physician should weigh multiple factors: stage of hypertension, target-organ disease, cardiovascular risk factors, cost, compliance, side effects, and comorbid conditions. In general, the higher the BP, the greater the damage to target organs; and the greater the risk factors for cardiovascular disease, the sooner treatment should be initiated. For example, patients with severe hypertension and encephalopathy require emergent treatment, whereas those with mild hypertension may attempt lifestyle modifications before drug therapy is initiated.

Lifestyle Modifications

Obesity, sedentary lifestyle, excessive sodium intake, high daily alcohol consumption, and inadequate intake of vitamins and minerals such as potassium, calcium, magnesium, and folate can contribute to the development of hypertension. Smoking is also important as a major contributor to cardiovascular disease in patients with hypertension. Lifestyle modifications, including weight reduction, adoption of the Dietary Approaches to Stop Hypertension (DASH) eating plan, dietary sodium reduction, increased physical activity, and moderation of alcohol consumption can decrease BP, enhance antihypertensive drug efficacy, and reduce cardiovascular disease risk (Table 2-4). Such healthy lifestyle habits are essential for the prevention and control of hypertension.

Pharmacologic Treatment

Several classes of drugs effectively lower BP and reduce the complications of hypertension. The most commonly prescribed antihypertensive drugs include diuretics, β-blockers,

Table 2-4 Lifestyle Modifications to Manage Hypertension*

Modification	Recommendation	Approximate Systolic BP Reduction, Range
Weight reduction	Maintain normal body weight (BMI, 18.5–24.9)	5–20 mm Hg/10 kg weight loss
Adoption of DASH eating plan	Consume a diet rich in fruits, vegetables, and low-fat dairy products with a reduced content of saturated and total fat	8–14 mm Hg
Dietary sodium reduction	Reduce dietary sodium intake to no more than 100 mEq/L (2.4 g sodium or 6 g sodium chloride)	2–8 mm Hg
Physical activity	Engage in regular aerobic physical activity such as brisk walking (at least 30 minutes per day, most days of the week)	4–9 mm Hg
Moderation of alcohol consumption	Limit consumption to no more than 2 drinks per day (1 oz or 30 mL ethanol [eg, 24 oz beer, 10 oz wine, or 3 oz 80-proof whiskey]) in most men and no more than 1 drink per day in women and lighter-weight persons	2–4 mm Hg

BMI = body mass index, calculated as weight in kilograms divided by the square of the height in meters, BP = blood pressure, DASH = Dietary Approaches to Stop Hypertension
*For overall cardiovascular risk reduction, stop smoking. The effects of implementing these modifications are dose- and time-dependent and could be higher for some individuals.

Adapted with permission from Chobanian AV, Bakris GL, Black HR, et al; National High Blood Pressure Education Program Coordinating Committee. The Seventh Report of the Joint National Committee on Prevention, Detection, Evaluation, and Treatment of High Blood Pressure: the JNC 7 report. *JAMA.* 2003;289(19):2564. ©2003 American Medical Association.

Other Modifications to Manage Hypertension*

Adequate sleep	Sleep deprivation increases risk twofold in middle-aged adults who sleep ≤5 hours a night.
Treatment of obstructive sleep apnea (OSA)	Reduce weight, apply CPAP (continuous positive airway pressure); surgery may be needed in more severe cases.

*For overall cardiovascular risk reduction, stop smoking.

ACE inhibitors, angiotensin II receptor blockers (ARB), and, more recently, calcium channel blockers (CCBs). Tables 2-5 and 2-6 list these and other types of oral antihypertensive drugs.

Numerous studies have confirmed the efficacy of diuretics in preventing the cardiovascular complications of hypertension. A thiazide-type diuretic is the preferred choice for initial therapy in most patients with hypertension, used either alone or in combination with other classes of antihypertensive medications. The use of other antihypertensive drugs as initial therapy is indicated in high-risk conditions such as heart failure, post-MI, high coronary disease risk, diabetes mellitus, and chronic kidney disease, and for recurrent stroke prevention (Table 2-7). In some cases, when BP is more than 20/10 mm Hg above goal, cautiously initiating treatment with 2 drugs may be appropriate. Figure 2-2 provides an algorithm for the treatment of hypertension.

Table 2-5 Oral Antihypertensive Drugs

Class	Drug (Trade Name)	Usual Dose, Range, mg/d*	Daily Frequency
Thiazide diuretics	Chlorothiazide (Diuril)	125–500	1
	Chlorthalidone (generic)	12.5–25	1
	Hydrochlorothiazide (Microzide, HydroDIURIL)	12.5–50	1
	Indapamide (Lozol)	1.25–2.5	1
	Metolazone (Mykrox)	0.5–1.0	1
	Metolazone (Zaroxolyn)	2.5–5	1
	Polythiazide (Renese)	2–4	1
Loop diuretics	Bumetanide (Bumex)	0.5–2	2
	Furosemide (Lasix)	20–80	2
	Torsemide (Demadex)	2.5–10	1
Potassium-sparing diuretics	Amiloride (Midamor)	5–10	1–2
	Triamterene (Dyrenium)	50–100	1–2
Aldosterone-receptor blockers	Eplerenone (Inspra)	50–100	1–2
	Spironolactone (Aldactone)	25–50	1–2
β-Blockers	Atenolol (Tenormin)	25–100	1
	Betaxolol (Kerlone)	5–20	1
	Bisoprolol (Zebeta)	2.5–10	1
	Metoprolol (Lopressor)	50–100	1–2
	Metoprolol extended release (Toprol-XL)	50–100	1
	Nadolol (Corgard)	40–120	1
	Propranolol (Inderal)	40–160	2
	Propranolol long-acting (Inderal LA)	60–180	1
	Timolol (Blocadren)	20–40	2
β-Blockers with intrinsic sympathomimetic activity	Acebutolol (Sectral)	200–800	2
	Penbutolol (Levatol)	10–40	1
	Pindolol (generic)	10–40	2
ACE inhibitors	Benazepril (Lotensin)	10–40	1–2
	Captopril (Capoten)	25–100	2
	Enalapril (Vasotec)	2.5–40	1–2
	Fosinopril (Monopril)	10–40	1
	Lisinopril (Prinivil, Zestril)	10–40	1
	Moexipril (Univasc)	7.5–30	1
	Perindopril (Aceon)	4–8	1–2
	Quinapril (Accupril)	10–40	1
	Ramipril (Altace)	2.5–20	1
	Trandolapril (Mavik)	1–4	1
Angiotensin II antagonists	Candesartan (Atacand)	8–32	1
	Eprosartan (Teveten)	400–800	1–2
	Irbesartan (Avapro)	150–300	1
	Losartan (Cozaar)	25–100	1–2
	Olmesartan (Benicar)	20–40	1
	Telmisartan (Micardis)	20–80	1
	Valsartan (Diovan)	80–320	1

(Continued)

Table 2-5 *(continued)*

Class	Drug (Trade Name)	Usual Dose, Range, mg/d*	Daily Frequency
Calcium channel blockers: nondihydropyridines	Diltiazem extended release (Cardizem CD, Dilacor XR, Tiazac)	180–420	1
	Diltiazem extended release (Cardizem LA)	120–540	1
	Verapamil (Covera-HS Verelan PM)	120–360	1
	Verapamil immediate release (Calan, Isoptin)	80–320	2
	Verapamil long-acting (Calan SR, Isoptin SR)	120–360	1–2
Calcium channel blockers: dihydropyridines	Amlodipine (Norvasc)	2.5–10	1
	Felodipine (Plendil)	2.5–20	1
	Isradipine (DynaCirc CR)	2.5–10	2
	Nicardipine sustained release (Cardene SR)	60–120	2
	Nifedipine long-acting (Adalat CC, Procardia XL)	30–60	1
	Nisoldipine (Sular)	10–40	1
α_1-Blockers	Doxazosin (Cardura)	1–16	1
	Prazosin (Minipress)	2–20	2–3
	Terazosin (Hytrin)	1–20	1–2
Combined α- and β-blockers	Carvedilol (Coreg)	12.5–50	2
	Labetalol (Normodyne, Trandate)	200–800	2
Central α_2-agonists and other centrally acting drugs	Clonidine (Catapres)	0.1–0.8	2
	Clonidine patch (Catapres-TTS)	0.1–0.3	1 weekly
	Guanfacine (generic)	0.5–2	1
	Methyldopa (Aldomet)	250–1000	2
	Reserpine (generic)	0.05–0.25	1†
Direct vasodilators	Hydralazine (Apresoline)	25–100	2
	Minoxidil (Loniten)	2.5–80	1–2
Direct renin inhibitor	Aliskiren (Tekturna)‡	150–300	1

ACE = angiotensin-converting enzyme.

*Dosages may vary from those listed in the *Physicians' Desk Reference,* which may be consulted for additional information. Many of the drugs in this table are available in generic formulations.

†0.1-mg dose may be given every other day to achieve this dosage.

‡Aliskiren is an oral renin inhibitor that effectively lowers BP when used either alone or with other antihypertensive agents. It is the first new class of antihypertensive drug approved by the FDA in more than a decade, and its role in the management of patients with hypertension is yet to be established.

Adapted with permission from Chobanian AV, Bakris GL, Black HR, et al; National High Blood Pressure Education Program Coordinating Committee. The Seventh Report of the Joint National Committee on Prevention, Detection, Evaluation, and Treatment of High Blood Pressure: the JNC 7 report. *JAMA.* 2003;289(19):2565–2566. ©2003 American Medical Association.

Table 2-6 Combination Drugs for Hypertension

Combination Type	Fixed-Dose Combination, mg*	Trade Name
ACE inhibitor and CCB	Amlodipine/benazepril HCl (2.5/10, 5/10, 5/20,10/20)	Lotrel
	Enalapril maleate/felodipine (5/5)	Lexxel
	Trandolapril/verapamil (2/180, 1/240, 2/240, 4/240)	Tarka
ACE inhibitor and diuretic	Benazepril/hydrochlorothiazide (5/6.25, 10/12.5, 20/12.5, 20/25)	Lotensin HCT
	Captopril/hydrochlorothiazide (25/15, 25/25, 50/15, 50/25)	Capozide
	Enalapril maleate/hydrochlorothiazide (5/12.5, 10/25)	Vaseretic
	Lisinopril/hydrochlorothiazide (10/12.5, 20/12.5, 20/25)	Prinzide
	Moexipril HCl/hydrochlorothiazide (7.5/12.5, 15/25)	Uniretic
	Quinapril HCl/hydrochlorothiazide (10/12.5, 20/12.5, 20/25)	Accuretic
ARB and diuretic	Candesartan cilexetil/hydrochlorothiazide (16/12.5, 32/12.5)	Atacand HCT
	Eprosartan mesylate/hydrochlorothiazide (600/12.5, 600/25)	Teveten HCT
	Irbesartan/hydrochlorothiazide (75/12.5, 150/12.5, 300/12.5)	Avalide
	Losartan potassium/hydrochlorothiazide (50/12.5, 100/25)	Hyzaar
	Telmisartan/hydrochlorothiazide (40/12.5, 80/12.5)	Micardis HCT
	Valsartan/hydrochlorothiazide (80/12.5, 160/12.5)	Diovan HCT
β-Blocker and diuretic	Atenolol/chlorthalidone (50/25, 100/25)	Tenoretic
	Bisoprolol fumarate/hydrochlorothiazide (2.5/6.25, 5/6.25, 10/6.25)	Ziac
	Metoprolol tartrate/hydrochlorothiazide (50/25, 100/25)	Lopressor HCT
	Nadolol/bendroflumethiazide (40/5, 80/5)	Corzide
	Propranolol LA/hydrochlorothiazide (40/25, 80/25)	Inderide
	Timolol maleate/hydrochlorothiazide (10/25)	Timolide
Centrally acting drug and diuretic	Methyldopa/hydrochlorothiazide (250/15, 250/25, 500/30, 500/50)	Aldoril
	Reserpine/chlorothiazide (0.125/250, 0.25/500)	Diupres
	Reserpine/hydrochlorothiazide (0.125/25, 0.125/50)	Hydropres
Diuretic and diuretic	Amiloride HCl/hydrochlorothiazide (5/50)	Moduretic
	Spironolactone/ hydrochlorothiazide (25/25, 50/50)	Aldactazide
	Triamterene/hydrochlorothiazide (37.5/25, 50/25, 75/50)	Dyazide, Maxzide

ACE = angiotensin-converting enzyme, ARB = angiotensin II receptor blocker, CCB = calcium channel blocker, HCl = hydrochloride, HCT = hydrochlorothiazide, LA = long-acting.

*Some drug combinations are available in multiple fixed doses. Each drug dose is reported in milligrams.

Adapted with permission from Chobanian AV, Bakris GL, Black HR, et al; National High Blood Pressure Education Program Coordinating Committee. The Seventh Report of the Joint National Committee on Prevention, Detection, Evaluation, and Treatment of High Blood Pressure: the JNC 7 report. *JAMA*. 2003;289(19):2567.

Table 2-7 Compelling Indications for Individual Drug Classes

High-Risk Condition	Diuretic	β-Blocker	ACE Inhibitor	ARB	CCB	Aldosterone Antagonist
Heart failure	•	•	•	•		•
Post–myocardial infarction		•	•			•
High coronary disease risk	•	•	•		•	
Diabetes	•	•	•	•	•	
Chronic kidney disease			•	•		
Recurrent stroke prevention	•		•			

ACE = angiotensin-converting enzyme, ARB = angiotensin II receptor blocker, CCB = calcium channel blocker

Adapted with permission from Chobanian AV, Bakris GL, Black HR, et al; National High Blood Pressure Education Program Coordinating Committee. The Seventh Report of the Joint National Committee on Prevention, Detection, Evaluation, and Treatment of High Blood Pressure: the JNC 7 report. *JAMA.* 2003;289(19):2568. ©2003 American Medical Association.

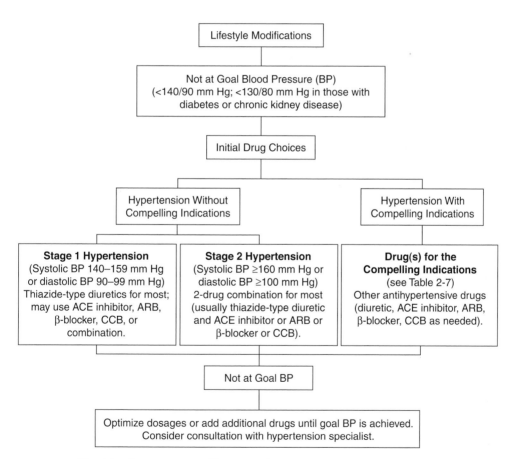

Figure 2-2 Algorithm for treatment of hypertension. *(Adapted with permission from Chobanian AV, Bakris GL, Black HR, et al; National High Blood Pressure Education Program Coordinating Committee. The Seventh Report of the Joint National Committee on Prevention, Detection, Evaluation, and Treatment of High Blood Pressure: the JNC 7 report. JAMA. 2003;289(19):2564. ©2003 American Medical Association.)*

Antihypertensive Drugs

Diuretics

Diuretics are categorized by their site of action in the kidney and are divided into thiazide, loop, and potassium-sparing types.

Thiazide diuretics increase the sodium load on the kidney's distal tubules and initially decrease plasma volume and cardiac output through natriuresis. As the renin-angiotensin-aldosterone system compensates for plasma volume, cardiac output returns to normal and peripheral vascular resistance is lowered.

Loop diuretics act on the ascending loop of Henle and block sodium resorption, causing an initial decrease in plasma volume. As with thiazide diuretics, BP is eventually reduced because of decreased peripheral vascular resistance. Loop diuretics are used primarily in treating patients with renal insufficiency. They are not as helpful for long-term use in patients with good renal function.

Potassium-sparing diuretics may competitively block the actions of aldosterone to prevent potassium loss from the distal tubule, or they may act directly on the distal tubule to inhibit aldosterone-induced sodium resorption in exchange for potassium. They are often used as adjuncts to the thiazides or loop diuretics to counteract potassium depletion.

Adverse effects of diuretics vary according to class. Thiazide diuretics can cause weakness, muscle cramps, impotence, hypokalemia, hyperglycemia, hyperlipidemia, hyperuricemia, hypercalcemia, hypomagnesemia, hyponatremia, azotemia, and pancreatitis. Long-term use of diuretics has been associated with type 2 diabetes. Therefore, their use in younger patients and those with diabetic risks should be limited. On a positive note, they may also slow the demineralization that occurs with osteoporosis. Loop diuretics can cause ototoxicity, as well as electrolyte abnormalities such as hypokalemia, hypocalcemia, and hypomagnesemia. Potassium-sparing diuretics can cause hyperkalemia, renal calculi, renal tubular damage, and gynecomastia. Diuretics are particularly effective in individuals with salt-sensitive hypertension such as older and black patients.

β-Blockers

There are 2 types of β-adrenergic receptor sites: β_1 is present in vascular and cardiac tissue, and β_2 is found in the bronchial system. Circulating or locally released catecholamines stimulate β sites, resulting in vasoconstriction, bronchodilation, tachycardia, and increased myocardial contractility. β-blockers inhibit these effects. They also decrease plasma renin, reset baroreceptors to facilitate lower BP, induce release of vasodilatory prostaglandins, decrease plasma volume, and may have a CNS-mediated antihypertensive effect.

β-Blockers are divided into those that are nonselective (β_1 and β_2), those that are cardioselective (primarily β_1), and those that have intrinsic sympathomimetic activity (ISA). The cardioselective agents may be prescribed with caution in patients with pulmonary disease, diabetes, or peripheral vascular disease, but at higher doses they lose their β_1 selectivity and can cause adverse effects in these patients. Those with ISA minimize the bradycardia caused by other β-blockers. β-Blockers with α-blocking properties such as carvedilol or labetalol have additional vasodilatory effects caused by selective $α_1$-receptor blockade.

Adverse effects of β-blockers include bronchospasm, bradycardia, heart failure, masking of insulin-induced hypoglycemia, insomnia, fatigue, depression, impotence, impaired peripheral circulation, impaired exercise tolerance, nasal congestion, and hypertriglyceridemia (except β-blockers with ISA). Angina pectoris and increased BP can be precipitated by abrupt cessation of β-blocker therapy. β-Blockers generally should be avoided in patients with asthma, reactive airways disease, or second-degree or third-degree heart block. β-Blockers are beneficial in the treatment of atrial fibrillation and tachyarrhythmias, migraine, thyrotoxicosis, and essential tremor.

Angiotensin-Converting Enzyme Inhibitors

Angiotensin-converting enzyme catalyzes the conversion of angiotensin I to angiotensin II. Angiotensin II, a potent vasoconstrictor, is the primary vasoactive hormone of the renin-angiotensin-aldosterone system, and it plays a major role in the pathophysiology of hypertension. ACE inhibitors block the conversion of angiotensin I to angiotensin II, resulting in vasodilation with decreased peripheral vascular resistance and natriuresis. They also decrease aldosterone production and increase levels of vasodilating bradykinins. Some ACE inhibitors stimulate production of vasodilatory prostaglandins. The efficacy of ACE inhibitors is enhanced when they are used together with diuretics; they can reduce hypokalemia, hypercholesterolemia, hyperglycemia, and hyperuricemia caused by diuretic therapy. ACE inhibitors are beneficial in patients with left ventricular dysfunction and with kidney disease. They may also help to improve insulin sensitivity.

Adverse effects of ACE inhibitors include a dry cough (5%–20% of patients), angioneurotic edema, hypotension, hyperkalemia, abnormal taste, leukopenia, proteinuria, and renal failure in patients with preexisting renal insufficiency. ACE inhibitors should be avoided in patients with a history of angioedema, and they are contraindicated in pregnancy because of the adverse effects on fetal renal function and fetal death.

Angiotensin II Receptor Blockers

Angiotensin II receptor blockers (ARBs) inhibit the vasoconstrictor and aldosterone-secreting effects of angiotensin II by selectively blocking angiotensin II receptors that are found in such tissues as vascular smooth muscle and the adrenal gland, resulting in decreased peripheral vascular resistance. ARBs are effective in managing hypertension in a variety of situations, including in patients with heart failure who are unable to tolerate ACE inhibitors. ARBs also have been associated with a reduced incidence of new-onset diabetes and, like ACE inhibitors, improve insulin sensitivity.

The side effects of ARBs are similar to those occurring with ACE inhibitors, although less common. The cough caused by ACE inhibitors generally does not occur with ARBs, and angioedema is rare. Like ACE inhibitors, ARBs are contraindicated in pregnancy.

Calcium Channel Blockers

Calcium channel blockers block the entry of calcium into vascular smooth-muscle cells, resulting in reduced myocardial contractility and decreased systemic vascular resistance. CCBs are divided into dihydropyridine and nondihydropyridine types.

Adverse effects of CCBs vary according to the agent but include constipation, headache, fatigue, dizziness, nausea, palpitations, flushing, edema, gingival hyperplasia, arrhythmias, and cardiac ischemia. Because of their negative inotropic effects, CCBs generally should be avoided in patients with cardiac conduction abnormalities or heart failure associated with left ventricular dysfunction and in the setting of acute MI. CCBs may be helpful in Raynaud syndrome and in some arrhythmias.

α_1-Blockers

α_1-Adrenergic antagonists block postsynaptic α-receptors, resulting in arterial and venous vasodilation. Selective α_1-blockers have replaced older nonselective agents in the treatment of hypertension. These agents are not as effective as diuretics, CCBs, and ACE inhibitors, but they may be prescribed as adjunct therapy in selected cases.

Adverse effects include "first-dose effect," in which BP is decreased more with the initial dose than with subsequent doses; orthostatic hypotension; headache; dizziness; and drowsiness.

Combined α-Adrenergic and β-Adrenergic Antagonists

Combined α-adrenergic and β-adrenergic antagonists block the action of catecholamines at both α-adrenergic and β-adrenergic receptor sites. Side effects are similar to those of other α-adrenergic and β-adrenergic antagonists.

Centrally Acting Adrenergic Agents

Centrally acting adrenergic drugs are potent antihypertensive agents that stimulate presynaptic α_2-adrenergic receptors in the central nervous system, causing decreased sympathetic tone, decreased cardiac output, and peripheral vascular resistance.

Adverse effects include fluid retention, dry mouth, drowsiness, dizziness, orthostatic hypotension, rash, impotence, positive direct antibody (Coombs) test, positive ANA test, hepatitis, heart failure in patients with decreased left ventricular dysfunction, and severe rebound hypertension when the drug is abruptly discontinued.

Methyldopa continues to be widely used in pregnancy because of its proven safety. Older centrally acting sympatholytic agents (eg, reserpine) have significant side effects and are now seldom used.

Direct Vasodilators

Direct-acting vasodilators such as minoxidil and hydralazine decrease peripheral vascular resistance by direct arterial vasodilation. They are generally reserved for special situations, such as pregnancy or intractable hypertension. They should be avoided or used with caution in patients with ischemic heart disease.

Adverse effects include headache, tachycardia, edema, nausea, vomiting, a lupuslike syndrome, and hypertrichosis. Because of the sympathetic hyperactivity and the sodium and fluid retention caused by direct vasodilators, they are often used in conjunction with diuretics or β-blockers.

Combination Therapy

Combination therapy usually includes small doses of a diuretic, which potentiates the effects of other drugs such as ACE inhibitors, ARBs, and β-blockers. This therapy may improve compliance and reduce target BP more quickly. Another advantage is that low-dose therapy with 2 antihypertensive agents is associated with fewer side effects than is higher-dose therapy with a single agent.

Direct Renin Inhibitors

Aliskiren is the first orally active renin inhibitor launched to treat hypertension. It has a high specificity for renin and has a long half-life (approximately 24 hours), which makes it ideal for once-daily treatment of hypertension. Direct renin inhibitors (DRIs) are more likely to be effective in younger white patients, who, in general, have a more active renin system, and in any patients receiving diuretics or CCBs in whom the renin system has been activated. The main side effect is diarrhea at higher doses.

Parenteral Antihypertensive Drugs

Parenteral antihypertensive therapy is indicated for immediate reduction of BP in hypertensive emergencies.

Sodium nitroprusside (Nitropress), a direct arterial and venous vasodilator, is the drug of choice for most hypertensive emergencies. Nitroglycerin (generic) may be preferable in patients with severe coronary insufficiency or advanced kidney or liver disease. Labetalol (Normodyne, Trandate) is also effective and is the drug of choice in hypertensive emergencies that occur in pregnancy. Esmolol (Brevibloc) is a cardioselective β-adrenergic antagonist that can be used in hypertensive emergencies when β-blocker intolerance is a concern; it is also useful in treating aortic dissection. Phentolamine (generic) is effective in managing hypertension with acute drug intoxication or withdrawal. Nicardipine (Cardene) is an IV calcium antagonist used for postoperative hypertension. Enalaprilat (Vasotec IV) is an IV ACE inhibitor that can be effective, although unpredictable results have been reported with its use. Diazoxide (Hyperstat) and hydralazine (generic) are used infrequently now, but hydralazine does have a long-established safety profile and may be useful in pregnancy-related hypertensive emergencies.

Future Treatments and Targets for Hypertension

Recently, data from the Conduit Artery Function Endpoint (CAFE) study showed that different classes of antihypertensive drugs have different effects on brachial versus central aortic systolic and pulse pressures and that central pressures may be a better predictor of cardiovascular outcomes in response to treatment. The Strong Heart Study has also shown that central aortic pressures may be a better predictor of target end-organ damage and outcomes than are conventional brachial pressures.

Thus, it is worth mentioning several new drugs, such as soluble guanylate cyclase (sGC) activators, that would lower central aortic pressures. These increase cyclic guanosine monophosphate levels in target tissues, resulting in vasodilation and an antiproliferative effect. A recent report found that such an activator lowered BP and inhibited cardiac hypertrophy in rats with angiotensin II–induced hypertension. This new drug may also potentially reduce large-artery stiffness, lowering central aortic systolic pressures beyond the benefits observed on brachial BP.

Other experimental agents, known as *advanced glycation cross-link breakers,* target vascular wall thickness and its effects on BP. We know that increased large-artery stiffness occurs with aging and disease and is associated with increased brachial systolic pressure. This is due to the accumulation of advanced glycation end products (AGEs) within the vascular wall. AGEs also impair endothelial function, which also leads to arterial stiffness. Thus, targeting these molecules to reduce their levels or indeed their presence in vascular walls may have an effect on decreasing vessel stiffness and lowering BP.

Other, more intriguing studies have involved attempts to develop a vaccine for hypertension and the use of acupuncture in its treatment.

Masuyama H, Tsuruda T, Kato J, et al. Soluble guanylate cyclase stimulation on cardiovascular remodeling in angiotensin II-induced hypertensive rats. *Hypertension.* 2006;48(5):972–978.

Williams B, Lacy PS, Thom SM, et al; CAFE Investigators; Anglo-Scandinavian Cardiac Outcomes Trial Investigators. Differential impact of blood pressure-lowering drugs on central aortic pressure and clinical outcomes: principal results of the Conduit Artery Function Evaluation (CAFE) study. *Circulation.* 2006;113(9):1213–1225.

Special Considerations

Ischemic Heart Disease

For patients with hypertension and stable angina pectoris, a β-blocker is generally the initial drug of choice; alternatively, CCBs can be used. ACE inhibitors and β-blockers are recommended as first-line drugs in hypertensive patients with acute coronary syndromes (unstable angina or MI). In patients with post-MI, β-blockers, ACE inhibitors, and potassium-sparing diuretics (aldosterone antagonists) are beneficial.

Heart Failure

In asymptomatic patients with ventricular dysfunction, ACE inhibitors and β-blockers are recommended. In patients with symptomatic ventricular dysfunction or end-stage heart failure, ACE inhibitors, β-blockers, ARBs, aldosterone antagonists, and loop diuretics are useful.

Diabetes and Hypertension

To achieve a BP goal of less than 130/80 mm Hg, patients usually need 2 or more antihypertensive drugs. Thiazide diuretics, β-blockers, ACE inhibitors, ARBs, and CCBs reduce cardiovascular complications in patients with diabetes. ACE inhibitors and ARBs are beneficial for those with diabetic nephropathy.

Chronic Renal Disease

Aggressive treatment, often with 3 or more drugs, is needed to achieve a BP goal of less than 130/80 and to prevent deterioration of renal function and cardiovascular complications in patients with chronic renal disease. ACE inhibitors and ARBs favorably alter the progression of diabetic and nondiabetic nephropathy. For cases of advanced renal disease, loop diuretics may be useful in combination with other drug classes.

Cerebrovascular Disease

The combination of an ACE inhibitor and a thiazide diuretic lowers the risk of recurrent stroke. The optimal BP level during an acute stroke remains undetermined, but consensus favors intermediate control in the range of 160/100 mm Hg until patient stabilization is achieved.

Obesity and the Metabolic Syndrome

Obesity (body mass index ≥30) is a risk factor for the development of hypertension and has become a major concern in the United States, where an estimated 122 million adults are overweight or obese. Closely related to obesity is the *metabolic syndrome,* defined as the presence of 3 or more of the following conditions: abdominal obesity, glucose intolerance, BP of 130/85 mm Hg or higher, hypertriglyceridemia, or low HDL-C level. Patients with these conditions should adopt healthy lifestyle habits and use drug therapy if necessary.

Sleep Disorders

Obstructive sleep apnea frequently coexists with obesity and appears to be an independent risk factor for hypertension and other cardiovascular diseases.

Left Ventricular Hypertrophy

Left ventricular hypertrophy is a risk factor for cardiovascular disease, but it can undergo regression with treatment of hypertension. All antihypertensive drug classes, except the direct vasodilators, are effective in treating left ventricular hypertrophy.

Peripheral Arterial Disease

The risk of peripheral arterial disease parallels that of ischemic heart disease in patients with hypertension. All classes of antihypertensive agents are useful in treating hypertensive patients with peripheral arterial disease.

Orthostatic Hypotension

Orthostatic hypotension is a postural drop in systolic BP of more than 10 mm Hg associated with dizziness or fainting. It occurs more frequently in older patients with systolic hypertension, in patients with diabetes, and in those taking diuretics, vasodilators, and certain psychotropic drugs. In these individuals, BP should be monitored while they are in the upright position, medication dosages should be carefully titrated, and volume depletion should be avoided.

Hypertension in Older Patients

Hypertension is present in the majority of individuals older than age 65. Treatment recommendations for this group are generally the same as for others with hypertension. In older patients with isolated systolic hypertension, a diuretic with or without a β-blocker, or a dihydropyridine CCB alone, is the preferred treatment.

Antihypertensive drug therapy in older patients can produce side effects such as dizziness and hypotension that increase the risk of falls. Appropriate precautions should be taken to reduce risks and enhance patient safety.

Dementia occurs more commonly with hypertension. In some patients, antihypertensive therapy may slow the progression of cognitive impairment.

Women and Pregnancy

Women taking oral contraceptives should have regular BP checks, as use of oral contraceptives increases the risk of hypertension. Hypertension in women who are pregnant potentially increases maternal and fetal morbidity and mortality. Also, the possibility of adverse effects of antihypertensive drugs on fetal development must be considered. Hypertension in women who are pregnant may be classified as follows:

- *preeclampsia or eclampsia:* preeclampsia—pregnancy, hypertension, proteinuria, generalized edema, and possibly coagulation and liver function abnormalities after 20 weeks' gestation; eclampsia—those same abnormalities plus generalized seizures
- *chronic hypertension:* BP of more than 140/90 mm Hg before 20 weeks' gestation
- *chronic hypertension with superimposed preeclampsia or eclampsia*
- *transient hypertension:* hypertension without proteinuria or CNS manifestations during pregnancy; the return of normal BP within 10 days of delivery

Methyldopa, β-blockers, and vasodilators are the recommended agents for treatment of hypertension in pregnancy. ACE inhibitors and ARBs are contraindicated in pregnancy because of teratogenic effects; they should also be avoided in women who are likely to become pregnant.

Children and Adolescents

Considerable advances have been made in the detection, evaluation, and management of hypertension in children and adolescents. Current evidence indicates that primary hypertension in the young occurs more commonly than previously recognized and has substantial long-term health implications. There is little doubt that obesity in young people predicts the risk of developing hypertension and associated metabolic risk factors. Hypertension in this group is defined as average systolic BP and/or diastolic BP that is in the 95th percentile or higher for gender, age, and height on 3 or more occasions. BP between the 90th percentile and the 95th percentile in childhood is now designated as *prehypertension* and is an indication for lifestyle modifications. It is recommended that children older than 3 years who are seen in a medical setting should have their BP measured.

Hypertensive children and adolescents are frequently overweight, and some have sleep disorders. Secondary hypertension occurs more commonly in children than in adults.

Indications for antihypertensive drug therapy in children include uncontrolled hypertension despite nonpharmacologic measures, symptomatic hypertension, secondary hypertension, hypertensive target-organ damage, and hypertension with diabetes. Acceptable drug choices for treating hypertension in children include diuretics, β-blockers, ACE inhibitors, ARBs, and CCBs.

Minority Populations

Significant racial and ethnic disparities in awareness, treatment, and control of hypertension exist in the United States. BP control rates are lowest in Mexican Americans and Native Americans. The prevalence and severity of hypertension are increased in blacks, in whom β-blockers, ACE inhibitors, and ARBs are less effective than are diuretics and CCBs in lowering BP. In general, treatment of hypertension is similar in all demographic groups; unfortunately, in many minority patients, socioeconomic and lifestyle factors continue to be barriers to treatment.

Withdrawal Syndromes

Hypertension can be associated with withdrawal from drugs such as alcohol, cocaine, amphetamines, and opioid analgesics. Withdrawal syndromes can occur with acute drug intoxication or as the result of abrupt discontinuation of a drug after chronic use. Phentolamine, sodium nitroprusside, and nitroglycerin are all effective in the acute management of these situations. β-Blockers should not be used in this setting, as unopposed α-adrenergic stimulation can exacerbate the hypertension.

Monoamine oxidase inhibitors taken with certain drugs or with tyramine-containing foods can cause accelerated hypertension by increasing catecholamines. Phentolamine, sodium nitroprusside, and labetalol are effective for treating this type of hypertension.

Abrupt discontinuation of antihypertensive therapy can cause severe rebound hypertension. This occurs most commonly with centrally acting adrenergic agents (particularly clonidine) and with β-blockers, but it can occur with other drug classes as well, including diuretics. When an acute withdrawal syndrome occurs and parenteral antihypertensive treatment is needed, sodium nitroprusside is the drug of choice.

Hypertensive Crisis

Patients with severe BP elevation and acute target-organ damage (eg, encephalopathy, MI, unstable angina, pulmonary edema, stroke, head trauma, eclampsia, or aortic dissection) should be hospitalized for emergency parenteral antihypertensive therapy. Patients with marked BP elevation but without target-organ damage may not require hospitalization, but they should be treated urgently with combination oral antihypertensive agents. Identifiable causes of hypertension should be sought, and these patients should be carefully monitored for target-organ damage.

◉ **Ophthalmic considerations**   Retinal vascular complications (hypertensive retinopathy, retinal vein occlusions, retinal arterial occlusions), glaucoma, ischemic optic neuropathy, microvascular cranial nerve palsies, and stroke-related disorders of the afferent and efferent visual system are commonly associated with hypertension. Moreover, ophthalmic surgical patients with poorly controlled hypertension may be more susceptible to operative and perioperative complications.

There is strong evidence that certain signs of hypertensive retinopathy, independent of other risk factors, are associated with increased cardiovascular risk. Based on these reported associations, a simplified classification of hypertensive retinopathy was proposed in 2004 (Table 2-8).

The JNC 7 report emphasizes that hypertension control is possible only if patients are motivated to take their prescribed medications and to maintain healthy lifestyle habits. Motivation improves when individuals develop empathy with and trust in their physicians. As members of the health care team, ophthalmologists have an important role in the detection, monitoring, and shared management of patients with hypertension.

Centers for Disease Control and Prevention (CDC). Racial/ethnic disparities in prevalence, treatment, and control of hypertension—United States, 1999–2002. *MMWR Morb Mortal Wkly Rep.* 2005;54(1):7–9.

Chobanian AV, Bakris GL, Black HR, et al; National Heart, Lung, and Blood Institute Joint National Committee on Prevention, Detection, Evaluation, and Treatment of High Blood Pressure; National High Blood Pressure Education Program Coordinating Committee. The Seventh Report of the Joint National Committee on Prevention, Detection, Evaluation, and Treatment of High BP: the JNC 7 report. *JAMA.* 2003;289(19):2560–2572.

Masuyama H, Tsuruda T, Kato J, et al. Soluble guanylate cyclase stimulation on cardiovascular remodeling in angiotensin II-induced hypertensive rats. *Hypertension.* 2006;48(5):972–978.

Table 2-8 Classification of Hypertensive Retinopathy With Systemic Associations

Grade of Retinopathy	Retinal Signs	Systemic Associations
None	No detectable signs	None
Mild	Generalized and/or focal arteriolar narrowing, arteriovenous nicking, opacity ("copper wiring") of arteriolar wall, or a combination of these signs	Modest association with risk of stroke, coronary artery disease, and death
Moderate	Hemorrhage (blot, dot, or flame-shaped), microaneurysm, cotton-wool spot, hard exudates, or a combination of these signs	Strong association with stroke, cognitive decline, and death from cardiovascular causes
Malignant	Signs of moderate retinopathy plus swelling of the optic disc	Strong association with death

Adapted from Wong TY, Mitchell P. Hypertensive retinopathy. *N Engl J Med.* 2004;351(22):2314. ©2004 Massachusetts Medical Society.

Medical Knowledge Self Assessment Program (MKSAP) 14, *Nephrology*. Philadelphia: American College of Physicians; 2006.

National High Blood Pressure Education Program Working Group on High Blood Pressure in Children and Adolescents. The fourth report on the diagnosis, evaluation, and treatment of high blood pressure in children and adolescents. *Pediatrics*. 2004;114(2 Suppl 4th report):555–576.

Sarafidis PA, Bakris GL. Resistant hypertension: an overview of evaluation and treatment. *J Am Coll Cardiology*. 2008;52(22):1749–1757.

Williams B. The year in hypertension. *J Am Coll Cardiol*. 2008;51(18):1803–1817.

Wong TY, Mitchell P. Hypertensive retinopathy. *N Engl J Med*. 2004;351(22):2310–2317.

CHAPTER 3

Cerebrovascular Disease

Recent Developments

- Intravenous recombinant tissue plasminogen activator (tPA) is strongly recommended for carefully selected patients who can be treated within 4½ hours of onset of ischemic stroke, as it improves neurologic outcomes.
- Carotid endarterectomy (CEA) is beneficial for symptomatic patients with recent nondisabling carotid artery ischemic events and ipsilateral 70%–99% carotid artery stenosis. CEA is not beneficial for symptomatic patients with 0%–29% or 100% stenosis. The potential benefit of CEA for symptomatic patients with 30%–69% stenosis is uncertain.
- Patients with acute ischemic stroke presenting within 48 hours of symptom onset should be given aspirin (160–325 mg/day) to prevent recurrent stroke, reduce stroke mortality, and decrease morbidity, provided contraindications such as allergy and gastrointestinal bleeding are absent and recombinant tPA was not or will not be used as treatment.
- Subcutaneous unfractionated heparin may be considered for deep venous thrombosis (DVT) prophylaxis in at-risk patients with acute ischemic stroke.
- Statin use reduces the risk of stroke and other coronary events in patients with coronary artery disease and in those who have had an ischemic stroke of atherosclerotic origin.

Introduction

Stroke is the third leading cause of death in developed countries, ranking behind heart disease and cancer. In the United States, approximately 795,000 strokes occur annually, with a mortality rate exceeding 20%. About 610,000 of these are first attacks. Stroke is the leading cause of long-term disability in America today.

There are 2 primary types of stroke: ischemic stroke and hemorrhagic stroke. For extensive discussion of the ophthalmic manifestations of cerebrovascular disease, see BCSC Section 5, *Neuro-Ophthalmology*.

Cerebral Ischemia

Cerebral ischemia results from interference with circulation to the brain. Usually, cerebral circulation is maintained by a very efficient collateral arterial system that includes the

2 carotid and the 2 vertebral arteries, anastomoses in the circle of Willis, and collateral circulation in the cerebral hemispheres. However, atheromas and congenital arteriovenous (AV) malformations can lead to a reduction in cerebral blood flow. This reduction may be generalized or localized. However, longer interruptions in cerebral blood flow can result in permanent neurologic deficits, depending on the extent and duration of the cerebral ischemia.

There are varying degrees of ischemia, which may be classified by severity and duration. A *transient ischemic attack (TIA)* is a focal loss of neurologic function of sudden onset, persisting for less than 24 hours and clearing without residual signs. Most TIAs last only a few minutes, and the symptoms are primarily associated with insufficiency of the internal carotid, middle cerebral, or vertebrobasilar arterial territories. A *completed stroke* is an ischemic event that produces a stable permanent neurologic disability. Most ischemic strokes consist of small regions of complete ischemia in conjunction with a larger area of incomplete ischemia. This ischemic but not infarcted area has been termed the *penumbra*. The penumbra is dynamic, resulting in changes to the once passive approach to treating patients with acute cerebral ischemia.

Emboli or thrombi caused by atherosclerosis, hypertension, or diabetes mellitus and located in large, medium, and small arteries account for the majority of strokes. Strokes caused by emboli of cardiac origin account for 20% of the total. Mural thrombi forming on the endocardium in conjunction with myocardial infarction (MI) account for 8%–10% of the total stroke incidence. Atrial fibrillation, mitral stenosis, mitral valve prolapse, and atrial myxoma are other cardiac conditions associated with intracranial embolism.

Nonarteriosclerotic causes of thrombotic occlusion leading to TIA and stroke include aortic dissection and inflammatory arteritis (eg, collagen vascular disease, giant cell arteritis, meningovascular syphilis, acute and chronic meningitis, and moyamoya disease).

Ischemia must be distinguished from hypoxemia (decreased oxygenation or oxygen-carrying capacity), which can be caused by carbon monoxide poisoning, chronic obstructive pulmonary disease, profound anemia, or pulmonary emboli. Ischemia can also be caused by increased viscosity of the blood due to pregnancy and the postpartum period, use of oral contraceptives, postoperative and posttraumatic states, hyperviscosity syndromes, polycythemia, and sickle cell disease.

Although cerebral ischemia can occur as a result of embolus or thrombus in any artery, common sites include the middle cerebral artery and its branches, the tortuous portion of the internal carotid artery extending from the carotid canal to its bifurcation in the anterior and middle cerebral arteries (carotid siphon), basilar artery, and small perforating arteries that can cause lacunar strokes.

Clinical manifestations of cerebral ischemia reflect the functions associated with the area of ischemia and include paresis, paresthesia, vision loss, language disturbances, vertigo, diplopia, ataxia, dysarthria, headache, nausea, and vomiting.

Diagnosis and Management

The diagnosis of ischemic stroke and TIAs should be differentiated from the diagnosis of diabetic and convulsive seizures, migraine, vertigo, and neoplasms. Although the presentation of stroke is usually characteristic, the diagnosis should be differentiated from that of other conditions that may mimic strokes, such as multiple sclerosis, subdural hematoma, cranial nerve palsy, encephalitis, hypoglycemia, seizures, brain tumor, hypertensive encephalopathy, syncope, migraine, and functional disorder.

A detailed history, including the time and duration of onset, is important. Also, an assessment of risk factors is critical for treating a patient. Nonmodifiable risk factors include age older than 60 years, male gender, and family history or prior history of stroke or TIAs. Modifiable risk factors include diabetes mellitus, hypertension, hyperlipidemia, cardiac arrhythmias, smoking, alcohol use, illicit drug use, migraine, and hypercoagulable states.

The clinical severity of a stroke can be determined using the National Institutes of Health Stroke Scale, which assesses level of consciousness, gaze, visual fields, facial strength, motor function of the arms and legs, ataxia, sensation, language, dysarthria, and inattention. The assessment is on a 0–42 scale, with *0* being normal function and *42* being the most severe functional impairment. For more information on the National Institutes of Health Stroke Scale refer to www.strokeassociation.org, where one can be trained and certified online in its usage.

Diagnostic Studies

For practical purposes, diagnostic studies may be separated into those done in an acute setting, such as in the emergency room, and those done in a more subacute setting, such as in a stable inpatient or stable outpatient setting. Acute testing assesses the patient's clinical stability and the possibility of stroke mimics or conditions that could contribute to stroke; the tests should include blood glucose, complete blood count, blood chemistry, coagulation studies such as PT/aPTT (prothrombin time/activated partial prothrombin time), international normalized ratio, troponins, and ECG. Ideally, all suspected cases of stroke and TIA should receive prompt *computed tomography (CT)* of the brain. The scan should be completed without contrast because contrast and blood appear similar on CT, and this similarity can result in misinterpretation of the image. CT is very sensitive to the presence of intracranial hemorrhage.

Once the acute investigations are complete, the next types of imaging studies to consider include *magnetic resonance imaging (MRI), magnetic resonance cerebral angiography, CT angiography,* and *conventional catheter angiography.* MRI is often more sensitive than CT in detecting an evolving stroke within hours of its onset, whereas CT results may be negative for up to several days after an acute cerebral infarct. These techniques can distinguish between acute and chronic infarction and help date hemorrhagic infarction; they can also evaluate for unsuspected space-occupying lesions. Magnetic resonance cerebral angiography or CT angiography may be needed to examine the intra- and extracranial vessels for stenoses or to identifiy an aneurysm. Carotid duplex ultrasonography may be used to evaluate the patency of the extracranial carotid arteries, and transcranial Doppler ultrasonography can evaluate the intracranial arteries. *Diffusion-weighted MRI, apparent diffusion coefficient (ADC) mapping,* and *perfusion-weighted MRI* are useful in evaluating early cerebral ischemia and regional blood flow. Early detection of these conditions by such techniques may allow for early treatment, which may be beneficial in salvaging tissue at risk. *Cerebral arteriography* is usually required only if the cause is unclear or if intra-arterial thrombolysis or surgical intervention is being strongly considered.

Investigation of the systemic arteries and the heart is essential in determining the cause of cerebral ischemia. Differences between upper limb pulse rates and blood pressure (BP) may indicate serious subclavian disease. Multiple bruits may suggest widespread arterial disease but may be present without significant occlusion. Evidence for a cardioembolic source should be pursued aggressively, especially in younger normotensive persons with cerebral ischemia and in older patients, for whom atrial fibrillation is in the differential diagnosis. Electrocardiography and telemetry or Holter monitoring should be routine to exclude cardiac dysrhythmia and occult MI. Echocardiography is often helpful in excluding intracardiac emboli. Transesophageal Doppler echocardiography is most sensitive in this regard. Lumbar puncture rarely is required to evaluate stroke or TIA, unless meningovascular syphilis, meningitis, or subarachnoid hemorrhage is a serious consideration.

Treatment

Treatment of ischemic stroke and TIA includes reduction of risk factors when possible. Hypertension should be controlled in the outpatient setting, although BP reduction during acute ischemic stroke may cause harmful decreases in local perfusion. Control of both hyperlipidemia and diabetes is indicated. Cigarette smoking and excessive alcohol consumption should be eliminated.

Controlled studies have *not* demonstrated the effectiveness of anticoagulants in the treatment of acute stroke. Intravenous heparin is not helpful in patients with acute stroke and should not be used in an urgent setting. Subcutaneous heparin can be used in ischemic stroke to prevent DVT. Because of the associated risk of hemorrhage in the ischemic area, there is no consensus on the best time to start oral anticoagulant therapy for patients with atrial fibrillation.

Antiplatelet therapy with aspirin is beneficial in all patients with ischemic stroke and for those with cardioembolic stroke who cannot tolerate long-term use of anticoagulant drugs. Low doses of aspirin (50–325 mg daily) cause less gastrointestinal discomfort than higher doses and reduce the incidence of recurrent ischemic stroke. Clopidogrel (Plavix) is an inhibitor of adenosine diphosphate (ADP)-induced platelet activation that reduces the relative risk of stroke by 7.3% compared with aspirin. Plavix is generally well tolerated, although thrombocytopenic purpura has been rarely reported. Aggrenox is a combination of aspirin and extended-release dipyridamole. It reduces the risk of stroke in patients who have had TIA or ischemic stroke by 23% compared to aspirin alone.

Studies have further investigated the role of thrombolytic agents for treatment of acute ischemic stroke. The National Institute of Neurological Disorders and Stroke (NINDS) Recombinant Tissue Plasminogen Activator Stroke study supports the use of recombinant tPA for treating acute ischemic stroke in patients who meet certain eligibility requirements, if treatment is initiated within 3 hours after the onset of symptoms. Tissue plasminogen activator is administered intravenously. However, use of this agent incurred a 6.4% risk of symptomatic intracerebral hemorrhage. Additional thrombolytic studies have provided similar results. More recently, stroke centers across the country have been using intra-arterial tPA with success. With the intra-arterial approach, the window of opportunity may extend from 3 to 6 hours, and less tPA is needed, as it is directly delivered to the clot. Ancrod, a fibrinogenolytic enzyme derived from snake venom, has also been shown to improve functional outcomes after stroke but is used less frequently.

In 2004, the FDA approved a new device called the Merci Retriever for mechanical embolus removal in moderate to severe cerebral ischemia. It is a corkscrew-like device designed to reopen occluded vessels by extracting occlusive thrombi. Although its effectiveness was not examined in a randomized controlled trial, it provides an additional treatment option for significantly disabled patients in the acute setting.

Flint AC, Duckwiler GR, Budzik RF, Liebeskind DS, Smith WS; MERCI and Multi MERCI Writing Committee. Mechanical thrombectomy of intracranial internal carotid occlusion: pooled results of the MERCI and Multi MERCI Part I trials. *Stroke.* 2007;38(4):1274–1280.

Carotid Occlusive Disease

Asymptomatic carotid bruits occur in 4% of the population over age 40. The annual stroke rate in patients with an asymptomatic bruit is 1.5%. This same population has an annual mortality rate of 4%, primarily from complications of heart disease. Bruit is more a marker for the presence of arteriosclerotic disease than a predictor of stroke. Patients with asymptomatic carotid bruits should be screened for risk factors related to atherosclerosis: hypertension, smoking, and hypercholesterolemia. The degree and severity of stenosis should be determined by noninvasive studies. Patients with asymptomatic carotid stenosis have a 2% annual risk of ipsilateral stroke.

In the Asymptomatic Carotid Atherosclerosis Study, patients with asymptomatic stenosis of greater than 60% were randomized to either CEA or medical treatment. Although the estimated 5-year risk of stroke was 53% lower (5.1% vs 11.0%) for the CEA group, the only significant difference was in the frequency of TIA or minor stroke ipsilateral to the CEA. No significant differences were discerned between the medical and surgical groups with regard to major ipsilateral stroke or death, and the benefits disappear with an operative risk of greater than 3%. Therefore, patients with asymptomatic carotid stenosis of greater than 80% may be considered for elective CEA; patients with less than 80% stenosis may be considered for repeat carotid imaging at intervals of 6–12 months and followed up for disease progression. Aspirin (325 mg daily) and risk factor reduction are also required in this patient group.

No hard data are currently available from which to make a clear recommendation about an appropriate course of therapy for asymptomatic carotid stenosis ≤80%. It appears that a trial of aspirin (325 mg/day) or Aggrenox should be the initial approach for all patients. Clopidogrel therapy may be considered for patients unable to take aspirin. CEA should be considered only if the surgeon has a perioperative morbidity rate of less than 3% and if any of the following conditions exist:

- Antiplatelet therapy proves to be ineffective.
- Stenosis appears to be progressive.
- The patient has no operative risk factors.

Patients with TIA or previous stroke in the territory of carotid stenosis are judged to be symptomatic. The risk of stroke within a year of onset of symptoms is 8% in patients with TIA; the risk thereafter is approximately 6% per year, with a 5-year risk of 35%–50%.

In the North American Symptomatic Carotid Endarterectomy Trial, CEA was evaluated in patients with a recent (within 120 days) hemispheric or retinal TIA or a recent nondisabling stroke who had high-grade (70%–99%) stenosis in the ipsilateral carotid artery. All the patients received optimal medical care, including antiplatelet therapy with aspirin, as well as treatment of hypertension, hyperlipidemia, or diabetes, when appropriate. The surgical group experienced lower rates of ipsilateral stroke (9.0% vs 26.0%), any stroke (12.6% vs 27.6%), major or fatal stroke (3.7% vs 13.1%), and death from all causes (4.6% vs 6.3%) over the 2-year follow-up period. The perioperative mortality rate was only 0.6%, and the perioperative rate of major stroke or death was 2.1%. The benefit of surgery for reducing the risk of ipsilateral stroke increased with higher degrees of stenosis: 12% risk reduction for 70%–79% stenosis; 18% risk reduction for 80%–89% stenosis; and 26% risk reduction for 90%–99% stenosis. The European Carotid Surgery Trial also demonstrated a statistically significant benefit for CEA in selected patients with greater than 70% stenosis. However, there is still uncertainty regarding CEA for symptomatic stenosis in the range of 50%–69%.

Ocular and cerebral conditions associated with carotid stenosis include transient monocular visual loss (TMVL), TIAs, and stroke. The ophthalmologist is often the first physician to see a patient with TMVL, which is usually embolic, having either a carotid or a cardiac source. The annual stroke rate among patients with isolated TMVL, retinal infarcts, or TIAs is approximately 2%, 3%, and 8%, respectively. Untreated patients with TMVL, retinal infarcts, or TIAs have a 30% risk of MI and an 18% risk of death over a 5-year period. A cardiac source of embolization should be excluded for all patients presenting with isolated TMVL. The best procedure for accomplishing this is transesophageal cardiac ultrasonography combined with ambulatory Holter monitoring.

If evidence suggests that a carotid lesion is the cause of the TMVL, or if venous stasis retinopathy is present, duplex scanning should be performed to determine the presence of vessel wall disease or carotid stenosis.

The risks of major morbidity and mortality with CEA are proportional to the severity of neurologic illness and comorbid factors such as ischemic heart disease. The risks for patients with symptomatic unilateral high-grade stenosis and favorable comorbidity are 1%–3% in the hands of capable surgeons. The long-term restenotic rate following CEA is approximately 10% at 5 years.

In summary, patients with symptomatic carotid stenosis exceeding 70% should be considered for CEA unless there is acute stroke, maximal neurologic defect, or other medical contraindication to surgery. The major perioperative morbidity and mortality rates for the surgical team should not exceed 6%.

The following approach to a patient presenting with a cerebral or retinal TIA should be considered:

- emergency room evaluation or hospital admission if the event occurred within the previous 48 hours
- patient evaluation for the presence of risk factors associated with atherogenesis: hypertension, diabetes mellitus, obesity, hyperlipidemia, and smoking
- institution of appropriate medical therapy
- evaluation by appropriate testing for the presence of a cardiac source of emboli
- determination using duplex ultrasonography of the possibility of carotid stenosis

If ipsilateral carotid stenosis exceeds 70%, if bilateral carotid stenosis greater than 50% is present, or if long-term evidence indicates progressive disease, CEA should be considered—but only if the surgeon's perioperative stroke and death rate is less than 6%. Otherwise, antiplatelet therapy with aspirin (325 mg/day), Aggrenox, or clopidogrel should be initiated. A patient presenting with TIA symptoms who has previously undergone CEA should be evaluated and treated similarly. Special attention should be paid to evaluating early restenosis and thrombosis.

As an additional note, elevated plasma homocysteine levels have been linked to extracranial carotid stenosis and, directly, to an increased risk of stroke and occlusive vascular disease, but so far, there is no evidence that dietary supplements with vitamins or minerals have any direct effect on stroke prevention, as indicated by the VITAmins VITATOPS study.

Intracranial Hemorrhage

Intracranial hemorrhage constitutes approximately 15% of acute cerebrovascular disorders. Bleeding from aneurysms of the arteries composing the circle of Willis, bleeding from arterioles damaged by hypertension or arteriosclerosis, and trauma are the most common causes of intracranial hemorrhage. Although there are many causes of intracranial hemorrhage, the anatomical location of the bleeding greatly influences the clinical picture. By location, hemorrhages can be grouped into the following general categories:

- subarachnoid hemorrhage
- intracerebral hemorrhage
- intraventricular hemorrhage

A variety of vascular malformations within and on the surface of the brain parenchyma may present with seizures and headaches. Arteriovenous malformations (AVMs) produce symptoms more commonly than do other types of cerebrovascular malformations.

Arterial "berry" aneurysms are round or saccular dilatations characteristically found at arteriole bifurcations on the circle of Willis and its major branches or connections. Intracranial aneurysms occur in all age groups but most commonly rupture in the fifth, sixth, and seventh decades of life. Approximately 85% of congenital berry aneurysms develop in the anterior part of the circle of Willis derived from the internal carotid artery in its major branches. The most common site is at the origin of the posterior communicating artery from the internal carotid artery. Such an aneurysm typically presents with headache and third nerve palsy involving the pupil. Vascular malformations within and on the surface of the brain parenchyma constitute approximately 7% of cases with subarachnoid hemorrhage. Four varieties are recognized:

1. capillary telangiectasia
2. cavernous angioma
3. venous angioma
4. AVM

Capillary telangiectasias are most commonly discovered as incidental postmortem findings in the brainstem. Cavernous angiomas are rare vascular disorders that may appear sporadically or exhibit autosomal dominant inheritance. Venous angiomas are cerebrovascular abnormalities often associated with the Sturge-Weber syndrome, but they may be found in otherwise healthy individuals. These lesions are best identified by MRI.

Findings that suggest an AVM as the cause of subarachnoid hemorrhage include a history of previous focal seizures, slow stepwise progression of focal neurologic signs, and, occasionally, recurrent unilateral throbbing headache resembling migraine. In addition to meningeal irritation and focal neurologic signs reflecting bleeding, a bruit may be present over the orbit or skull in approximately 40% of patients.

Hypertensive intracerebral hemorrhages are often catastrophic events. Headache is the predominant feature at the onset in 40%–50% of hemorrhages. Restlessness and vomiting are more common with hemorrhage than with infarction. Generalized seizures are common with intracerebral hemorrhage and are less frequent with subarachnoid hemorrhage or cerebral infarction. The most important clues in the diagnosis of intracranial hemorrhage are explosive headache onset, history of high BP, and early decline of the level of consciousness with evidence of a focal neurologic deficit.

Immediate CT examination demonstrates blood in the subarachnoid space in approximately 95% of the cases of ruptured aneurysm within 24 hours of headache onset. CT scans identify the size and location of intracerebral hemorrhages, as well as the degree of surrounding edema and the amount and location of any distortion of the brain. If subarachnoid hemorrhage is suspected and CT results are negative, lumbar puncture is indicated. CT should always be carried out first to rule out a mass lesion. Cerebral arteriography remains the definitive procedure for identifying an aneurysm or AVM.

Control and maintenance of BP are mandatory in treating ruptured aneurysms. Surgical intervention is best accomplished by placing a small clip or ligature across the neck of the sac. Coil embolization of the aneurysm is an alternative procedure that may be used. If the aneurysm cannot be directly obliterated, surgical ligation of a proximal vessel may be necessary. Symptomatic AVMs sometimes can be dissected and removed, depending on their location. Proton-beam irradiation remains controversial. Ligation of the feeding vessels, coupled with balloon catheter embolization, may be carried out. Results of surgical drainage or clot removal of parenchymal intracerebral hemorrhages are mostly unsatisfactory.

Adams H, Adams R, Del Zoppo G, Goldstein LB; Stroke Council of the American Heart Association; American Stroke Association. Guidelines for the early management of patients with ischemic stroke: 2005 guidelines update a scientific statement from the Stroke Council of the American Heart Association/American Stroke Association. *Stroke.* 2005;36(4):916–923.

Adams RJ, Albers G, Alberts MJ, et al; American Heart Association; American Stroke Association. Update to the AHA/ASA recommendations for the prevention of stroke in patients with stroke and transient ischemic attack. *Stroke.* 2008;39(5):1647–1652.

Brott T, Bogousslavsky J. Treatment of acute ischemic stroke. *N Engl J Med.* 2000;343(10): 710–722.

Moore WS, Barnett HJ, Beebe HG, et al. Guidelines for carotid endarterectomy: a multidisciplinary consensus statement from the ad hoc Committee, American Heart Association. *Stroke.* 1995;26(1):188–201.

The authors would like to thank Renee B. Van Stavern, MD, for her contributions to this chapter.

CHAPTER 4

Acquired Heart Disease

Recent Developments

- Atherosclerotic *coronary artery disease (CAD)* remains by far the number one killer in the United States and around the world.
- Markers of inflammation, such as high-sensitivity C-reactive protein (CRP), are strong risk factors for CAD.
- Primary prevention of CAD at a public health level requires lifestyle changes, including reduced intake of saturated fat and cholesterol, increased physical activity, and weight control.
- Smoking remains the number one preventable risk factor for *cardiovascular disease (CVD)* worldwide.
- Recent trials suggest that, regardless of cholesterol level, any patient at significant risk for vascular events should be given a statin.
- Heart failure is increasing in prevalence as the aging population increases.
- Primary *percutaneous coronary intervention (PCI)* performed by experienced operators is superior to thrombolysis for the treatment of acute *myocardial infarction (MI)*.
- Stenting, either bare-metal (BMS) or drug-eluting (DES), is now widely used in patients with acute MI and for prevention of MI in selected patients, and requires some postprocedure period of *dual antiplatelet therapy (DAT)*.
- Prophylactic *implantable cardioverter-defibrillators (ICDs)* are indicated for patients who have survived a cardiac arrest or an episode of hemodynamically unstable ventricular tachycardia. ICDs are also indicated for severe left ventricular dysfunction after MI. ICDs are not indicated for patients who do not have a reasonable expectation of survival with an acceptable functional status of at least 1 year.
- Pharmacologic adjuncts for the management of *acute coronary syndromes (ACSs)* include low-molecular-weight heparin and glycoprotein IIb/IIIa inhibitors.

Ischemic Heart Disease

Atherosclerotic CAD is by far the number one killer not only in the United States but also in the world. It is estimated that every minute, 1 person dies in the United States because of CAD. The number of women who die from CVD is 10 times the number of women who die of breast cancer.

Pathophysiology

Abnormal cholesterol intake and metabolism are central factors in ischemic heart disease (IHD). The "fatty streak" is an accumulation under the endothelium of the coronary arteries of lipids and lipid-laden macrophages, called "foam" cells, which organize in a plaque. As the plaque becomes calcified, the lumen of the vessel narrows. The plaque can also become unstable and rupture. This rupture leads to turbulence and activation of the coagulation cascade, causing intravascular thrombosis. The result is partial or complete vessel occlusion, which causes the symptoms of unstable angina or MI.

Ischemia is defined as a local, temporary oxygen deprivation associated with inadequate removal of metabolites caused by reduced tissue perfusion. IHD is typically caused by decreased perfusion of the myocardium secondary to stenotic or obstructed coronary arteries. The balance between arterial supply and myocardial demand for oxygen determines whether ischemia occurs. Significant coronary stenosis, thrombosis, occlusion, reduced arterial pressure, hypoxemia, or severe anemia can impede the supply of oxygen to the myocardium. On the demand side, an increase in heart rate, ventricular contractility, or wall tension (which is determined by systolic arterial pressure, ventricular volume, and ventricular wall thickness) may cause increased utilization of oxygen. When the demand for oxygen exceeds the supply, ischemia occurs. If this ischemia becomes prolonged, infarction and myocardial necrosis result. The necrotic process begins in the subendocardium, usually after approximately 20 minutes of coronary obstruction, and progresses to transmural and complete infarction in 4–6 hours.

Risk Factors for Coronary Artery Disease

The majority of patients with CAD have some identifiable risk factors. These risk factors are evident when epidemiologic studies are performed and include a positive family history, male gender, lipid abnormalities, diabetes mellitus, hypertension, physical inactivity, obesity, and smoking. Many of these risk factors may be modified, such as smoking. Although the number of people who smoke is decreasing in the United States, it is estimated that 25% of men and 21% of women smoke. The risk of CAD can be decreased by 50% in just 1 year after an individual stops smoking. Also included among preventable risk factors are lipid abnormalities. Higher low-density-lipoprotein (LDL) and lower high-density-lipoprotein (HDL) levels increase the risk of CAD. (See Chapter 5, Hypercholesterolemia, for a discussion of hyperlipidemia and global cardiometabolic risk.) In addition, obesity is being reported more often in the United States (20% of the population). A diet low in saturated fat is widely accepted and promoted as a way of reducing weight in obese men and women. Eating fish rich in omega-3 fatty acids may help protect against vascular disease. Markers of inflammation are also strong risk factors for CAD. High sensitivity C-reactive protein is the best marker and is now available for clinical use. C-reactive protein levels less than 1, between 1 and 3, and greater than 3 mg/mL identify patients at low, medium, and high risk, respectively, for future cardiovascular events.

Cardiovascular disease is the leading cause of death in women, accounting for one third of all deaths, and kills more women than men each year. The average lifetime risk of CAD in women is very high, nearly 1 in 2. In contrast to men, a 50-year-old woman with a single additional risk factor has a substantially increased lifetime risk for CAD. Fortunately, most CVD in women is modifiable with the recommendations previously discussed; optimizing modifiable risk is of crucial importance in women.

Clinical Syndromes

Clinical presentations of IHD include angina pectoris (stable angina; variant, or Prinzmetal, angina), the acute coronary syndromes (unstable angina, acute MI), congestive heart failure (CHF), sudden cardiac death (SCD), and asymptomatic IHD.

Angina pectoris

The cardinal symptom in patients with IHD is angina pectoris, usually manifested as precordial chest pain or tightness that is often triggered by physical exertion, emotional distress, or eating. Angina pectoris is usually due to atherosclerotic heart disease. Coronary vasospasm may occur at the site of a lesion or even in otherwise normal coronary arteries. Angina typically lasts 5–10 minutes and is usually relieved by rest, nitroglycerin, or both. Patients may present with pain radiating into other areas, including the jaw, arm, neck, shoulder, back, chest wall, or abdomen.

Occasionally, angina may be misinterpreted as indigestion or musculoskeletal pain. The level of physical activity that results in angina pectoris is clinically significant and is useful in determining the severity of CAD, treatment, and prognosis. Myocardial ischemia may be painless in diabetic patients and women, which often delays the diagnosis until the disease is more advanced. The pain associated with MI is similar to that of angina, but it is usually more severe and more prolonged.

Stable angina pectoris   Angina is considered stable if it responds to rest or nitroglycerin and if the patterns of frequency, ease of onset, duration, and response to medication have not changed substantially over 3 months.

Variant (Prinzmetal) angina   Variant angina occurs at rest and is not related to physical exertion. The ST segment is elevated on electrocardiography during the anginal episodes, which are caused by coronary artery spasm. Underlying atherosclerosis is present in 60%–80% of cases, and thrombosis and occlusion may result during the episodes of coronary spasm.

Acute coronary syndrome

Acute coronary syndrome comprises the spectrum of unstable cardiac ischemia, from unstable angina to acute MI. Plaque rupture is considered to be the common underlying event. Unstable angina and acute MI should be considered closely related events, clinically differentiated by the presence or absence of markers of myocardial injury.

If a coronary thrombus is occlusive and if it persists, MI can result. The location and extent of the infarction depend on the anatomical distribution of the occluded vessel, the presence of additional stenotic lesions, and the adequacy of collateral circulation. If the patient has chest pain at rest, unstable angina is the diagnosis. If the ischemia is severe enough to cause myocardial necrosis, infarction results. *Acute MI* is further differentiated into *non–ST-segment elevation MI (NSTEMI)* and *ST-segment elevation MI (STEMI)*. This electrocardiogram (ECG) distinction identifies patients most likely to benefit from acute reperfusion therapy.

In NSTEMI, the ECG typically demonstrates ST-segment depression, T-wave inversion, or both. If it is established that no biochemical marker of myocardial necrosis has been released, the patient may be considered to have experienced unstable angina. When clinical evidence of necrosis is detected by cardiac enzyme testing, the diagnosis is NSTEMI, a condition midway between unstable angina and STEMI. Plaque rupture in unstable angina and NSTEMI is typically accompanied by a less obstructive thrombus or lesser amounts of fibrin formation compared with what occurs in STEMI.

If plaque rupture results in a completely occlusive thrombus, a *Q-wave* infarction may occur. Typically, ST-segment elevation is apparent on the ECG. Necrosis involving the full or nearly full thickness of the ventricular wall in the distribution of the affected artery ultimately occurs, leading to Q waves on the ECG. The goal of early therapy and intervention is to prevent the progression to a transmural Q-wave infarction.

Myocardial infarction may occur suddenly, without warning, in a previously asymptomatic patient or in a patient with stable or variant angina; MI may also follow a period of unstable angina. Patients commonly experience chest pain, nausea, vomiting, diaphoresis, weakness, anxiety, dyspnea, lightheadedness, and palpitations. Nearly 25% of myocardial infarcts are painless; painless MI is more common in persons with diabetes and with increasing age. These patients may present with CHF or syncope. Symptoms may begin during or after exertion or at rest.

The clinical findings in IHD vary and depend on the location and severity of myocardial ischemia or injury. Approximately half of all infarctions involve the inferior myocardial wall, and most of the remaining half involve the anterior regions. Examination may reveal pallor, coolness of the extremities, low-grade fever, signs of pulmonary congestion and increased central venous pressure (if left ventricular dysfunction is present), an S_3 or S_4 gallop, an apical systolic murmur (caused by papillary muscle dysfunction), hypertension, or hypotension. The ECG may demonstrate a variety of ST-segment and T-wave changes and arrhythmias.

Subendocardial (NSTEMI, nontransmural) infarcts usually result in a smaller region of myocardial injury and cause less ventricular dysfunction and heart failure. However, the patient with an NSTEMI infarction may be considered to have an incomplete infarction, with potential for reocclusion of the affected artery. Not surprisingly, these patients experience a greater incidence of post-MI angina and reinfarction during the initial hospitalization and during the first 6 months following the infarction. Approximately 20% experience an acute Q-wave infarction within 3 months. Although the in-hospital prognosis for patients with non–Q-wave infarction is better than that for patients with Q-wave infarction, the prognosis at 6–12 months tends to equalize. As such, patients with non–Q-wave infarction constitute a specific subgroup requiring aggressive diagnostic evaluation and treatment. Detection and dilation or bypass of a high-grade coronary stenosis may prevent subsequent reinfarction.

Approximately 60% of patients who die of cardiac disease expire suddenly before reaching the hospital. However, the prognosis for those hospitalized with MI has become remarkably good. In some studies using thrombolytic therapy or PCI, the mortality rate has been in the range of 5%–8%. Mortality is affected by a wide variety of factors, such as the degree of heart failure, myocardial damage, severity of the underlying atherosclerotic process, heart size, and previous ischemia.

Immediate coronary angiography and primary PCI (including stenting) of the infarct-related artery have been shown to be superior to thrombolysis when done by experienced operators in high-volume centers with rapid time from first medical contact to intervention ("door-to-balloon"). If this time is kept under 90 minutes, outcome is improved and is superior to that of thrombolysis. This intervention, in conjunction with the platelet glycoprotein IIb/IIIa antagonist abciximab (ReoPro), is now widely used in patients with acute MI.

The complications of MI depend on its severity and may include CHF, rupture of the ventricular wall, pericarditis, and arrhythmias. Regional and global ventricular contractile dysfunction may result in CHF or pulmonary edema. Mild to moderate heart failure occurs in nearly 50% of patients following MI; and severe heart failure, in approximately 15%. Cardiogenic shock, which results in a dramatic fall in systemic blood pressure, is observed in 10% of patients with MI and carries a mortality rate of more than 75%. Rupture of the ventricular septum or a papillary muscle is uncommon, with each occurring in about 5% of patients. Rupture of the left ventricular wall, which may occur at any time within 2 weeks of MI, has been found to be the cause of sudden death in about 9% of autopsies after acute MI. Some patients experience post-MI pericarditis, characterized by a pericardial friction rub 2–3 days after infarction. When this rub is accompanied by fever, arthralgia, and pleuropericardial pain, the diagnosis is most likely *post-MI*, or *Dressler*, *syndrome*. This condition is treated with aspirin, nonsteroidal anti-inflammatory agents, or corticosteroids. Injury along the conduction pathways of the atria or ventricles may result in bradycardia, heart block, supraventricular tachycardias, or ventricular arrhythmias. Arrhythmias often exacerbate ischemic injury by reducing the perfusion pressure in the coronary arteries. Most acute deaths from MI result from arrhythmia.

An important aim of a good cardiac program is to enable patients to return to their usual jobs after discharge from the hospital. Approximately 80%–90% of patients with uncomplicated MI can return to work within 2–3 months. Patients are advised to modify or eliminate their risk factors for atherosclerosis. Dietary programs, reduction of physiologic and psychological stress, and cardiac rehabilitation benefit many patients.

Congestive heart failure secondary to ischemic heart disease
Congestive heart failure is discussed later in this chapter.

Sudden cardiac death
Sudden cardiac death is defined as unexpected nontraumatic death that occurs within 1 hour after onset of symptoms in clinically stable patients. A disproportionate number of sudden deaths occur in the early morning hours. SCD is usually caused by a severe arrhythmia, such as ventricular tachycardia, ventricular fibrillation, profound bradycardia, or asystole. SCD may result from MI, occur during an episode of angina, or occur without warning in a patient with frequent arrhythmias secondary to underlying IHD or ventricular dysfunction. Other causes of SCD are Wolff-Parkinson-White syndrome,

long QT syndrome, torsades de pointes, atrioventricular block, aortic stenosis, myocarditis, cardiomyopathy, ruptured or dissecting aortic aneurysm, and pulmonary embolism. There is evidence that prophylactic ICDs are the preferred first-line therapy for patients who have survived a cardiac arrest or an episode of hemodynamically unstable ventricular tachycardia. Results from the Multicenter Automatic Defibrillator Implantation Trial II (MADIT II) demonstrate that ICDs are also the preferred first-line therapy for severe left ventricular dysfunction after MI.

Asymptomatic ischemic heart disease

Asymptomatic patients with IHD are at particular risk for unexpected MI, life-threatening arrhythmias, and SCD. These patients may develop advanced CAD and experience multiple infarcts before the correct diagnosis is made and appropriate treatment is initiated. Older persons, women, and individuals with diabetes are more likely to have painless ischemia. Approximately 25% of MIs may be asymptomatic and detected on a subsequent ECG. A patient who has unexplained dyspnea, weakness, arrhythmias, or poor exercise tolerance requires cardiac testing to evaluate for the presence of undiagnosed IHD.

Noninvasive Cardiac Diagnostic Procedures

Noninvasive diagnostic testing in IHD includes ECG, serum enzyme measurements, echocardiography, various types of stress testing, and imaging studies such as *positron emission tomography (PET)* and *cardiac magnetic resonance imaging (MRI)*.

Electrocardiography

The ECG may appear normal between episodes of ischemia in patients with angina. During angina, the ST segments often become elevated or depressed by up to 5 mm. T waves may be inverted; they may become tall and peaked; or inverted T waves may normalize. These ECG findings, when associated with characteristic anginal pain, are virtually diagnostic of IHD. However, absence of ECG changes does not exclude, with certainty, myocardial ischemia.

During MI, QT-interval prolongation and peaked T waves may appear. The ST segments may be depressed or elevated. ST-segment elevation may persist for several days to weeks, then return to normal. T-wave inversion appears in the leads corresponding to the site of the infarct. Q waves or a reduction in the QRS amplitude appears with the onset of myocardial necrosis. Q waves are typically absent in a subendocardial (nontransmural) infarction. These findings usually occur in the ECG leads related to the site of the infarct and may be accompanied by reciprocal ST depression in the opposite leads. Tachycardia and ventricular arrhythmias are most common within the first few hours after the onset of infarction. Bradyarrhythmias such as heart block are more common with inferior infarction; ventricular tachycardia and fibrillation are more common with anteroseptal infarction.

Serum enzyme testing

Cardiac enzymes are released into the bloodstream when myocardial necrosis occurs and are therefore valuable in differentiating MI from unstable angina and noncardiac causes of chest pain. With the advent of assays for cardiac-specific troponins, serum enzyme testing has also proven useful in identifying patients with ACS at greatest risk for adverse outcomes.

Cardiac-specific troponins are accepted as the most sensitive and specific biochemical cardiac marker in ACS. Cardiac isoforms of troponins (troponins T and I) are important regulatory elements in myocardial cells and, unlike creatine kinase MB (CK-MB), are not normally present in the serum of healthy persons. Troponins T and I have been shown to be more cardiac-specific and sensitive than CK-MB, allowing for more accurate diagnosis of cardiac injury. Moreover, unlike with CK-MB, levels of troponins T and I are not elevated in patients with skeletal muscle injury. Troponin levels remain elevated from 3 hours to 14 days after MI (long after CK-MB levels have normalized). Therefore, for patients who delay seeking medical attention for MI, troponin assays are the test of choice. The greater sensitivity of the cardiac troponin assay allows for the detection of lesser amounts of myocardial damage. In fact, mildly elevated troponin levels may be found in patients with NSTEMI who otherwise would be considered to have unstable angina. However, troponin T is a less sensitive marker than is CK-MB in the early stages of infarction (6–12 hours).

Apart from their diagnostic value, troponin levels also confer prognostic information. It has been demonstrated that patients with an ACS who present with normal CK-MB and elevated troponin T levels have an increased risk of death, recurrent nonfatal infarction, and need for revascularization with PCI or *coronary artery bypass grafting (CABG)*. Similarly, studies have shown that patients with elevated troponin levels at the time of hospital admission are at increased risk for death, cardiogenic shock, or CHF. Finally, a quantitative relationship between the amount of troponin I measured and the risk of death in patients who present with ACS has been demonstrated. Patients who are at greatest risk for adverse outcomes can be identified in the emergency room setting, allowing for more appropriate medical decisions and therapeutic triage.

Until recently, CK-MB isoenzyme was the principal serum cardiac marker used in the evaluation of ACS. Although not as sensitive or specific as the troponins, CK-MB by mass assay remains a useful marker for detecting more than minor myocardial damage. Three isoenzymes of CK can be identified. The MB isoenzyme is relatively specific for myocardium, although it constitutes only about 15% of the total CK released after infarction. Serial plasma samples should be drawn for CK-MB and CK isoenzymes after the onset of chest pain. CK-MB levels begin to rise approximately 4 hours after MI, peaking between 12 and 24 hours, and return to normal within 36–48 hours after an initial MI. CK without isoenzymes is nonspecific, and levels can also be elevated following injury to skeletal muscles or the brain (perioperative or traumatic).

Serum myoglobin is the first marker to rise following myocardial damage, and levels can be elevated between 1 and 20 hours after infarction. Although myoglobin might appear to be ideal for early detection of MI, its performance is not consistent and its specificity for cardiac events is poor. Therefore, myoglobin should not be the only diagnostic marker used to identify patients with MI, but its early appearance with myocardial injury makes its absence useful in ruling out myocardial necrosis.

Echocardiography

Echocardiography employs 1- and 2-dimensional ultrasound and color flow Doppler techniques to image the ventricles and atria, the heart valves, left ventricular contraction and wall-motion abnormalities, left ventricular ejection fraction, and the pericardium. Patients with IHD, particularly following infarction, commonly have regional wall-motion abnormalities that correspond to the areas of myocardial injury. Other, less-frequent complications of infarction, such as mitral regurgitation from papillary muscle injury, ventricular septal defect, ventricular aneurysm, ventricular thrombus, and pericardial effusion, can also be detected with echocardiography. Color flow Doppler provides information on the flow of blood across abnormal valves, pressure differences within the chambers, intracardiac shunts, and cardiac output.

Exercise echocardiography (stress echocardiography) is useful for imaging cardiac valve and wall-motion abnormalities and ventricular dysfunction induced by ischemia during exercise. Predischarge exercise stress echocardiography provides useful prognostic information following acute MI.

Exercise stress testing

Patients with angina may have normal findings on clinical examination, ECG, and echocardiography between episodes of ischemia. Standardized exercise tests have been developed to induce myocardial ischemia under controlled conditions. The ECG, heart rate, blood pressure, and general physical status of the patient are monitored during the procedure. The end point in angina patients is a symptom or sign of cardiac ischemia, such as chest pain, dyspnea, ST-segment depression, arrhythmia, or hypotension. The level of exercise required to induce ischemia is inversely correlated with the likelihood of significant CAD. False-positive and false-negative results occur, and the sensitivity increases with the number of coronary arteries involved. A modified exercise stress test is also performed in patients with a recent MI to help determine functional status and prognosis.

Radionuclide scintigraphy and scans

The sensitivity of exercise testing can be increased via radionuclide techniques. Several agents are available for injection, including thallium-201, technetium-99m sestamibi, and tetrofosmin. Other techniques include thallium-201 myocardial and technetium-99 pyrophosphate (Tc-99) scintigraphy, or blood-pool isotope scans.

Thallium accumulates in normal myocardium and reveals a perfusion defect in areas of myocardial ischemia. Thallium scans have a high sensitivity and specificity for CAD. Reversible thallium/technetium-99m sestamibi defects are those that are present during exercise but resolve during rest. This correlates with myocardial ischemia. In contrast, a fixed thallium/sestamibi defect is present during both exercise and rest and represents a region of prior infarction/nonviable tissue. For patients unable to exercise vigorously enough to reach the required heart rates, a thallium scan or echocardiogram in conjunction with a pharmacologic stress test using intravenous adenosine, dipyridamole, or dobutamine may provide information similar to that of an actual exercise examination. Tomographic imaging of myocardial perfusion is possible with thallium-201 via a technique called *single-photon emission computed tomography (SPECT),* which provides better imaging of infarcts, improved detection of multivessel disease, and reduced severity of artifacts.

A number of other imaging technologies are available and may add clinically useful information. PET scans can accurately differentiate metabolically active myocardium from scar. *Coronary CT angiography (CCTA)* is useful in evaluating occlusive vascular disease and is most useful in ruling out atherosclerotic disease. *Electron beam CT* is useful in quantifying coronary artery calcification, which correlates with atherosclerosis and is highly sensitive but not specific. CT scanning can provide excellent resolution and may provide an alternative to angiography in some patients; disadvantages include significant radiation exposure and the use of contrast. Finally, cardiac MRI provides excellent imaging, and perfusion testing is possible with gadolinium. MRI may be contraindicated in some patients with ICDs or pacemakers. Recent studies by Mosca and colleagues suggest that imaging studies may be more sensitive than stress tests in detecting and assessing CAD in women.

Invasive Cardiac Diagnostic Procedures

Coronary arteriography and *ventriculography* provide valuable information about the presence and severity of CAD and about ventricular function. These techniques can indicate the specific areas of coronary artery stenosis or occlusion, the number of involved vessels, the ventricular systolic and diastolic volumes, the ejection fraction, and regional wall-motion abnormalities. *Multiple gated acquisition (MUGA)* can also be obtained for these purposes. This information helps the cardiologist and cardiac surgeon plan appropriate treatment for the patient. *Intravascular ultrasound imaging* is an evolving invasive modality for studying the intraluminal coronary anatomy and may be particularly useful in evaluating the effects of stents or angioplasty.

Coronary artery stenosis is hemodynamically significant when the arterial lumen diameter is narrowed by more than 50% or the cross-sectional area is reduced by more than 75%. Common indications for coronary arteriography are ACS, post-MI angina, stable angina unresponsive to medical therapy or revascularization, a markedly positive exercise stress test result, and a recent MI in a patient younger than 40 years. The technique may also be useful in evaluating valvular heart disease, ventricular septal defect, papillary muscle dysfunction, cardiomyopathy of unknown cause, or unexplained ventricular arrhythmias.

Management of Ischemic Heart Disease

The goals of management for the patient with CAD are to reduce the frequency of or eliminate angina, prevent myocardial damage, and prolong life. The first line of attack should include eliminating or reducing risk factors for atherosclerosis. Smoking cessation, dietary modification, weight loss, exercise, and improved control of diabetes and hypertension are critical steps. Recent studies by Fraker and colleagues have reported actual regression of atherosclerotic lesions following intensive lipid-lowering therapy, and statins should be considered for CAD patients. Antiplatelet therapy with daily aspirin has also been advocated for all patients with CAD because it significantly reduces the risk of MI.

Women, unlike men and unless they are in a high-risk group, do not appear to benefit from aspirin in reducing MI risk. Aspirin does, however, provide protection against stroke and is recommended for all women age 65 and older. Hormone therapy, antioxidant vitamin supplements, and folic acid therapy do not appear to provide any benefit in preventing CVD in women.

Treatment of stable angina pectoris

Medical management of angina pectoris is designed to deliver as much oxygen as possible to the potentially ischemic myocardium, to reduce the oxygen demand to a level where symptoms are eliminated or reduced to a comfortable level, or both. Oxygen delivery through the coronary arteries may be maximized via coronary vasodilators. Nitroglycerin or other nitrates, which are the drugs of choice, may be given sublingually for acute episodes of angina. Long-acting, orally administered nitrates or topically applied nitroglycerin ointments or transdermal patches may be administered for prevention and long-term control of angina. The systemic effects of nitrates include venous dilation and a decline in arterial pressure; these physiologic effects contribute to the therapeutic effects. Oxygen demands can be reduced by decreasing heart rate and contractility.

The best agents for reducing heart rate and contractility are the *β-adrenergic blockers,* which are useful in managing both stable and unstable angina. Their favorable properties have made them the first line and mainstay of treatment for these patients. β-Blockers are also the only antianginal agents demonstrated to prolong life in CAD patients. The *slow-channel calcium-blocking agents* (diltiazem, nifedipine, verapamil, nicardipine, and amlodipine) are effective in treating chronic angina and may be useful in preventing episodes of coronary spasm, but they should be considered third-line agents, as some studies suggest associated increased mortality rates. β-Adrenergic blockers and calcium channel blockers (particularly verapamil) must be used with caution when left ventricular dysfunction is present. *Ranolazine* (Ranexa), a new antianginal agent, provides symptomatic relief without reducing blood pressure or heart rate but does not appear to change the rate of MI or death in controlled trials. Myocardial oxygen requirements can also be reduced by decreasing ventricular wall tension through controlling systemic hypertension and by reducing the ventricular volume with venous dilators such as nitrates. In addition, routine administration of aspirin reduces the likelihood of thrombus formation. Patients intolerant of aspirin may be treated with *clopidogrel* (Plavix), and ACS patients benefit from DAT with both agents. Improving the oxygen-carrying capacity of the blood by treating anemia or coexisting pulmonary disease provides some additional benefit. Patients in whom medical therapy is unsuccessful may be candidates for revascularization with either PCI or CABG.

Revascularization may improve coronary blood flow, control angina, and increase exercise tolerance. In high-risk patients, the risk of infarction is reduced and long-term survival is enhanced. Revascularization is indicated in otherwise healthy patients with advanced left main CAD, left ventricular dysfunction with 3-vessel disease, angina not responsive to medical treatment, and patients on medical therapy with ischemia on exercise testing. Revascularization procedures include PCI with or without stenting and CABG.

PCI was developed as an alternative to surgical revascularization. Angioplasty involves passing a balloon catheter into a stenosed vessel and inflating the balloon at the site of the narrowing to widen the lumen. Although 85%–90% of vessels can be opened with PCI, the rate of restenosis is approximately 25%–40% at 6 months. The insertion of a wire-mesh *stent* at the time of PCI improves patency and reduces the risk of restenosis by nearly 50%. Drug-eluting stents (DESs) are superior to bare-metal stents (BMSs) in preventing restenosis but are also more likely to lead to late stent thrombosis. Stent thrombosis may result in MI or death, so patients receiving stents should receive a platelet IIb/IIIa receptor antagonist (abciximab, eptifibatide or tirofiban) along with heparin, aspirin, and clopidogrel at the time of stenting (Table 4-1). Dual antiplatelet therapy (DAT; aspirin +

Table 4-1 Summary of the Current ACC/AHA Guideline Recommendations for Medical Management of Acute Coronary Syndromes (ACS) and Acute Myocardial Infarction (AMI)[1]

Medication	Acute Therapies ACS	Acute Therapies AMI	Discharge Therapies
Aspirin (ASA)	IA	IA	IA
Clopidogrel in ASA-allergic patients	IA	IC	IA
Clopidogrel, intended medical management	IA	—	IA
Clopidogrel, or IIb/IIIa inhibitor, up front (prior to catheterization)	IA		
Clopidogrel, early catheterization/ percutaneous coronary intervention (catheterization/percutaneous coronary intervention [cath/PCI])	IA (prior to or at time of PCI)	IB	IA
Heparin (unfractionated or low-molecular-weight)	IA	IA[2]	—
β-Blockers	IB	IA	IB
Angiotensin-converting enzyme (ACE) inhibitors	IB[3]	IA/IIaB[4]	IA
GP IIb/IIIa inhibitors for intended early cath/PCI			
Eptifibatide/tirofiban	IA	—	—
Abciximab	IA	IIaB[5]	—
GP IIb/IIIa inhibitors for high-risk patients without intended early cath/PCI			
Eptifibatide/tirofiban	IIaA	—	—
Abciximab	IIIA	—	—
Lipid-lowering agent[6]	—	—	IA
Smoking cessation counseling	—	—	IB

ACC/AHA = American College of Cardiology/American Heart Association, PCI = percutaneous coronary intervention.

[1] Class I indicates treatment is useful and effective, IIa indicates weight of evidence is in favor of usefulness/efficacy, class IIb indicates weight of evidence is less well established, and class III indicates intervention is not useful/effective and may be harmful. Type A recommendations are derived from large-scale randomized trials, and B recommendations are derived from smaller randomized trials or carefully conducted observational analyses.

[2] As a class IIb, low-molecular-weight heparin (best studied is enoxaparin with tenecteplase) can be considered an acceptable alternative to unfractionated heparin for patients less than 75 years old who are receiving fibrinolytic therapy provided significant renal dysfunction is not present.

[3] For patients with persistent hypertension despite treatment, diabetes mellitus, congestive heart failure, or any left ventricular dysfunction.

[4] IA for patients with congestive heart failure or ejection fraction <0.40, IIa for others, in absence of hypotension (systolic blood pressure <100 mm Hg); angiotensin receptor blocker (valsartan or candesartan) for patients with ACE inhibitor intolerance.

[5] As early as possible before primary PCI.

[6] For patients with a low-density lipoprotein cholesterol level >100 mg/dL.

From Bashore TM, Granger CB, Hranitzky P, Patel MR. Heart disease. In: *Current Medical Diagnosis and Treatment 2009*. Lange Current Series. McPhee SJ, Papadakis MA (eds). 48th ed. New York: McGraw-Hill; 2009:318, Table 10-4.

clopidogrel) should continue for at least 1 month poststenting for a BMS and at least 1 year for a DES. DAT should not be stopped during this period, and elective surgery should be postponed unless the patient can continue on DAT. Patients intolerant of aspirin may use clopidogrel alone. A new drug under consideration by the FDA, prasugrel, appears to have a superior anticoagulant effect to clopidogrel but more risk of serious bleeding.

PCI is recommended for patients with lesions amenable to passing a catheter; patients with a 1- or 2-vessel disease, with no involvement of the left anterior descending coronary artery; and nondiabetic patients with a good ejection fraction with multivessel disease. Diabetic patients do well with PCI if the procedure is paired with a stent and a glycoprotein IIb/IIIa agent. PCI and CABG have similar mortality rates, but patients undergoing PCI are more likely to require repeat procedures.

When angioplasty is inappropriate or ineffective and medical therapy has failed to control symptoms in severe multivessel disease, CABG may be considered. CABG is the treatment of choice in patients with high-risk disease (ie, those with significant left main, proximal left anterior descending, or 3-vessel disease, especially if accompanied by left ventricular dysfunction), because it is superior to medical therapy in preventing infarction and prolonging survival. A shunt is installed from the aorta to the diseased coronary artery, bypassing the area of obstruction, and increases blood flow, thereby eliminating angina and often reducing the risk of infarction and cardiac death or preventing these altogether. CABG has also been shown to increase left ventricular function, improve quality of life, and increase life expectancy compared with medical treatment for patients with significant high-risk disease. Saphenous veins are most commonly used as the bypass material, but use of the internal mammary artery has become the standard for the left anterior descending artery because of its improved long-term patency rate. Some patients now receive "off-the-pump bypass surgery," in which the grafts are sewn onto the beating heart. This technique avoids the adverse effects of cardiopulmonary bypass, which include memory, cognitive, and other neurologic deficits.

Anderson JL, Adams CD, Antman EM, et al. ACC/AHA 2007 guidelines for the management of patients with unstable angina/non–ST-elevation myocardial infarction. *J Am Coll Cardiol.* 2007;50(7):e1–e157.

Canadian Cardiovascular Society, American Academy of Family Physicians, American College of Cardiology, et al. 2007 focused update of the ACC/AHA 2004 guidelines for the management of patients with ST-elevation myocardial infarction. *J Am Coll Cardiol.* 2008;51(2): 210–247.

Fraker TD Jr, Fihn SD; 2002 Chronic Stable Angina Writing Committee, et al. 2007 chronic angina focused update of the ACC/AHA 2002 guidelines for the management of patients with chronic stable angina. *J Am Coll Cardiol.* 2007;50(23):2264–2274.

King SB III, Smith SC Jr, Hirshfeld JW Jr, et al. 2007 focused update of the ACC/AHA/SCAI 2005 guideline update for percutaneous coronary intervention. *J Am Coll Cardiol.* 2008;51(2): 172–209.

Mosca L, Banka CL, Benjamin EJ, et al. Evidence-based guidelines for cardiovascular disease prevention in women: 2007 update. *Circulation.* 2007;115(11):1481–1501.

Treatment of acute coronary syndromes

Patients with an ACS are admitted to a hospital or a chest pain observation unit for monitoring and treatment. They are initially treated aggressively with anti-ischemic pharmacotherapy. Once these initial measures are instituted, further management and triage of patients with an ACS is based on the presence or absence of ST-segment elevation. Patients with ST-segment elevation ACS are given reperfusion therapy with either thrombolysis or catheter-based interventions; patients with a non–ST-segment elevation ACS may be appropriately followed up with either medical treatment alone or a more aggressive interventional approach. The use of a risk stratification table (TIMI, GRACE, PURSUIT) may help identify high-risk patients and determine subsequent management. Acute therapy of ACS and MI patients, as well as recommended therapy at the time of discharge, is summarized in Table 4-1.

Management of non–ST-segment elevation ACS   In general, myocardial oxygen demands are managed with medications and supplemental oxygen. Patients are given dual anti-platelet therapy (DAT) (160–325 mg of aspirin and 75 mg of clopidogrel), which is effective in reducing the mortality of MI. The first dose of aspirin should be chewed rather than swallowed to achieve rapid blood levels. If the patient is neither hypotensive nor bradycardic, nitroglycerin may be administered, either sublingually or intravenously. Intravenous administration permits careful titration, allowing control of anginal symptoms without causing excessive hypotension. Nitrates should be used with caution in patients on erectile-dysfunction medications, who can experience profound hypotension. When nitroglycerin does not provide pain relief, morphine sulfate may be administered. β-Blocker therapy reduces myocardial oxygen demands and should be considered for all patients with evolving MI if no contraindication exists.

For patients not receiving reperfusion therapy, β-blocker therapy provides a survival benefit, particularly for high-risk patients (older patients and those with previous MI and mild pulmonary venous congestion). When β-blockers cannot be used, heart rate–slowing calcium antagonists (eg, verapamil or diltiazem) offer an alternative. However, rapid-release, short-acting dihydropyridine-type calcium channel blockers (eg, nifedipine) should be avoided if adequate concurrent β-blockade in ACS is absent; controlled trials suggest that, in this setting, the risk of MI and cardiac death is increased. Moreover, the risk of cardiac death is significantly increased when calcium channel blockers are used in the setting of left ventricular failure.

Angiotensin-converting enzyme (ACE) inhibitors such as captopril (Capoten), enalapril (Vasotec), lisinopril (Prinivil), and ramipril (Altace), given orally during the acute phase of MI, have been demonstrated to decrease the risk of immediate mortality when initiated within the first 24 hours of acute MI. ACE inhibitors are beneficial with or without concomitant reperfusion therapy. Patients receiving the greatest benefit are those in high-risk groups, including those with anterior infarctions, evidence of left ventricular systolic dysfunction, mild CHF, and previous MI. ACE inhibitors are contraindicated in patients with hypotension and should be used with caution in patients with renal insufficiency. If CHF or pulmonary edema is present, management should include vasodilators, diuretics, digoxin, or other inotropic agents.

Antithrombin therapy, which involves a variety of agents, including unfractionated heparin (UFH); low-molecular-weight heparins, including enoxaparin (Lovenox); the direct thrombin inhibitors (hirudin and bivalirudin); and the factor Xa inhibitor fondaparinux (Arixtra), is beneficial in ACS. Controlled studies have yet to determine the optimal regimen, although fondaparinux and enoxaparin appear slightly better than UFH. Fondaparinux appears to cause fewer bleeding complications than the other agents, but the anticoagulation is more difficult to reverse due to a longer half-life, so UFH may be superior if surgery is anticipated within 24 hours. The direct thrombin inhibitors are not currently recommended in ACC/AHA guidelines.

The glycoprotein IIb/IIIa receptor is present on the surface of platelets. When platelets are activated, this receptor increases its affinity for fibrinogen and other ligands, resulting in platelet aggregation. This mechanism constitutes the final and obligatory pathway for platelet aggregation. The platelet glycoprotein IIb/IIIa receptor antagonists tirofiban (Aggrastat), abciximab (ReoPro), and eptifibatide (Integrilin) act by preventing fibrinogen binding and thereby preventing platelet aggregation. Platelets are involved in the development of both ACS and complications after PCI. Glycoprotein IIb/IIIa inhibitors have been shown to reduce the risk of death and MI in patients with non–ST-segment elevation ACS, as well as after coronary angioplasty and stenting. In addition to PCIs, glycoprotein IIb/IIIa inhibitors are indicated in the treatment of non–ST-segment elevation ACS. However, the benefit in these patients is less than that observed with PCIs.

Once unstable angina and NSTEMI have been managed as described, patients may be evaluated with either a conservative noninvasive approach or an early invasive (angiographic) strategy, depending on their level of risk for adverse outcome. In the initial conservative strategy, coronary angiography is reserved for patients with evidence of recurrent ischemia (angina or ST-segment changes at rest or with minimal activity) or a strongly positive stress test result despite vigorous medical therapy. In the invasive strategy, patients without clinically obvious contraindications to coronary revascularization are routinely recommended for coronary angiography and angiographically directed revascularization. Controlled trials have shown the superiority of an invasive approach in managing ACS patients, particularly patients with refractory angina or hemodynamic instability, or patients at elevated risk as measured by bedside risk stratification tools (TIMI, GRACE). The decision to proceed from diagnostic angiography to revascularization is influenced not only by the coronary anatomy but by a number of additional factors, including anticipated life expectancy, ventricular function, comorbidity, functional capacity, severity of symptoms, and quantity of viable myocardium at risk.

Management of ST-segment elevation ACS   Modern therapy for evolving Q-wave MI involves rapid and effective reperfusion, because necrosis is a time-dependent process. Optimal myocardial salvage requires that nearly complete reperfusion be achieved as soon as possible: maximal benefit, within 1 hour of symptom onset; significant benefit, within 6 hours of symptom onset; some benefit, 6–12 hours after symptom onset. The benefit of reperfusion therapy after 12 hours of symptom onset has not been established.

Methods of reperfusion include thrombolysis and catheter-based PCIs (balloon angioplasty with or without stent placement). Initial medical management prior to and following reperfusion therapy should include aspirin, clopidogrel, morphine (for pain), and β-blockers if no contraindications exist. Nonsteroidal agents besides aspirin should not be used acutely or during hospitalization, as they increase the risk of CHF and death. Other adjuncts to therapy may include low-molecular-weight heparins and glycoprotein IIb/IIIa inhibitors.

Numerous clinical trials have demonstrated the superiority of early PCI over thrombolysis, particularly if performed in the first 90 minutes following medical contact. Hospitals without PCI capability should transfer the patient to a PCI facility if the procedure can be done within 90 minutes. Otherwise, thrombolytic therapy should be started within 30 minutes of first medical contact. PCI following full-dose thrombolytics carries significant risks but may be done in high-risk patients or if thrombolytic therapy has failed ("rescue PCI"). Totally occluded arteries generally do not benefit from PCI.

Thrombolysis Patients with a STEMI treated with thrombolytics in the first 3 hours show a 50% reduction in mortality; those treated at 12 hours show a 10% reduction. Several intravenous thrombolytic agents are available that effectively lyse coronary thrombi and restore coronary blood flow in most patients. *Tissue plasminogen activators (tPAs),* including alteplase (Activase), reteplase (Retavase), and tenecteplase (TNKase) are the most commonly used thrombolytics because they are more effective in opening arteries and reducing mortality than is streptokinase. The efficacy of these 3 tPA agents is similar, but administering reteplase (2 bolus injections) and tenecteplase (1 weight-adjusted bolus) is easier and may encourage earlier intervention. When any tPA is used, intravenous heparin should be administered concurrently.

Major bleeding complications occur in up to 5% of patients undergoing thrombolytic therapy. The major disadvantage of tPA is a slightly greater risk of intracranial hemorrhage compared with that of streptokinase. Although most studies have restricted the use of these drugs to patients aged 75 or younger, older patients experience distinctly more infarction mortality and therefore may benefit from thrombolytic therapy. Contraindications include known sites of potential bleeding, a history of prior cerebrovascular accident, recent surgery, or prolonged cardiopulmonary resuscitation efforts. Thrombolysis should not be used in NSTEMI due to decreased benefits and, possibly, increased hemorrhagic risks.

Congestive Heart Failure

The epidemiologic magnitude of CHF is staggering. Approximately 5 million patients in the United States have CHF, and there are 500,000 new cases per year. Many of the patients consulting an ophthalmologist belong to the older population, a group especially prone to this condition. If the heart cannot meet the metabolic demands of the metabolizing tissues, heart failure is the diagnosis. The cardiac pump may be in failure, or it may be near normal but unable to keep up with demand. The direct result of heart failure is circulatory failure.

Symptoms and signs of CHF may occur when the heart is not able to pump a sufficient amount of blood for a prolonged period to meet the body's requirements. *Compensated CHF* refers to patients whose clinical manifestations of CHF have been controlled by treatment. *Decompensated CHF* represents heart failure with symptoms that are not under control. *Refractory CHF* exists when previous therapeutic measures have failed to control the clinical manifestations of the syndrome. Pulmonary edema usually results from severe left ventricular failure with increased pulmonary capillary pressure, causing parenchymal and intra-alveolar fluid accumulation in the lung. Heart failure is often preventable with early detection and intervention, and this is emphasized by new guidelines and classifications that recognize 4 stages of heart failure, including stages for those at risk and those with no current signs of CHF. Figure 4-1 illustrates the stages and recommended therapy at each stage. The New York Heart Association has also developed a classification for heart failure symptoms, ranging from class I (no symptoms) to class IV (symptoms at rest).

Symptoms

Heart failure causes a variety of symptoms, depending on the severity of ventricular dysfunction. Symptoms may result from inadequate tissue perfusion caused by pump failure or from the failing heart's inability to empty adequately, leading to edema and fluid accumulation in the lungs, extremities, and other sites. The most frequent symptoms of left ventricular failure are dyspnea with exertion or at rest, orthopnea, paroxysmal nocturnal dyspnea, diaphoresis, generalized weakness, fatigue, anxiety, and lightheadedness. With more severe CHF, the patient may also experience a productive cough; copious pink, frothy sputum; and mental confusion. Angina may also occur if the CHF results from IHD. Right-sided heart failure may occur separately from or secondary to chronic left-sided heart failure. Patients with right-sided heart failure typically develop peripheral edema.

Clinical Signs

Examination findings in acute left ventricular failure may include respiratory distress, use of the respiratory accessory muscles, pinkish sputum or frank hemoptysis, coarse rales on pulmonary auscultation, expiratory wheezes, a rapid heart rate, an S gallop, diaphoresis, and deterioration in mental status. Blood pressure is often markedly elevated but may be reduced during MI. Long-standing cases of CHF show signs of right ventricular failure, especially elevated central venous pressure, pedal edema, hepatomegaly, and cyanosis. In some patients, pleural effusion or ascites may be detected.

Diagnostic Evaluation

The history and clinical examination are the most important components in the diagnostic assessment of CHF. Helpful diagnostic studies in evaluating CHF and its underlying causes include chest radiograph, ECG, blood gases, hemoglobin level, serum electrolytes, and urinalysis. Measurement of serum B-type natriuretic peptide (BNP), a peptide associated with reduced left ventricular ejection fraction and increased left ventricular filling pressure, may be helpful in determining the underlying cause and guiding the treatment of CHF. If the primary mechanism of heart failure is unclear, additional tests may prove useful in selected patients. Such tests may include echocardiography, exercise stress testing, cardiac nuclear imaging studies, coronary arteriography, right-sided and left-sided heart catheterization, Holter monitoring, pulmonary function tests, and thyroid function tests.

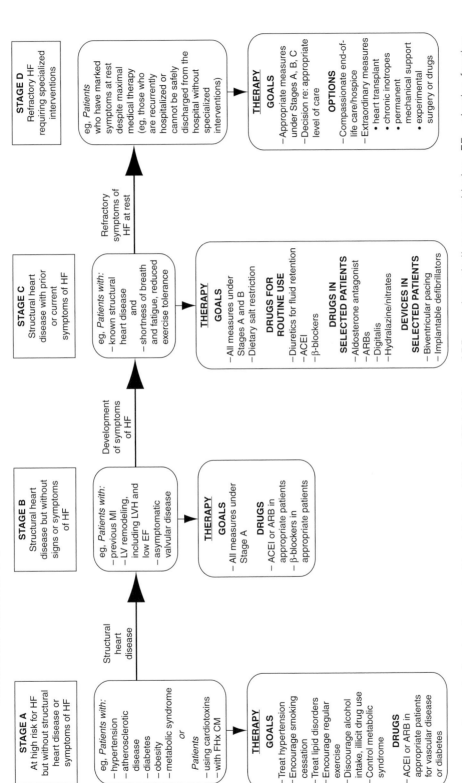

Figure 4-1 Stages in the development of heart failure. *ACEI* = ACE inhibitors, *ARB* = angiotensin II receptor blocker, *EF* = ejection fraction, *FHx CM* = family history of cardiomyopathy, *HF* = heart failure, *LV* = left ventricular, *LVH* = left ventricular hypertrophy, *MI* = myocardial infarction. *(From Hunt SA: American College of Cardiology; American Heart Association Task Force on Practice Guidelines. ACC/AHA 2005 guideline update for the diagnosis and management of chronic heart failure in the adult. J Am Coll Cardiol. 2005;46(6):e1-e82.)*

The ECG may reveal acute ischemic changes, acute or old MI, ventricular hypertrophy, chamber enlargement, and atrial fibrillation or other arrhythmias. Typical chest radiographic findings are prominent pulmonary vessels, interstitial or alveolar pulmonary edema, cardiomegaly, and pleural effusions. Patients with severe pump failure may have abnormal serum electrolytes owing to poor renal perfusion. Abnormalities in the blood or urine may help detect severe anemia or renal failure as a precipitating factor in CHF. Abnormal liver enzymes are common if venous congestion is present as a result of right ventricular failure.

Echocardiography and other cardiac studies can help differentiate the many cardiac causes of CHF, including IHD, valvular heart disease, cardiomyopathies, and cardiac arrhythmias. Coronary angiography can be helpful in identifying patients with cardiac ischemia and CHF, where revascularization may lead to symptomatic improvement.

Ejection fraction (EF) is the calculated percentage of blood ejected by the ventricle during a single or average contraction. In patients without CHF, the EF is more than 0.50. An EF of 0.40–0.50 indicates mild impairment; 0.25–0.40, moderate impairment; and less than 0.25, severe impairment. Ejection fraction can be measured using echocardiography, radionuclide ventriculography, and contrast ventriculography. Echocardiography is the most useful and least invasive method of determining and sequentially following EF and the systolic state of the ventricles.

Etiology

As was noted previously, IHD is the most common cause of CHF. Cumulative injury to the ventricular myocardium from ischemia and infarction can lead to impaired ventricular systolic and diastolic function, and, ultimately, pump failure. Additional causes of systolic dysfunction include valvular heart disease (primarily aortic stenosis and aortic or mitral regurgitation), cardiomyopathies (which may be idiopathic or which may have metabolic, infectious, toxic, or connective tissue causes) and myocarditis (from viral or inflammatory diseases).

Diseases that impair the relaxation and filling properties of the left ventricle can result in diastolic dysfunction. Such disorders include infiltrative diseases (eg, amyloidosis, sarcoidosis, and metastatic disease) and left ventricular hypertrophy (which can be caused by arterial hypertension, idiopathic hypertrophic subaortic stenosis, and coarctation of the aorta).

Systolic dysfunction and diastolic dysfunction often occur simultaneously in the common causes of CHF—namely, IHD, valvular disease, and the congestive cardiomyopathies. Some of the causes of high-cardiac-output heart failure are severe anemia, hyperthyroidism, arteriovenous fistulas, beriberi, and Paget disease.

In high-output failure, the demand for oxygen is so great that the heart eventually fails because it cannot maintain the excessive cardiac output indefinitely. In some patients, heart failure may be more complex—for example, a patient with IHD may develop CHF after becoming severely anemic. Pure right ventricular failure may result from chronic pulmonary disease, pulmonary hypertension, tricuspid or pulmonary valve disease, right ventricular infarction, or constrictive pericarditis.

Pathophysiology and Clinical Course

The left and right ventricles function as pumping chambers, and their action can be subdivided into a *systolic,* or contraction, phase and a *diastolic,* or relaxation, phase. During systole, the ventricular muscle actively contracts, developing pressure and ejecting blood into the aorta or pulmonary artery for forward perfusion. During diastole, the ventricular muscle actively and passively relaxes and allows a refilling of the ventricle from the corresponding atrium. Either or both of these phases may become impaired, leading to dysfunction of systole, diastole, or both. Some of the symptoms and clinical signs of CHF can be distinguished as being attributable to systolic or diastolic impairment. Treatment varies, depending on which type of dysfunction predominates.

Systolic dysfunction

The ability of the heart to contract and eject blood is determined by preload, afterload, and contractility. *Preload* refers to the amount of stretch to which muscle fibers are subjected at the end of diastole, or refilling. Preload is determined by blood volume and venous return. Excessive preload is often called *volume overload.* Up to a point, as the preload increases, the force of contraction also increases, allowing adequate emptying of the ventricle.

Afterload is the amount of tension or force in the ventricular muscle mass just after onset of contraction, as the ventricle begins emptying. Clinically, afterload represents the pressure that the ventricle must withstand during contraction. Thus, the aortic pressure determines afterload for the left ventricle, whereas the pulmonary artery pressure determines afterload for the right. Even a normal ventricle may fail with extremely high preload or afterload.

Contractility refers to the intrinsic ability of the myocardial fibers to contract, independent of the preload or afterload conditions. Contractility can be adversely affected by metabolic, ischemic, or other structural derangement of the myocardial cells. Abnormal intracellular modulation of calcium ions is a key component in heart failure. Clinical disorders that affect preload, afterload, or contractility result in systolic dysfunction— and therapy directed toward improving these parameters can be used to treat systolic dysfunction.

Diastolic dysfunction

Several of the disorders that impair the diastolic, or relaxation, properties of the ventricle were listed previously among the causes of CHF. Diastolic dysfunction causes elevated filling pressures in the ventricles and atria. In the left ventricle, diastolic dysfunction causes pulmonary venous hypertension and its clinical manifestations, such as dyspnea on exertion, orthopnea, and paroxysmal nocturnal dyspnea. Clinical signs of diastolic dysfunction are pulmonary edema with rales, lung congestion visible on chest radiograph, and hypoxemia.

The clinical course of CHF may follow a downward spiral of left ventricular systolic and diastolic dysfunction, ventricular dilation, and a decline in the EF, followed by right-sided heart failure. A continuous reduction in cardiac output and tissue perfusion may be accompanied by increasing pulmonary and systemic venous congestion. Appropriate treatment may slow or even halt progression in some patients. BNP, which is synthesized in the cardiac ventricles and whose release is directly proportional to ventricular volume expansion and pressure overload, may indicate the course of CHF. Levels of BNP correlate with left ventricular pressure, the amount of dyspnea, and the state of neurohumoral modulation. In addition, BNP levels correlate well with the New York Heart Association classification system of CHF.

Medical and Nonsurgical Management

Appropriate treatment at each stage of CHF is summarized in Figure 4-1. In general, most symptomatic patients should be treated with a combination of a diuretic and an ACE inhibitor. Diuretics, whether oral thiazide or loop diuretics, reduce the blood volume and thus preload. More severely affected CHF patients should receive a loop diuretic (furosemide, bumetanide, torsemide) either orally or by IV. Hypokalemia may result from the use of these agents, necessitating the use of potassium-sparing agents (spironolactone, triamterene, amiloride), but these agents tend to be less potent diuretics. Spironolactone also reduced mortality in the RALES study by presumably acting as a neurohormonal antagonist.

> Hauben M, Reich L, Gerrits CM, Madigan D. Detection of spironolactone-associated hyperkalaemia following the Randomized Aldactone Evaluation Study (RALES). *Drug Saf.* 2007;30(12):1143–1149.

Systolic dysfunction

Reducing afterload is the most effective way to manage systolic dysfunction in most clinical situations. Reducing vascular resistance and lowering arterial blood pressure decrease the burden on the left ventricle and enhance contraction and ejection. Regardless of the baseline values, lowering blood pressure (while maintaining adequate tissue perfusion) is the mainstay of treatment of systolic dysfunction. The most effective drugs for reducing afterload in current clinical practice are the ACE inhibitors, including captopril (Capoten), enalapril (Vasotec), lisinopril (Prinivil), and ramipril (Altace). These drugs effectively decrease the clinical manifestations of CHF and have been demonstrated in clinical trials to lower both mortality and morbidity rates among patients with CHF. These beneficial effects can be seen in patients with idiopathic dilated cardiomyopathy, as well as in those with diminished left ventricular function after an MI. Asymptomatic patients with reduced EFs may also benefit from ACE inhibitors, as these drugs may slow or prevent progression to stage C of CHF (see Fig 4-1). *Angiotensin II receptor blockers (ARBs)*, including candesartan (Atacand) and valsartan (Diovan), may be useful as alternatives to ACE inhibitors when side effects such as hypotension are not tolerated.

Patients with CHF have an increased adrenergic drive that is associated with a worsened prognosis. High levels of norepinephrine are both arrhythmogenic and cardiotoxic. The use of β-blockers such as carvedilol (Coreg), bisoprolol, and metoprolol has clearly been shown to improve heart failure symptoms and to reduce all-cause mortality and the risk of hospitalization in patients with CHF. Stable patients with mild, moderate, or severe heart failure should be treated with a β-blocker unless noncardiac contraindications exist. However, as many as 6% of patients may not tolerate even small amounts of a β-blocker.

Therefore, initial doses must be very low, with gradual and careful upward titration over 3–6 months.

Other drugs that reduce afterload by lowering blood pressure and peripheral vascular resistance are hydralazine, clonidine, and calcium channel blockers. However, calcium channel blockers have generally been found to be of little benefit in patients with CHF. In fact, diltiazem (Cardizem) was associated with increased mortality when used in patients with CHF. Amlodipine (Norvasc) is the only calcium channel blocker shown to be safe in patients with CHF and is therefore the calcium channel blocker of choice in patients with CHF and ongoing angina or hypertension not controlled by other means. α-Adrenergic blockers such as prazosin or doxazosin can also be considered for patients who cannot tolerate ACE inhibitors because of renal dysfunction or other relative contraindications. Hospitalized patients with more severe CHF, particularly pulmonary edema, may require more aggressive afterload reduction with intravenous agents such as nitroprusside, nitroglycerin, or enalapril.

For patients with systolic dysfunction, the contractility of the left ventricle can be enhanced with inotropic agents. *Digoxin,* or *digitalis,* the time-honored drug for increasing contractility, and once a mainstay of treatment, has safety and toxicity concerns. Thus, digoxin is now reserved largely for patients who remain symptomatic despite the use of diuretics and ACE inhibitors or for patients with CHF and atrial fibrillation requiring rate control. With the exception of digoxin, oral inotropic agents have not proven safe or effective in patients with chronic CHF, although intravenous inotropic agents play a key role in treating patients hospitalized for worsening heart failure. Three intravenous inotropic agents are FDA approved as therapy for acute exacerbations of CHF: the adrenergic agonist dobutamine, the phosphodiesterase inhibitor milrinone, and the dopaminergic/adrenergic agonist dopamine. These IV agents show no benefit in long-term use but may be useful in patients with low cardiac output, in patients not responsive to IV diuretics, and for patients awaiting cardiac transplantation. For patients on these potent drugs, close monitoring of blood pressure, heart rate, cardiac output, and urine production is required.

Diastolic dysfunction

Diastolic function can be improved by reducing preload, which in turn lowers filling pressures in the ventricle. Preload can be reduced by reducing circulating blood volume, by increasing the capacitance of the venous bed, and by improving systolic function to more effectively empty the ventricle. Diuretics are the most effective agents for reducing blood volume. Oral thiazide or loop diuretics are effective for long-term diuresis, but, as noted earlier, intravenous loop diuretics such as furosemide or bumetanide are more potent for severe CHF or pulmonary edema. Venous capacitance can be increased by administering venous dilators, particularly the nitrates. Intravenous furosemide and morphine also have some venodilation effects, partially explaining their effectiveness in treating pulmonary edema. Any of the measures previously discussed that improve systolic function also indirectly enhance diastolic function by reducing the residual blood volume in the ventricle following contraction.

Other approaches to CHF

Other strategies for managing CHF include seeking underlying causes or the contributing factors responsible for the failure and correcting them, if possible. Precipitating factors can include excessive salt or fluid intake, poor medication compliance, excessive activity, obesity, pulmonary infection or embolism, MI, renal disease, anemia, thyrotoxicosis, and arrhythmias.

Intermittent arrhythmias may seriously compromise ventricular function. Tachyarrhythmias may aggravate ischemia; bradyarrhythmias may decrease cardiac output and blood pressure further. As previously discussed, β-blockers should be considered in these patients and all patients with CHF for their effects on overall prognosis and particularly SCD. Amiodarone was not beneficial in the SCD-HeFT trial, and most other antiarrhythmic agents are contraindicated in CHF because they may decrease cardiac function and be paradoxically proarrhythmic. ICDs can be useful adjuncts to medical therapy in patients with CHF, cardiomyopathy, and an EF ≤35%, and they improved mortality in both the MADIT II and SCD-HeFT trials. Biventricular pacing also improves mortality rates and decreases rehospitalization rates in patients with CHF and a wide QRS complex by improving contraction efficiency. Patients with heart block and other severe bradyarrhythmias may also require cardiac pacing.

Patients with a dilated cardiomyopathy and atrial fibrillation should be treated with warfarin (Coumadin) unless specific contraindications exist. Many physicians also prescribe warfarin for patients with a dilated cardiomyopathy, low EF, and normal sinus rhythm, if no contraindications exist.

Other measures that can help in managing CHF are restricting dietary sodium, avoiding fluid overload by carefully monitoring oral and intravenous fluid intake, controlling pain and anxiety, treating concomitant metabolic or pulmonary diseases, and providing supplemental oxygen to hypoxemic patients. Finally, all patients with CHF should receive an influenza vaccination and the pneumococcal vaccine.

Bardy GH, Lee KL, Mark DB, et al; Sudden Cardiac Death in Heart Failure Trial (SCD-HeFT) Investigators. Amiodarone or an implantable cardioverter-defibrillator for congestive heart failure. *N Engl J Med.* 2005;352(3):225–237.

Invasive or Surgical Management

Depending on the underlying causes, other surgical procedures that may benefit patients with CHF include percutaneous balloon valvuloplasty, mitral commissurotomy, mitral or aortic valve replacement, left ventricular aneurysmectomy, and pericardectomy. Patients with CAD, the leading cause of CHF, may benefit from coronary revascularization by either CABG or PCI. Cardiac transplantation has become an effective surgical treatment for patients with refractory CHF. Many transplant centers have achieved a 5-year survival rate above 75%. The use of corticosteroids and immunosuppressive agents, such as cyclosporine, tacrolimus (Prograf), sirolimus (Rapamune), azathioprine, and mycophenolate (CellCept), has reduced transplant rejection and mortality. Implantable ventricular assist devices may help to maintain patients awaiting cardiac transplantation.

Finally, as many of these patients are older with multiple comorbidities, palliative care directed only at symptomatic improvement should also be considered.

Hunt SA; American College of Cardiology, American Heart Association Task Force on Practice Guidelines. ACC/AHA 2005 guideline update for the diagnosis and management of chronic heart failure in the adult. *J Am Coll Cardiol.* 2005;46(6):e1–e82.

Disorders of Cardiac Rhythm

Abnormalities of cardiac rhythm can vary widely from asymptomatic premature atrial complexes or mild sinus bradycardia to life-threatening ventricular tachycardia or fibrillation. Disorders of cardiac rhythm can be categorized into several groups, including bradyarrhythmias and conduction disturbances, ectopic or premature contractions, and the tachyarrhythmias.

Although many rhythm and conduction disturbances are caused by underlying IHD, they are also attributable to valvular heart disease, myocarditis, cardiomyopathy, congenital aberrant conduction pathways, pulmonary disease, toxic or metabolic disorders, neurogenic causes, and cardiac trauma.

The electrical impulse that initiates each heartbeat normally begins in the *sinoatrial (SA) node* and is conducted down through the atria and ventricles, resulting in a coordinated series of contractions of these chambers. The SA node is the primary pacemaker of the heart. It controls the heart rate and is influenced by neural, biochemical, and pharmacologic factors. If the SA node function is depressed or absent, secondary pacemakers in the *atrioventricular (AV) junction, the bundle of His,* or the *ventricular muscle* can generate stimuli and maintain the heartbeat. Normally, stimulus formation in these secondary pacemaker sites is slower than is that in the SA node. However, abnormal stimuli can also be generated at any of these sites at a rapid pace, resulting in tachycardia.

Bradyarrhythmias and Conduction Disturbances

A *bradyarrhythmia* is any rhythm resulting in a ventricular rate of less than 60 beats per minute (bpm). Table 4-2 illustrates the most common types of bradyarrhythmias and conduction disturbances and their typical ECG findings, causes, associations, and treatment. These bradyarrhythmias and conduction blocks are generally asymptomatic, although they may cause light-headedness or syncope in rare cases. Treatment is generally not necessary except in cases of syncope or hemodynamic instability, as noted in Table 4-2.

Premature Contractions

The principal types of premature contractions are *premature atrial complexes (PACs), premature junctional complexes (PJCs),* and *premature ventricular complexes (PVCs).* These complexes result from ectopic premature depolarization arising from the atria (PAC), the AV node or proximal His/Purkinje system (PJC), or the ventricles (PVC) (Table 4-3). Patients often experience no symptoms or may have a sensation of "skipped beats." Often no treatment is necessary, although β-blockers or calcium channel blockers can be helpful in

Table 4-2 Bradyarrhythmias: Heart Rate <60 bpm

Arrhythmia	ECG Findings	Causes/Associations	Treatment
Sinus bradycardia	<60 bpm Normal P, QRS	↑ vagal tone, ischemia, SA node disease, antiarrhythmic drugs	Usually none
Sinus arrest	Single or multiple beats dropped	↑ vagal tone, ↓ potassium, sick sinus syndrome, antiarrhythmic drugs	Discontinue inciting drug atropine if unstable; possibly pacemaker
AV junctional rhythm	QRS normal P abnormal, may follow QRS	SA node depressed or nonfunctional	Usually none; evaluate for unknown heart disease
1st-degree AV block	PR interval >0.20 sec	↑ vagal tone, β-blocker, calcium channel blocker, digoxin, ischemia	Discontinue inciting drug, especially digoxin; pacer if PR >0.3 sec
2nd-degree AV block (Wenckebach)	PR interval gradually ↑, then nonconducted; irregular pulse	Acute MI, autonomic lability in adolescence	Usually none; atropine, pacer if necessary
2nd-degree AV block (Mobitz II)	QRS dropped at regular intervals; slow, regular pulse	MI, ischemia more likely to go on to complete block	Pacemaker; avoid atropine—may worsen
3rd-degree AV block	P waves and QRS are asynchronous	Ischemia, drug toxicity, endocarditis, infiltrative	Atropine, isoproterenol, pacemaker
L anterior fascicular block	Left axis deviation	MI, pulmonary embolism (PE), cardiac surgery or cath	Usually none
L posterior fascicular block	Inferior and right axis deviation	Ischemia, myocarditis, valvular disease	Usually none
Complete LBBB	Left axis deviation, notched broad QRS	May mask typical ECG findings in MI	Usually none; heart disease evaluation
Complete RBBB	No axis deviation, wide QRS	PE, ischemia, cardiac surgery, chest trauma, cor pulmonale	Usually none, unless other pathology present

↑ = increase.

Table 4-3 Premature Contractions

Type	ECG Findings	Causes/Associations
Premature atrial contraction (PAC)	P waves appear different from normal sinus P waves	Infection, inflammation, ischemia; tobacco, alcohol, caffeine; drug toxicity; ↑ catecholamines; electrolyte imbalance
Premature junctional contraction (PJC)	Premature normal QRS with inverted P wave	Similar to PAC
Premature ventricular contraction (PVC)	Widened/blurred QRS; T wave opposite polarity	Electrolyte imbalance, heart disease, ↑ thyroid; uncertain association with SCD

symptomatic patients. The correction of underlying abnormalities (drug toxicity, electrolyte imbalance, hyperthyroid) is often curative.

Premature ventricular complexes typically require no therapy. However, frequent or complex PVCs in the presence of cardiac disease are markers of an increased risk of SCD. Symptomatic patients requiring treatment are best treated with β-blockers (class II) (Table 4-4) because class I and III drugs appear to worsen the arrhythmias in 5%–20% of patients.

Tachyarrhythmia

Tachyarrhythmia is defined as a heart rate in excess of 100 bpm. Tachycardias are distinguished as being supraventricular or ventricular, depending on the mechanism and site of origin. *Narrow complex tachycardias* are almost exclusively supraventricular in origin; *wide complex tachycardias* may be either supraventricular or ventricular in origin. Correct identification of the origin and mechanisms of the tachycardia is critical to selecting appropriate treatment. The patient with a supraventricular tachycardia (Table 4-5) often describes palpitations and in some cases may be syncopal. Symptoms often correlate with a higher ventricular rate. The category of supraventricular tachycardias includes paroxysmal atrial tachycardia, AV junctional tachycardia, atrial flutter, and atrial fibrillation. The exact site of the pacing focus may be difficult to determine when the heart rate is

Table 4-4 **Vaughan Williams Classification of Antiarrhythmic Drugs**

Class	Drugs	Mechanism of Action	Indications for Use
Class Ia	Disopyramide, procainamide, quinidine	Sodium channel blockers slow conduction velocity, prolong APD	SVT and VT prevent ventricular fibrillation; symptomatic PVCs
Class Ib	Lidocaine, mexilitine, phenytoin, tocainide	Shorten APD, no effect on conduction velocity	VT, symptomatic PVCs, prevent VF
Class Ic	Flecanide, propafenone, moricizine	Slow conduction velocity, may mildly prolong APD	Refractory SVT, VT, or VF
Class II	Esmalol, metoprolol, propranolol	β-blockers block β-adrenergic receptors	SVT, prevent VF
Class III	Amiodarone, sotalol, dofetilide, ibutilide, azimilide, N-acetyl procainamide	Prolong APD, no effect on conduction	Amiodarone: VT, VF, SVT, AF Sotalol: VT, AF Dofetilide/ ibutilide: AF, atrial flutter
Class IV	Verapamil, diltiazem	Nondihydropyridine slow calcium channel blockers	SVT

AF = atrial fibrillation, APD = action potential duration, PVC = premature ventricular contraction, SVT = supraventricular tachycardia, VF = ventricular fibrillation, VT = ventricular tachycardia.

Modified from Arnsdorf MF, Makielski JC. Myocardial action potential and action of antiarrhythmic drugs. In: *UpToDate,* Basow DS (ed), Waltham, MA. Available at www.uptodate.com. Accessed 2008.

Table 4-5 Supraventricular Tachyarrhythmias: Heart Rate >100 bpm

Arrhythmia	ECG Findings	Causes/Associations	Treatment
Sinus tachycardia	>100 bpm, normal P and QRS	↑ sympathetic tone, ↓ vagal tone, ↑ catecholamines, pain, hypovolemia, MI, PE, hypoxemia	Treat underlying cause; β-blockers if needed
Paroxysmal supra-ventricular tachycardia	>140 bpm, regular, P waves abnormal, QRS normal or narrow	Emotional stress, cardiac or lung disease, caffeine, drugs, alcohol, thyrotoxicosis	Valsalva maneuvers, carotid sinus massage, IV adenosine, verapamil, digoxin or β-blockers; occasionally, cardioversion
AV junctional tachycardia	60–130 bpm, P waves dissociated from QRS or inverted, QRS normal or wide	Ischemia, postop; myocarditis, digoxin toxicity	Treat underlying cause, IV lidocaine, β-blockers; AV overdrive pacing if unstable
Wolff-Parkinson-White	Wide, slurred QRS with upsloping delta wave; can resemble VT	Ventricular preexcitation via accessory pathway	Ablation of accessory pathway; class Ia, Ic, or III antiarrhythmic drugs; anticoagulation
Atrial flutter	Atrial rate 200–380; slower ventricular rate, "sawtooth" flutter waves	MI, ↑ thyroid, mitral stenosis, lung disease	β-Blockers, calcium channel blockers, digoxin, electrical cardioversion, ibutilide if recent onset; anticoagulation if chronic
Atrial fibrillation	Atrial rate 300–600; irregular waves, pulse; "irregularly irregular" ventricular rate	Similar to flutter; age (10% of patients over 80 have AF)	Rate control with β-blockers or calcium channel blockers; anticoagulation: warfarin; cardioversion drug or electrical; catheter ablation/MAZE surgery

↑ = increase, ↓ = decrease.

very rapid. The prognosis for supraventricular tachycardias is usually better than that associated with ventricular tachycardia. Supraventricular tachycardias may be paroxysmal or chronic, as with chronic atrial fibrillation. Causes include emotional stress, caffeine, alcohol, drugs, thyrotoxicosis, lung disease, and cardiac disease.

Special considerations: atrial fibrillation

Atrial fibrillation is caused by multiple simultaneous wavelets occurring in both the right and the left atria, resulting in a chaotic electrical rhythm with ineffective atrial contraction.

Cardiac output can be reduced markedly when the ventricular rate is very rapid, possibly resulting in CHF. Atrial thrombi may accumulate from stagnation of blood in the atrial appendages. These thrombi may embolize to the lungs, brain, or other organs. Anticoagulation is indicated for patients with chronic atrial fibrillation and chronic atrial flutter associated with valvular disease, cardiomyopathy, or cardiomegaly and before conversion to sinus rhythm is attempted. Several risk stratification tools have been devised to weigh the risk of embolism versus bleeding in these patients. For example, the CHADS2 measure, which estimates the risk of stroke, considers factors such as age, diabetes, CHF, hypertension, and previous stroke or embolic events to determine the optimal anticoagulation approach for each patient.

Conversion of atrial fibrillation can be attempted with quinidine, procainamide, ibutilide, or DC (direct-current) cardioversion. In many patients with chronic atrial fibrillation, maintenance therapy is directed toward controlling the ventricular rate, which can usually be accomplished with digoxin, verapamil, or β-blockers.

Other curative approaches have been developed for both atrial fibrillation and atrial flutter. These treatments include radiofrequency catheter ablation and the surgical Maze procedure. The Maze procedure interrupts all possible reentry circuits to the atrium with multiple incisions. A single uninterrupted pathway is left intact to allow normal conduction from the SA node to the AV node. Of the 178 patients who underwent the Maze procedure, 93% were free of arrhythmia; the rest were converted to sinus rhythm with medical therapy.

Calkins H, Brugada J, Packer DL, et al. HRS/EHRA/ECAS expert Consensus Statement on catheter and surgical ablation of atrial fibrillation: recommendations for personnel, policy, procedures and follow-up. A report of the Heart Rhythm Society (HRS) Task Force on catheter and surgical ablation of atrial fibrillation. *Heart Rhythm*. 2007;4(6):816–861.

Ventricular tachyarrhythmias

Ventricular tachycardia   The ventricular tachyarrhythmias include ventricular tachycardia (VT), torsade de pointes (a variant of VT), ventricular flutter, and ventricular fibrillation; they are summarized in Table 4-6. These arrhythmias may present with palpitations, heart failure, or syncope or may progress rapidly to SCD. VT occurs infrequently in young patients with no organic heart disease. Brief episodes of VT cause palpitations; prolonged attacks in patients with organic cardiac disease can lead to heart failure or cardiac shock. If the rate is not very high and there is no significant underlying heart disease, VT may be well tolerated; however, it may degenerate into ventricular fibrillation, resulting in hemodynamic collapse and death.

Treatment with immediate synchronized DC cardioversion is indicated for sustained VT associated with hemodynamic compromise, severe CHF, or ongoing ischemia or infarction. Pharmacologic cardioversion with IV procainamide or lidocaine and amiodarone may be attempted in patients with clinically stable VT. Amiodarone is probably the agent of choice for recurrent VT if its side effects are tolerated.

Electrophysiologic testing is often performed on patients with suspected or documented ventricular arrhythmias. In this procedure, direct transcatheter electrical stimulation of various sites in the ventricle induces arrhythmias. Given the efficacy and low risk

Table 4-6 Ventricular Tachycardias

Arrhythmia	ECG findings	Causes/Associations	Treatment
Ventricular tachycardia	Wide QRS, 100–250 bpm, 3 or more consecutive abnormal complexes for diagnosis	↓ potassium, ↓ magnesium, CAD, acute MI, cardiomyopathy; digoxin, quinidine, other drugs	*Stable:* lidocaine, procainamide, amiodarone *Unstable:* cardioversion *Recurrent:* amiodarone; if chronic or with structural heart disease, implantable defibrillator
Torsades de pointes	QRS amplitude and morphology changes, prolonged QT interval	Similar to above, plus antiarrhythmic drugs, phenothiazines, tricyclic antidepressants, antihistamines	Treat underlying cause; β-blockers, magnesium sulfate, overdrive pacing or cardioversion; do *not* use class Ia, Ic, or III antiarrhythmic drugs
Ventricular flutter	300 bpm, monomorphic "sine wave" appearance to QRS	CAD, hypoxia, antiarrhythmic drugs, attempts to convert other rhythms	Immediate DC cardioversion; consider implantable defibrillator
Ventricular fibrillation	250–400 bpm; rapid, uncoordinated ventricular contractions, highly variable QRS	MI, complete heart block, electrocution, anesthesia, digoxin, quinidine, antiarrhythmic drugs	Immediate DC cardioversion; consider defibrillator (ICD), amiodarone, sotalol

CAD = coronary artery disease, DC = direct current, ICD = implantable cardioverter-defibrillator, MI = myocardial infarction, ↓ = decrease.

associated with implantation, ICD therapy (in conjunction with antiarrhythmic drugs) has become the treatment of choice for patients with life-threatening ventricular arrhythmias. Less common therapies include ventricular aneurysmectomy, ventricular electrical mapping and resection of the arrhythmogenic focus, and radiofrequency catheter ablation.

Ventricular fibrillation Ventricular fibrillation (VF) is the most ominous of all the cardiac arrhythmias because it is fatal when untreated or when refractory to treatment. It is a major cause of SCD outside the hospital. The ventricular contractions are rapid and uncoordinated, resulting in ineffective ventricular pumping that soon leads to syncope, convulsions, and death if the VF is not interrupted. The prognosis is generally poor because each episode can be fatal.

Cardiopulmonary resuscitation efforts must be initiated emergently. Immediate unsynchronized DC cardioversion is the primary therapy. After successful cardioversion, continuous intravenous infusion of effective antiarrhythmic therapy should be maintained until any reversible causes have been corrected. The choice of chronic antiarrhythmic therapy depends on the conditions responsible for the initial VF episode. Primary VF occurring within the first 72 hours of an acute MI is not associated with an elevated risk of recurrence and does not require chronic antiarrhythmic therapy. However, VF without an identifiable and reversible cause requires chronic therapy in the form of either prophylactic antiarrhythmic drug therapy (eg, amiodarone, sotalol) or implantation of an automatic defibrillator.

Implantable cardioverter-defibrillators ICDs monitor the heart rhythm and, when a tachyarrhythmia is identified, deliver therapy. Their evolution has been impressive. Initially, a thoracotomy was necessary to implant an epicardial patch or patches. The overwhelming majority of patients receive a transvenous system, which significantly reduces the morbidity and mortality associated with the implantation of these devices. Current-generation ICDs are generally implanted in the prepectoral region (similar to pacemaker implantation). Although first-generation ICDs delivered only high-energy "defibrillating" shocks, current-generation devices provide tiered therapy, including antitachycardia-pacing algorithms, low-energy cardioversion for stable VT, high-energy cardioversion for VT or VF, single-chamber or dual-chamber bradycardic-pacing support, and stored diagnostic information for rhythm discrimination.

ICDs treat arrhythmias when they occur and do not prevent them. Most patients require concomitant antiarrhythmic therapy to reduce the frequency of device discharges or facilitate antitachycardia pacing by slowing the tachycardia rate. The development of an effective and safe antiarrhythmic prescription may be complex and requires the skills of a trained electrophysiologist. Generally, the acute management of life-threatening ventricular arrhythmias in these patients does not differ from that of other patients with similar rhythm disturbances. If the device fails to terminate an arrhythmia, cardiopulmonary resuscitation and external defibrillation should proceed normally. Three randomized prospective studies have demonstrated that automated ICDs are the preferred first-line therapy for patients who have survived a cardiac arrest or an episode of hemodynamically unstable VT. At 2-year follow-up, the automated ICD was associated with a 20%–30% relative reduction in the risk of death. The MUSTT and MADIT trials have also proven the benefit of ICDs used for primary prevention of sudden death in patients with CAD, reduced EFs, nonsustained VT, and inducible ventricular arrhythmias during electrophysiologic testing. Following an MI, ICDs appear to be the best available therapy for preventing SCD. An ICD should be considered for patients on optimal medical therapy, with left ventricular dysfunction from an MI at least 40 days previously and with an expected survival with a good functional status of at least 1 year. Ongoing trials may expand the role of ICDs in the primary prevention of sudden death.

Arnsdorf MF, Makielski JC. Myocardial action potential and action of antiarrhythmic drugs. In: *UpToDate*, Basow DS (ed), Waltham, MA. Available at www.uptodate.com. Accessed 2008.

Bashore TM, Granger CB, Hranitzky P, Patel MR. Heart disease. In: *Current Medical Diagnosis and Treatment 2009*. Lange Current Series. McPhee SJ, Papadakis MA (eds). 48th ed. New York: McGraw-Hill; 2009.

Epstein AE, DiMarco JP, Ellenbogen KA, et al. ACC/AHA/HRS 2008 guidelines for device-based therapy of cardiac rhythm abnormalities. *J Am Coll Cardiol*. 2008;51(21):e1–e62.

◉ **Ophthalmic considerations**   Many of the adult patients seen and treated by ophthalmologists are in the age group at risk for IHD and its many complications. These patients often undergo stressful eye surgery under local or general anesthesia, and ophthalmologists need to be cognizant of their risks of myocardial ischemia, MI, CHF, and arrhythmias. Similarly, ophthalmologists need to be aware of the association between proliferative diabetic retinopathy and IHD. This information should be given to the patient's primary medical care provider so that appropriate screening tests can be considered.

Cardiac complications of noncardiac surgery are a major cause of perioperative morbidity and mortality, with MI the most significant. Older age, preexisting CAD, and CHF are the principal risk factors for development of these complications.

Finally, ophthalmologists should be aware of the potential ocular side effects associated with medications commonly used in treating CVD. Following are the medications of clinical relevance:

- *Amiodarone.* Corneal microdeposits due to amiodarone probably occur in nearly all patients who use this drug for a long time. The corneal epithelial whorl-like deposition is indistinguishable from that due to chloroquine. Visual changes are unusual and most often consist of complaints of hazy vision or colored halos around lights. Occasionally, a patient may complain that bright lights, especially headlights at night, cause a significant glare problem. A side effect that has been seen secondary to photosensitivity reactions is discoloration (usually slate gray or blue) of periocular skin. A rare adverse effect is amiodarone optic neuropathy, which is characterized by an insidious onset, slow progression, bilateral visual loss, and protracted disc swelling that tends to stabilize within several months of discontinuing the medication. Patients on chronic amiodarone therapy should have a baseline ophthalmic examination, follow-up examinations every 6–12 months, and immediate evaluation of any new visual disturbances. Due to this drug's photosensitizing effects, UV-blocking spectacle lenses should be considered in selected cases of chronic lid disease or macular disease.
- *β-Blockers.* As with other β-adrenergic blocking agents, there is the possibility of a keratoconjunctivitis sicca–like syndrome with use of β-blockers, probably due to decreased lacrimation. Not all the listed possible ocular side effects have been reported with each agent; however, in general, these drugs may decrease tear secretion, possibly enhance migraine ocular scotomata, and may decrease IOP. Topical β-blockers, particularly timolol, may be less effective in lowering IOP in patients on systemic β-blockers. Visual disturbances and vivid visual hallucinations may also be associated with the systemic use of β-blockers.
- *Digoxin.* The glare phenomenon and disturbances of color vision are the most striking and the most common adverse ocular reactions

seen. These ocular side effects include decreased vision and problems with color vision, such as blue-yellow pattern defects; a yellow, green, blue, or red tinge to objects; and colored halos (mainly blue) around lights. Patients on digoxin may also describe yellow or green flickering vision, colored borders around objects, glare phenomena, light flashes, scintillating scotomata, a frosted appearance to objects, and formed visual hallucinations.

- *Angiotensin-converting enzyme inhibitors.* ACE inhibitors may cause angioedema involving the eye and orbit. The presumed mechanism is the disruption of bradykinin metabolism.

American Academy of Ophthalmology. www.aao.org.

American College of Cardiology. www.acc.org.

American Heart Association. www.americanheart.org.

Johnson LN, Krohel GB, Thomas ER. The clinical spectrum of amiodarone-associated optic neuropathy. *J Natl Med Assoc.* 2004;96(11):1477–1491.

Rosenman RH, Maser JD. Bizarre images and beta-adrenergic blocking agents: A unique case report. *J Psychoactive Drugs.* 1999;31(2):163–166.

Shaikh S, Shaikh N, Chun SH, Spin JM, Blumenkranz MS, Marmor MF. Retinal evaluation of patients on chronic amiodarone therapy. *Retina.* 2003;23(3):354–359.

UpToDate. www.uptodate.com.

CHAPTER 5

Hypercholesterolemia

Recent Developments

- Therapeutic lifestyle changes (TLC) remain an essential modality in the management of hypercholesterolemia.
- More aggressive management of cholesterol and risk factors has been emphasized by the US National Cholesterol Education Program (NCEP; www.nhlbi.nih.gov/about/ncep/index.htm).
- Numerous clinical trials have demonstrated that effective low-density-lipoprotein cholesterol (LDL-C) reduction substantially reduces the risk of coronary heart disease (CHD). For every 30-mg/dL change in LDL-C, the CHD risk is changed by 30%. An LDL-C goal of less than 70 mg/dL should be considered for very high risk patients.
- Statin therapy is recommended for the majority of dyslipoproteinemic adult patients with cardiometabolic risk (CMR).
- Apolipoprotein B (Apo-B) and non–high-density-lipoprotein cholesterol (non–HDL-C) levels should be used to guide adjustments of therapy for patients with CMR already on statin therapy.
- Use of statins in acute coronary syndromes reduces the risk of recurrent coronary events.
- Lipid-lowering therapy should be encouraged for elderly patients; they will derive equal or greater benefit compared with younger patients.

Introduction

Coronary heart disease is the leading cause of death in the United States, accounting for more deaths than all forms of cancer combined. Several major studies have confirmed earlier reports that lowering elevated LDL-C levels reduces the risk of CHD. The NCEP has provided 3 updates for treating elevated blood cholesterol levels in adults (Adult Treatment Panel [ATP] I, II, III). ATP I proposed a strategy for primary prevention of CHD in persons with high levels of LDL-C (>160 mg/dL) or borderline high levels of LDL-C (130–159 mg/dL) and multiple (at least 2) risk factors (discussed later in the chapter). ATP II added intensive management of LDL-C in persons with established CHD (target cholesterol <100 mg/dL). Table 5-1 lists the guidelines of ATP III, updated through 2004.

Table 5-1 Adult Treatment Panel III Classification of Total, LDL, and HDL Cholesterol and Triglycerides, mg/dL

Total cholesterol	
<200	Desirable
200–239	Borderline high
≥240	High
LDL cholesterol	
<100	Optimal
100–129	Near or above optimal
130–159	Borderline high
160–189	High
≥190	Very high
HDL cholesterol	
<40	Low: a major risk factor for heart disease
40–59	Borderline high: the higher the better
≥60	High: protective against heart disease
Triglycerides	
<150	Normal
150–199	Borderline high
200–499	High
≥500	Very high

Modified from Executive Summary of the Third Report of the National Cholesterol Education Program (NCEP) Expert Panel on Detection, Evaluation, and Treatment of High Blood Cholesterol in Adults (Adult Treatment Panel III). *JAMA.* 2001;285(19):2486–2497.

Lipoproteins, Cholesterol, and Cardiovascular Disease

Cholesterol and triglycerides are transported in the body by *lipoproteins.* The various classes of lipoprotein differ in the relative concentrations of their components: cholesterol, triglycerides, phospholipids, and proteins *(apolipoproteins).* Chylomicrons carry triglycerides following dietary lipid absorption, whereas *very-low-density lipoproteins (VLDLs)* produced by the liver carry most circulating triglycerides. LDL, or "bad cholesterol," originates from VLDL metabolism and is the primary carrier of cholesterol. HDL, or "good cholesterol," is the smallest and densest lipoprotein category. The result of the inflammatory interaction among these lipoproteins, macrophages, and the cellular components of the arterial wall is *atherosclerosis.* Although it is cholesterol levels that are typically measured, it is the lipoproteins that interact with the arterial wall, producing plaques. The narrowing of the arterial lumen by these plaques or the rupture of a plaque with subsequent thrombosis leads to stroke and cardiovascular disease (CVD), including myocardial infarction (MI) and peripheral vascular disease.

Risk Assessment

The cholesterol level of approximately half the US population puts these persons at significant risk. A fasting lipoprotein profile (total cholesterol, LDL-C, HDL-C, and triglyceride levels) determines an individual's risk status and should be obtained in all adults aged 21 and older at least once every 5 years. Typically, the LDL-C concentration is not measured directly but instead is estimated by the *Friedewald formula*:

LDL cholesterol = total cholesterol − VLDL cholesterol − HDL cholesterol

where the VLDL is assumed to be one fifth of total triglycerides. This formula is not valid if the triglyceride total exceeds 400 mg/dL. Although some assays measure LDL directly, they are generally unnecessary, and all recommendations are based on the estimated value approach. Table 5-1 shows the ATP III classification of cholesterol levels and triglycerides. According to American Heart Association (AHA) guidelines, the HDL ratio (ratio of total serum cholesterol to HDL-C) should be less than 5. Other CHD risk factors, such as hypertension, should be assessed and managed appropriately in all adults (Table 5-2).

Experimental studies directly support the central role of LDL in atherogenesis, and reduction of LDL-C levels is associated with a reduction in CVD risk. Conversely, HDL-C appears protective against atherosclerosis due to its anti-inflammatory properties and ability to transport cholesterol from vessel walls to the liver for disposal. In general, current guidelines recommend a high HDL and low LDL concentration to decrease CVD risk.

Once LDL-C goals have been reached, some residual CVD risk remains. Some authors have suggested that directly measuring Apo-B, an apoprotein found in all of the most atherogenic molecules, may be superior to other measures in assessing residual risk and directing subsequent treatment. In such an approach, reducing LDL levels would represent the primary goal of treatment, followed by reducing Apo-B levels to further decrease risk.

Table 5-2 Risk Factor Modification Treatment Goals

Risk Factor	Goal	Intervention
Blood pressure	BP <140/90 mm Hg BP <130/80 mm Hg with chronic kidney disease or diabetes	Weight control, increased physical activity, alcohol moderation, sodium reduction, medications
Smoking	Smoking cessation Avoid environmental tobacco smoke	Smoking cessation programs, nicotine replacement, bupropion, verenicline
Lipid management	LDL-C <100 mg/dL (optional goal <70 mg/dL if high CAD risk) Non–HDL-C ≤130 mg/dL	Diet low in saturated fat, weight control, increased physical activity, statins, niacin, fibrates
Diabetes mellitus	HbA$_{1c}$ <7%	Diet, weight control, oral hypoglycemic agents, insulin
Physical activity	30 minutes, 7 days/week Minimum 5 days/week	Walking, biking, swimming, gardening, household work
Weight management	BMI 18.5–24.9 kg/m^2 Waist circumference: ≤40 inches men; ≤35 inches women	Physical activity, caloric intake, behavioral programs, rimonabant

BMI = body mass index, BP = blood pressure, CAD = coronary artery disease, HDL-C = high-density-lipoprotein cholesterol, LDL-C = low-density-lipoprotein cholesterol.

From American College of Cardiology Foundation et al. ACCF/SCAI/SVMB/SIR/A SITN 2007 clinical expert consensus document on carotid stenting. *J Am Coll Cardiol*. 2007;49(1):126–170.

Management

In its simplest terms, the management of hypercholesterolemia consists of matching the intensity of LDL-lowering therapy with absolute risk: the higher the risk, the lower the target level. This approach is based primarily on data from recent clinical trials and epidemiologic studies, which have suggested that a direct relationship exists between the level of LDL-C and the risk of CHD. The ATP III guidelines suggest measuring fasting lipoprotein levels in patients with hypercholesterolemia/hyperlipidemia/hyperlipoproteinemia. The clinician should also assess the presence of other risk factors (see Table 5-2) and the presence of clinical atherosclerotic disease, including clinical cardiovascular disease, carotid or peripheral artery disease, or abdominal aortic aneurysm. The patient's 10-year risk for CVD is determined based on these factors on a scale from lower risk to high risk. LDL treatment goals are determined based on this risk level (Table 5-3).

Therapeutic lifestyle changes, including dietary modifications (Table 5-4), weight management, and increased physical activity, should be initiated. Typical steps are illustrated in Figure 5-1. If LDL goals are not achieved by TLC alone, drug therapy should be introduced and advanced, as illustrated in Figure 5-2. Specific drugs, doses, and side effects are presented in Table 5-5.

Once the LDL treatment goals have been reached, other lipid and nonlipid risk factors may be modified. Elevated triglycerides (see Table 5-1) may respond to increased physical activity or weight management but if the triglycerides are ≥200 mg/dL after the LDL goal is reached, a secondary goal of treatment would be for a non–HDL-C (total – HDL) level of 30 mg/dL higher than the LDL goal.

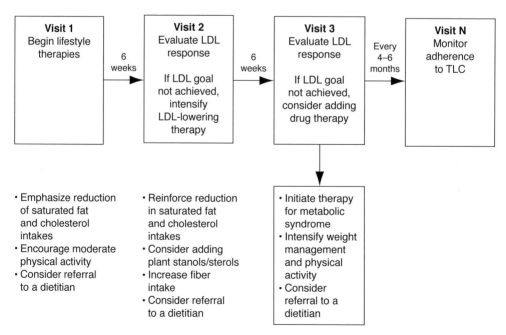

Figure 5-1 Model of steps in therapeutic lifestyle changes (TLC). *LDL* = low-density lipoprotein. *(From Executive summary of the third report of the National Cholesterol Education Program (NCEP) Expert Panel on Detection, Evaluation, and Treatment of High Blood Cholesterol in Adults (Adult Treatment Panel III). JAMA. 2001;285(19):2491.)*

Table 5-3 ATP III LDL-C Goals and Cutpoints for TLC and Drug Therapy in Different Risk Categories and Proposed Modifications Based on Recent Clinical Trial Evidence

Risk Category	LDL-C Goal	Initiate TLC	Consider Drug Therapy
High risk: CHD* or CHD risk equivalents† (10-year risk >20%)	<100 mg/dL (optional goal: <70 mg/dL)	≥100 mg/dL	≥100 mg/dL (<100 mg/dL: consider drug options)
Moderately high risk: 2+ risk factors‡ (10-year risk 10% to 20%)	<130 mg/dL	≥130 mg/dL	≥130 mg/dL (100–129 mg/dL: consider drug options)
Moderate risk: 2+ risk factors‡ (10-year risk <10%)	<130 mg/dL	≥130 mg/dL	≥160 mg/dL
Lower risk: 0–1 risk factor	<160 mg/dL	≥160 mg/dL	≥190 mg/dL (160–189 mg/dL: LDL-lowering drug optional)

*CHD includes history of myocardial infarction, unstable angina, stable angina, coronary artery procedures (angioplasty or bypass surgery), or evidence of clinically significant myocardial ischemia.

†CHD risk equivalents include clinical manifestations of noncoronary forms of atherosclerotic disease (peripheral arterial disease, abdominal aortic aneurysm, and carotid artery disease [transient ischemic attacks or stroke of carotid origin or >50% obstruction of a carotid artery]), diabetes, and 2+ risk factors with 10-year risk for hard CHD >20%.

‡Risk factors include cigarette smoking, hypertension (BP ≥140/90 mm Hg or on antihypertensive medication), low HDL-C (<40 mg/dL), family history of premature CHD (CHD in male first-degree relative <55 years of age; CHD in female first-degree relative <65 years of age), and age (men ≥45 years; women ≥55 years).

Modified from Grundy SM, Cleeman JI, Merz N, et al. Implications of recent clinical trials for the National Cholesterol Education Program Adult Treatment Panel III guidelines. *Am Coll Cardiol.* 2004;44(3):720–732.

Table 5-4 Nutrient Composition of the Therapeutic Lifestyle Changes Diet

Nutrient	Recommended Intake
Saturated fat*	<7% of total calories
Polyunsaturated fat	Up to 10% of total calories
Monounsaturated fat	Up to 20% of total calories
Total fat	25%–35% of total calories
Carbohydrate†	50%–60% of total calories
Fiber	20–30 g/d (soluble fiber 10–25 g/d)
Plant stanols/sterols‡	2 g/d
Protein	Approximately 15% of total calories
Cholesterol	<200 mg/dL
Total calories§	Balance energy intake and expenditure to maintain desirable body weight/prevent weight gain

*Trans fatty acids are another LDL-raising fat that should be kept at a low intake.

†Carbohydrates should be derived predominantly from foods rich in complex carbohydrates, including grains (especially whole grains), fruits, and vegetables.

‡Sitostanol/sterol esters inhibit intestinal absorption of dietary and biliary cholesterol and are available in grocery stores as regular and low-fat margarines.

§Daily energy expenditure should include at least moderate physical activity (contributing approximately 200 kcal/d).

Modified from Executive Summary of the Third Report of the National Cholesterol Education Program (NCEP) Expert Panel on Detection, Evaluation, and Treatment of High Blood Cholesterol in Adults (Adult Treatment Panel III). *JAMA.* 2001;285(19):2486–2497.

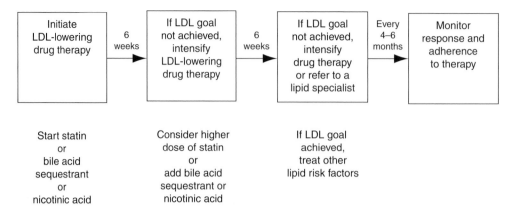

Figure 5-2 Progression of drug therapy in primary prevention. *LDL* = low-density lipoprotein. *(From Executive summary of the third report of the National Cholesterol Education Program (NCEP) Expert Panel on Detection, Evaluation, and Treatment of High Blood Cholesterol in Adults (Adult Treatment Panel III). JAMA. 2001;285(19):2492.)*

Brunzell JD, Davidson M, Furberg CD, et al. Lipoprotein management in patients with cardio-metabolic risk: consensus conference report from the American Diabetes Association and the American College of Cardiology Foundation. *J Am Coll Cardiol.* 2008;51(15):1512–1524.

Fletcher B, Berra K, Ades P, et al. Managing abnormal blood lipids: a collaborative approach. *Circulation.* 2005;112(20):3184–3209.

Rosenson RS. Overview of treatment of hypercholesterolemia. In: *UpToDate,* Basow DS (ed), Waltham, MA. Available at www.uptodate.com. Accessed 2008.

Special Issues

The Role of Statins

Statins are the first choice for medical therapy in virtually all patients whose LDL goals cannot be achieved by TLC alone. Multiple trials involving the use of statins have reinforced the value of LDL-lowering therapy in reducing CMR. Moreover, the statins are the only class of drugs to demonstrate improvement in overall mortality in primary and secondary prevention. In the Heart Protection Study (HPS), treatment with simvastatin reduced the risk of major vascular events in high-risk patients by 24%. The Myocardial Ischemia Reduction with Acute Cholesterol Lowering (MIRACL) study found that lowering lipids with atorvastatin, 80 mg/day, reduced the number of recurrent ischemic events in patients with acute coronary syndrome (ACS) in the first 16 weeks. Results from the PROVE IT study suggest that more intensive LDL-C–lowering therapy reduces the risk of major cardiovascular events in patients with the ACS, compared with less intensive treatment over the first 2 years.

Recent findings from the JUPITER trial suggest that statins, which are known to lower C-reactive protein (CRP) levels, in addition to their effects on hyperlipidemia, may decrease the risk of stroke, coronary artery disease (CAD), and death in apparently healthy persons without hyperlipidemia but with a CRP level >2.0 mg/L. The full implications of this study, which would dramatically increase the use of statins, are yet to be elucidated.

Table 5-5 Drugs Affecting Lipoprotein Metabolism

Drug Class	Agents and Daily Doses	Lipid/Lipoprotein Effects	Side Effects	Contraindications	Clinical Trial Results
HMG-CoA reductase inhibitors	Lovastatin (20–80 mg) Pravastatin (20–40 mg) Simvastatin (20–80 mg) Fluvastatin (20–80 mg) Atorvastatin (10–80 mg) Rosuvastatin (5–40 mg)	LDL ↓ 18%–55% HDL ↑ 5%–15% TG ↓ 7%–30%	Myopathy; increased liver enzymes	*Absolute*: active or chronic liver disease *Relative*: concomitant use of certain drugs*	Reduced major coronary events, CHD deaths, need for coronary procedures, stroke, and total mortality
Bile acid sequestrants	Cholestyramine (4–16 g) Colestipol (5–20 g) Colesevelam (2.6–3.8 g)	LDL ↓ 15%–30% HDL ↑ 3%–5% TG no change or increase	Gastrointestinal distress; constipation; decreased absorption of other drugs	*Absolute*: dysbetalipoproteinemia; TG >400 mg/dL *Relative*: TG >200 mg/dL	Reduced major coronary events, CHD deaths
Nicotinic acid	Immediate release (crystalline) nicotinic acid (1.5–3 g); extended-release nicotinic acid (Niaspan) (1–2 g); sustained-release nicotinic acid (1–2 g)	LDL ↓ 5%–25% HDL ↑ 15%–35% TG ↓ 20%–50%	Flushing; hyperglycemia; hyperuricemia (or gout); upper gastrointestinal distress; hepatotoxicity	*Absolute*: chronic liver disease; severe gout *Relative*: diabetes; hyperuricemia; peptic ulcer disease	Reduced major coronary events and possible total mortality
Fibric acids	Gemfibrozil (600 mg BID) Fenofibrate (200 mg) Clofibrate (1000 mg BID)	LDL ↓ 5%–20% (may be increased in patients with high TG) HDL ↑ 10%–20% TG ↓ 20%–50%	Dyspepsia; gallstones; myopathy; unexplained non-CHD deaths in WHO study	*Absolute*: severe renal disease; severe hepatic disease	Reduced major coronary events

CHD = coronary heart disease, HDL = high-density lipoprotein, HMG-CoA = 3-hydroxy-3-methylglutaryl coenzyme A, LDL = low-density lipoprotein, TG = triglycerides, ↓ = decrease, ↑ = increase.

*Cyclosporine, macrolide antibiotics, various antifungal agents, and cytochrome P-450 inhibitors (fibrates and niacin should be used with appropriate caution).

Modified from Executive Summary of the Third Report of the National Cholesterol Education Program (NCEP) Expert Panel on Detection, Evaluation, and Treatment of High Blood Cholesterol in Adults (Adult Treatment Panel III). *JAMA.* 2001;285(19):2486–2497.

Side effects of statin use are rare but can include elevated hepatic transaminases, diarrhea, liver failure, polyneuropathy, and myopathy. Simvastatin should not be started at or increased to a dose of 80 mg per day because of the high risk of muscle injury. The risk of myopathy is also increased when simvastatin is used in conjunction with other medications, including amiodarone and some calcium channel blockers. Cerivastatin (Baycol) was voluntarily withdrawn from the market after more than 30 reports of rhabdomyolysis and death related to this statin. Although these drugs are largely safe and effective, these serious side effects must be carefully monitored, especially in the first few months of treatment.

Ridker PM, Danielson E, Fonseca FA, et al; JUPITER Study Group. Rosuvastatin to prevent vascular events in men and women with elevated C-reactive protein. N Engl J Med. 2008;359(21):2195–2207.

Rouleau J. Improved outcome after acute coronary syndromes with an intensive versus standard lipid-lowering regimen: results from the Provastatin or Atorvastatin Evaluation and Infection Therapy-Thrombolysis in Myocardial Infarction 22 (PROVE IT-TIMI 22) trial. Am J Med. 2005;118(Suppl 12A):28–35.

Waters D, Schwartz GG, Olsson AG. The Myocardial Ischemia Reduction With Acute Cholesterol Lowering (MIRACL) trial: a new frontier for statins? Curr Control Trials Cardiovasc Med. 2001;2(3):111–114.

The Metabolic Syndrome

The metabolic syndrome comprises a constellation of lipid and nonlipid risk factors of metabolic origin. Diagnosis is based on the presence of 3 or more of the following risk determinants: increased abdominal obesity as measured by waist circumference (men: >102 cm, women: >88 cm), blood pressure ≥130/85 mm Hg, a fasting glucose ≥110 mg/dL, elevated triglycerides (≥150 mg/dL), and decreased HDL (men: <40 mg/dL, women: <50 mg/dL).

The metabolic syndrome is closely linked to insulin resistance. Excess body fat (particularly abdominal fat) and physical inactivity promote impaired responses to insulin, which may also occur as a genetic predisposition. The risk factors for metabolic syndrome are highly concordant; in aggregate, they increase the risk of CHD at any given LDL level. Management of the metabolic syndrome includes measures previously discussed for elevated LDL and triglycerides, as well as treatment of hypertension and the use of aspirin for CHD patients to reduce the prothrombotic state.

Grundy SM, Cleeman JI, Daniels SR, et al. Diagnosis and management of the metabolic syndrome. Circulation. 2005;112(17):2735–2752.

◎ **Ophthalmic considerations**   Hypercholesterolemia is a significant risk factor for ischemic heart disease, cerebrovascular disease, and peripheral vascular disease. The ophthalmologist may be the first physician to detect or recognize manifestations of atherosclerosis, particularly amaurosis fugax, retinal vascular emboli or occlusions, ischemic optic neuropathy, or cortical visual field deficits from a previous cerebral infarction. Detection of atherosclerosis may initiate a diagnostic evaluation that reveals significant carotid artery stenosis or CAD.

Patients with ocular hypertension or glaucoma being treated with topical β-blockers have small but significant changes in the serum levels of HDL and LDL when using these drugs. In a 12-week randomized clinical trial of 112 women aged 60 years and older, topical timolol 0.5% increased LDL-C by 3% and decreased HDL-C by 6%. In the same trial, topical carteolol 1% had no impact on LDL levels but increased HDL levels by 2%.

The relationship of statin use to AMD is unresolved. Several population-based studies (ARIC, MELBOURNE) have suggested that the use of statins is associated with a decreased risk of AMD, whereas other studies (Beaver Dam) and an epidemiologic meta-analysis suggest there is no change in AMD risk with statin use. The Blue Mountains Eye Study, a recent population-based study from Australia, and a retrospective case study from San Francisco suggest a decrease in late AMD changes such as indistinct soft drusen or CNV with the use of statins. Other studies have suggested an increase in the risk of developing wet AMD in individuals who smoke or have other cardiac risk factors. All of these studies are limited by either small sample size or lack of prospective data on the use of statins. Therefore, more data are required to assess the nature of this relationship.

The ACCORD Eye Study, a large prospective NEI study to assess the effects of tight control of glycemia, blood pressure, and dyslipidemia on the course of diabetic retinopathy, is now under way.

Corneal arcus, a nonreversible lipid deposit at the corneal limbus, is associated with age and hyperlipidemia. In the Blue Mountains Eye Study, the presence of arcus in persons aged 49 years and older was associated with higher total cholesterol and high triglyceride levels.

Finally, clinical experience has revealed that use of lovastatin and other HMG-CoA reductase inhibitors does not significantly increase the risk of cataracts.

American Academy of Ophthalmology. www.aao.org.

American College of Cardiology. www.acc.org.

American Heart Association. www.americanheart.org.

Chuo JY, Wiens M, Etminan M, Maberley DA. Use of lipid-lowering agents for the prevention of age-related macular degeneration: a meta-analysis of observational studies. *Ophthalmic Epidemiol.* 2007;14(6):367–374.

Hogg RE, Woodside JV, Gilchrist SE, et al. Cardiovascular disease and hypertension are strong risk factors for choroidal neovascularization. *Ophthalmology.* 2008;115(6):1046–1052.

Klein R, Knudtson MD, Klein BE. Statin use and the five-year incidence and progression of age-related macular degeneration. *Am J Ophthalmol.* 2007;144(1):1–6.

Mitchell P, Wang JJ, Cumming RG, House P, England JD. Long-term topical timolol and blood lipids: the Blue Mountains Eye Study. *J Glaucoma.* 2000;9(2):174–178.

Tan JS, Mitchell P, Rochtchina E, Wang JJ. Statins and the long-term risk of incident age-related macular degeneration: the Blue Mountains Eye Study. *Am J Ophthalmol.* 2007;143(4): 685–687.

CHAPTER 6

Pulmonary Diseases

Recent Developments

- Sildenafil (Viagra) has been shown to be effective in patients with pulmonary arterial hypertension.
- People with chronic obstructive pulmonary disease are more likely to develop pneumonia if they use inhaled corticosteroids.

Introduction

The lungs can be affected by numerous pathologic processes, including inflammation (allergic, infectious, autoimmune, occupational exposure, toxic), vascular insults, fibrosis, carcinoma, and changes secondary to cardiac or musculoskeletal problems. The functional consequences of the pathology can be divided into *obstructive* and *restrictive* ventilatory functions.

Symptoms of lung disease include dyspnea, cough, and wheezing. *Dyspnea* develops when the demand for gas exchange exceeds the capacity of the respiratory system, as in hypoxemia or hypercapnia. Dyspnea may also reflect the increased work of breathing as occurs with airway obstruction or reduced compliance of the lungs or chest. *Cough* develops when mucus, inflammatory debris, or irritants stimulate the bronchi, causing reflex clearing expectoration or when the lung parenchyma is infiltrated with fluid, cells, or fibrosis. *Wheezing* occurs when bronchospasm narrows the large airways and exhaled air is forced through narrowed passages.

Obstructive Lung Diseases

In obstructive lung disease, changes in the bronchi, bronchioles, and lung parenchyma can cause airway obstruction. Obstructive diseases can be separated into reversible and irreversible causes, although many obstructive lung diseases may have some degree of both reversible and irreversible obstruction. The Global Initiative for Chronic Obstructive Lung Disease (GOLD) is an international consortium that publishes a guide on the diagnosis, classification, and management of pulmonary disease that is regularly updated and can be downloaded from the Internet (www.goldcopd.com). GOLD offers a framework for the management of chronic obstructive pulmonary disease.

Reversible obstructive diseases are grouped under the term *asthma.* In asthma, the airways are hyperresponsive and develop an inflammatory response to various stimuli, although the specific cause and duration of the bronchospasm vary. In some persons, allergic IgE-mediated reactions to defined antigens cause bronchospasm. In many patients, however, the cause of abnormal airway reactivity is unknown. Precipitating factors may include exercise, aspirin, sulfites, tartrazine dye, emotional stress, cold air, environmental pollutants, or viral infection. Bronchial smooth muscle constriction, mucosal edema, excess mucus accumulation, and epithelial cell shedding all contribute to airway obstruction. This obstruction may be reversible spontaneously or with treatment.

Irreversible obstructive disease (sometimes known as *chronic obstructive pulmonary disease,* [COPD]) comprises a group of conditions in which forced expiratory flow is reduced in either a constant or a slowly progressive manner over months or years. COPD is the fourth leading cause of death in the United States. Some conditions, such as *cystic fibrosis* or *bronchiectasis,* either secondary to recurrent necrotizing bacterial infections or occurring as part of Kartagener syndrome, have an identifiable cause. However, most irreversible obstructive diseases, such as *emphysema, chronic bronchitis,* and *peripheral airway disease,* cannot be ascribed to specific conditions; rather, they represent an individual response to cigarette smoking and other airborne pollutants. For example, such responses occur in the setting of either α_1-antitrypsin deficiency (in certain forms of emphysema) or airway hyperactivity and mucus hypersecretion (as in bronchitis). The pathologic consequences of the abnormal response result in specific damage to lung tissue. Emphysema is characterized by pathologic enlargement of the terminal bronchiole air spaces and by destruction of the alveolar connective tissue septa. Bronchitis is characterized by hypertrophied mucous glands in the bronchi; in peripheral airway disease, only the small airways demonstrate fibrosis, inflammation, and tortuosity.

> The Global Initiative for Chronic Obstructive Lung Disease (GOLD). Global strategy for the diagnosis, management, and prevention of chronic obstructive pulmonary disease. Updated 2008. Available at www.goldcopd.com.

Restrictive Lung Diseases

The restrictive lung diseases encompass a diverse group of conditions that cause diffuse parenchymal damage. The physiologic consequences of this damage include a reduction in total lung volume, diffusing capacity, and vital capacity. Occasionally, patients without parenchymal involvement who have diseases of the chest wall, respiratory muscles, pleura, or spine may have similarly restricted lung volumes. A *fibrotic* parenchymal response can result from occupational exposure to various substances, including asbestos, silica dust, graphite, talc, coal, and tungsten. A *granulomatous* hypersensitivity reaction can develop in response to moldy hay, grains, birds, humidifiers, and cooling systems. Endogenous pulmonary disease can result from collagen vascular diseases, sarcoidosis, eosinophilic granuloma, Wegener granulomatosis, Goodpasture syndrome, alveolar proteinosis, idiopathic pulmonary hemosiderosis, idiopathic pulmonary fibrosis, and other idiopathic parenchymal diseases. Therapeutic agents such as phenytoin (Dilantin), penicillin, gold, methotrexate, and radiation can also cause pulmonary disease.

Evaluation

Although all patients with respiratory problems should be under the care of a capable internist or pulmonologist, ophthalmologists and other physicians should be aware of the methods used to diagnose and evaluate breathing disorders. The following should be considered:

- *Symptoms:* Symptoms include dyspnea, orthopnea, chronic cough, and chronic sputum production.
- *History:* History may reveal occupational exposure, family history, cigarette use.
- *Signs:* Signs include audible wheezing, cyanosis, finger clubbing, forced expiratory time greater than 4 seconds, increased anteroposterior diameter of the chest.
- *Laboratory studies:* Results may reveal elevated hematocrit and hypoxia or hypercapnia on arterial blood gas measurement.
- *Chest radiography:* Radiographic findings include parenchymal disease, hyperinflation, diaphragmatic flattening, increased retrosternal lucency, and pleural abnormalities.
- *Computerized tomography* of the chest can detect many abnormalities not seen on chest radiographs, such as small areas of adenopathy, pulmonary embolus, small nodules, infiltrative lung disease, and bronchiectasis.
- *Bronchoscopy, transbronchial biopsy,* and *bronchial lavage* are used to obtain culture material, cytology material, and pathologic specimens for analysis.
- *Pulmonary function tests* measure the mechanical and gas exchange functions of the lungs. The *forced expiratory volume over 1 second (FEV$_1$)* represents the volume exhaled in the first second of exhalation; the *forced vital capacity* represents the total volume that the patient can exhale. Both parameters and their serial rate of decline in a patient are objective measures of lung function as well as prognostic indicators of comorbidity and mortality from lung cancer and cardiovascular disease. An FEV$_1$/FVC ratio less than 70% of predicted suggests obstructive disease; total lung capacity less than 70% of predicted suggests restrictive disease.

Treatment

Treatment of pulmonary disease has 2 major goals: first, to favorably alter the natural history of the disease; and second, to improve the patient's symptoms and functional status and minimize associated problems.

Nonpharmacologic Treatment

Smoking cessation is the single most efficacious and cost-effective intervention in reducing the risk of COPD and slowing its progression. Ophthalmologists should not underestimate the impact of even a brief discussion about the impact of smoking and the beneficial effects of smoking cessation. Similarly, *avoiding precipitants* of airway obstruction is important in ameliorating asthmatic conditions. In patients with severe pulmonary hypertension and cor pulmonale, use of supplemental oxygen to maintain an arterial oxygen pressure above 60 mm Hg confers a modest reduction in pulmonary hypertension and improved survival. However, a patient receiving supplemental oxygen must be carefully monitored because such treatment may decrease the respiratory drive to eliminate carbon dioxide, aggravating the respiratory acidosis that may lead to carbon dioxide narcosis. *Breathing exercises* and *postoperative chest physiotherapy* have demonstrable short-term effects in improving respiratory function.

Noninvasive pressure support ventilation can be used to deliver increased airway pressure. Continuous positive airway pressure (CPAP) throughout the ventilation cycle improves alveolar oxygen exchange. In CPAP, a tight, well-fitting mask is placed over the patient's mouth and nose or just over the nose. Noninvasive pressure support ventilation is best applied to patients with respiratory failure who are expected to quickly respond to medical therapy. Mask CPAP treatment of cardiogenic pulmonary edema was first described more than 50 years ago and has been shown to be a useful adjunct, reducing the need for intubation. Noninvasive pressure support ventilation for acute respiratory failure requires an alert patient capable of protecting the airway and handling secretions. Intubation and standard ventilation are preferred for patients who require total ventilatory support because the mask may slip and effective ventilation may cease. Nasal CPAP can be used in the management of obstructive sleep apnea. Ophthalmologists should be aware that nasal CPAP has been reported to modestly increase intraocular pressure in patients with glaucoma.

Mojon DS, Hess CW, Goldblum D, et al. Normal-tension glaucoma is associated with sleep apnea syndrome. *Ophthalmologica*. 2002;216(3):180–184.

Phamacologic Treatment

Pharmacologic approaches include medications that are specific for the particular pulmonary condition and medications that improve the patient's symptoms and functional status. *Specific medications* directly alter the pathophysiologic mechanisms underlying pulmonary disease. Some examples include cyclophosphamide for Wegener granulomatosis, corticosteroids for sarcoidosis, and plasmapheresis with immunosuppressive drugs in Goodpasture syndrome.

Symptomatic medications are designed to reduce the obstructive or restrictive components affecting the patient's lung function. Medications used to treat symptomatic bronchospastic airway obstruction include bronchodilators, inhibitors of inflammation, and antibiotics during infection-precipitated airway closure (Table 6-1).

Bronchodilators, which include theophylline, β-adrenergic agonists, and anticholinergics, act primarily by relaxing the tracheobronchial smooth muscle. *β-Adrenergic agonists* activate bronchial smooth muscle resulting in bronchodilation. The selective β_2-adrenergics, which have greater bronchodilatory and less cardiostimulatory effects, are commonly used, often in metered-dose inhalers (they can also be administered orally or parenterally). These drugs have replaced the nonselective β-adrenergic agents such as isoproterenol. The short-acting β_2-agonists include fenoterol, salbutamol, tertbutaline,

Table 6-1 Drugs for the Treatment of Asthma

Short-acting β₂-selective adrenergic agents
  Albuterol (Proventil, Ventolin, AccuNeb, VoSpire ER, ProAir HFA)
  Pirbuterol acetate (Maxair)
Long-acting β₂-selective adrenergic agents
  Formoterol (Perforomist, Foradil Aerolizer)
  Terbutaline sulfate (Aerodur, Alloxygen, Arubendol, Asmaline, Astebron, Asthmasian,
    Asthmo-Kranit Mono, Asthmoprotect, Ataline, Brethaire, Brethine, Bricanyl)
Anticholinergics
  Ipratropium bromide (Atrovent)
  Oxitropium bromide
  Tiotropium (Spiriva)
Xanthine derivatives and combinations
  Theophylline (Aerolate, Marax, Quibron, Respbid, Theo-Dur, Theo-Time, TheoCap,
    Theochron, Uniphyl)
Combination short-acting β₂-agonist plus anitcholinergic in 1 inhaler
  Fenoterol/Ipratropium (Respimat)
  Albuterol/Ipratropium (Combivent)
Combination long-acting β₂-agonist plus corticosteroid in 1 inhaler
  Salmeterol/Fluticasone (Advair)
Leukotriene modifiers
  Zafirlukast (Accolate)
  Zileuton (Zyflo)
  Montelukast (Singulair)
Mast cell stabilizers
  Cromolyn sodium (Intal)
  Nedocromil sodium (Tilade)
Corticosteroids
  Beclomethasone dipropionate (Beclovent, Vanceril)
  Budesonide (Pulmicort)
  Flunisolide (AeroBid)
  Triamcinolone acetonide (Azmacort)
  Fluticasone (Flovent)

and isoetharine. These drugs differ in onset and duration of action. For example, isoetharine action begins within 1–3 minutes and lasts for 60–90 minutes. Common long-acting β₂-agonists include formoterol and salmeterol. Salmeterol, a particularly long-acting β₂-adrenergic, is helpful in maintenance treatment of asthma; it should not be used for acute exacerbations. Although epinephrine causes predominantly β-adrenergic stimulation in the lungs, it also causes peripheral α-adrenergic stimulation, resulting in vasoconstrictive hypertension and tachycardia. Epinephrine is most often administered subcutaneously to help control an acute asthma attack.

Anticholinergic agents directly relax smooth muscle by competing for acetylcholine at muscarinic nerve-ending receptors. Atropine and similar agents have been replaced by poorly absorbing atropinic congeners such as *ipratropium bromide, oxitropium bromide,* and *tiotropium*. These newer inhalation agents have few systemic and minimal cardiac effects. They have an additive bronchodilator effect when combined with submaximal doses of β-adrenergic agonists.

Inhibitors of inflammation include corticosteroids, leukotriene inhibitors, and cromolyn sodium. *Corticosteroids* not only suppress inflammation of the bronchioles but also potentiate the bronchodilator response to β-adrenergic receptors. *Inhaled corticosteroids* can be used chronically to reduce bronchial hyperreactivity; they are not used to manage acute attacks. *Systemic corticosteroids,* however, are highly effective in managing acute episodes. Systemic corticosteroids should be reserved for serious flare-ups to avoid adverse side effects. Leukotriene inhibitors suppress the effects of inflammatory mediators. They are especially useful for prophylaxis and chronic maintenance therapy in asthma. *Cromolyn sodium* prevents the release of chemical mediators from mast cells in the presence of IgE antibody and the specific antigen. *Immunotherapy* has been shown to be helpful for asthma triggered by a defined antigen.

Asthma treatment should be tailored to disease severity. Medication doses should be adequate to control symptoms rapidly and should later be reduced to the minimal level required to maintain control. The goals of therapy should include prevention of symptoms, reduction in frequency and severity of exacerbations, maintenance of normal (or near-normal) pulmonary function, maintenance of normal activity levels, and minimization of medication side effects. Maintenance medications include inhaled corticosteroids, chromones, leukotriene modifiers, long-acting β_2-agonists, anticholinergic agents, and oral corticosteroids. Appropriately used supplemental oxygen increases survival among patients with chronic respiratory failure and has a beneficial effect on pulmonary arterial pressure, polycythemia, exercise capacity, lung mechanics, and mental state.

Preoperative and Postoperative Considerations

Before operating on a patient with lung disease, the surgeon should consult with an internist or pulmonologist to carefully define the patient's functional respiratory status, especially with respect to the supine position. The patient's respiratory function should be maximized with medications and nonpharmacologic means, as appropriate. He or she should be sedated only if necessary and, in that case, should be carefully monitored for arterial gas values.

Campos MA, Wanner A. The rationale for pharmacologic therapy in stable chronic obstructive pulmonary disease. *Am J Med Sci.* 2005;329(4):181–189.

Fabbri L, Peters SP, Pavord I, et al. Allergic rhinitis, asthma, airway biology, and chronic obstructive pulmonary disease in AJRCCM in 2004. *Am J Respir Crit Care Med.* 2005;171(7): 686–698.

Martinez FJ, Standiford C, Gay SE. Is it asthma or COPD? The answer determines proper therapy for chronic airflow obstruction. *Postgrad Med.* 2005;117(3):19–26.

CHAPTER 7

Hematologic Disorders

Recent Developments

- Iron deficiency anemia remains the most common cause of anemia worldwide. It can be distinguished from anemia of chronic disease by using serum transferrin receptor assays.
- Allogenic bone marrow transplantation has become the treatment of choice for β-thalassemia major and has increased survival rates for this disease.
- The best screening test for paroxysmal nocturnal hemoglobinuria is now flow cytometry.
- Parental diagnosis is now available for couples at risk for producing a child with sickle cell anemia. Genetic counseling should be made available for such couples.
- Additional thrombotic risk factors (eg, factor V and prothrombin gene mutations, hyperhomocysteinemia) have been identified.
- Thrombophilia (the hypercoagulable state) is associated with recurrent fetal loss and preeclampsia.

Blood Composition

Formed elements—erythrocytes (red blood cells, or RBCs), white blood cells, and platelets—constitute approximately 45% of the total blood volume. The fluid portion, *plasma,* is about 90% water. The remaining 10% of the plasma consists of proteins (albumin, globulin, fibrinogen, and enzymes), lipids, carbohydrates, hormones, vitamins, and salts. If a blood specimen is allowed to clot, the fibrinogen is consumed and the resultant fluid portion is called *serum.*

Erythropoiesis

All blood cells originate from the uncommitted pluripotential stem cells. The latter give rise to lymphoid stem cells and myeloid stem cells. Myeloid stem cells are the precursors of RBCs, granulocytes, monocytes, and platelets. Hormones such as erythropoietin, thrombopoietin, and others initiate the differentiation of the various cellular elements. The life span of a circulating RBC is 100 days.

Anemia

Anemia is diagnosed in adults if the hemoglobin component is less than 13.5 g/dL in males and less than 12 g/dL in females. If anemia is suspected, a physical examination should concentrate on primary hematologic disease, such as lymphadenopathy or hepatosplenomegaly, and on bone tenderness. Congenital forms of anemia are suggested by the patient's personal and family history.

The most used classification of the anemias is based on RBC size. If the cell size is very small, *microcytic anemia* is the diagnosis. Possible causes are iron deficiency, thalassemia, and anemia of chronic disease. If the cell size is enlarged, *macrocytic anemia* is the diagnosis, and possible etiologies are vitamin B_{12} or folate deficiency *(megaloblastic)*, very high reticulocyte counts, and other causes such as drugs and alcohol.

Iron Deficiency Anemia

By far the most common type of anemia worldwide, *iron deficiency anemia* is diagnosed when serum ferritin is less than 30 μg/L. Every adult with iron deficiency anemia is suspected to be bleeding until proven otherwise. Menstrual blood loss in women plays a major role, as does gastrointestinal bleeding in both men and women. Aspirin can cause gastrointestinal bleeding.

The signs and symptoms of iron deficiency anemia are the same as those of the other anemias (pallor, cool skin, exercise intolerance or fatigue at rest, and so forth), but severe iron deficiency can cause mucosal changes, such as a smooth tongue, brittle nails, or cheilosis. Esophageal webs may also occur, as well as pica (which is, most commonly, a craving for ice chips). The most important part of the workup of iron deficiency anemia is detection of the occult source of blood loss. In the absence of this occult source, the preferred therapy is iron supplementation (oral or parenteral forms).

Anemia of Chronic Disease

A specific type of anemia can occur in chronic conditions such as chronic inflammation, infections, cancer, and liver disease. Chronic renal failure can also cause a more severe type of anemia, which is due to the resulting decrease in erythropoietin production. In this case, erythropoietin (epoetin alfa) can be used as treatment.

The Thalassemias

Thalassemia is a hereditary type of anemia characterized by reduction of the synthesis of hemoglobin chains alpha and beta. This leads to reduced hemoglobin synthesis and a microcytic hypochromic anemia. *α-Thalassemia* is due to a gene deletion, which causes reduced alpha hemoglobin chain synthesis. *β-Thalassemia* is caused by a point mutation rather than a deletion. In the absence of beta chains, the excess of alpha chains leads to instability in the RBC and hemolysis. The bone marrow becomes hyperplastic, and in severe cases this may lead to bone deformities and fractures. Transfusion and iron chelation are used for treatment so that iron overload can be minimized. Allogenic bone marrow transplantation has become the treatment of choice for β-thalassemia major, improving the survival rate of these patients to more than 80%.

Sideroblastic Anemia

If the incorporation of heme into protoporphyrin fails, hemoglobin synthesis is reduced; this condition is referred to as *sideroblastic anemia (SA)*. (A normal sideroblast is an erythroblast that has few granules of ferritin in the cytoplasm.) In SA, iron accumulates, particularly in the mitochondria, creating the "ring sideroblast." The causes of sideroblastic anemia are usually acquired and may include chronic alcoholism and lead poisoning. The primary form of SA may lead to leukemia.

Vitamin B$_{12}$ Deficiency

Vitamin B$_{12}$ comes from the diet and is available in all foods of animal origin. To be absorbed, it requires an intrinsic factor produced by the gastric parietal cells. This complex is absorbed in the terminal ileum and stored in the liver. It takes 3 years to deplete the reserves of vitamin B$_{12}$ in the liver. Strict vegetarians (vegans), patients with a history of abdominal surgery or gastrectomy, and persons with parasitic or pancreatic disease are at increased risk for vitamin B$_{12}$ deficiency. *Pernicious anemia* is an autoimmune disease that leads to lack of vitamin B$_{12}$ absorption due to atrophic gastritis. Megaloblastic anemia is the result. Often, leukopenia and thrombocytopenia accompany the anemia. Vitamin B$_{12}$ deficiency, even in the absence of hematologic changes, by itself can cause a neurologic syndrome, with peripheral nerves affected first; balance problems and alteration of cerebral function occur in more severe cases (dementia and neuropsychiatric changes). The diagnosis is confirmed by obtaining a serum level of vitamin B$_{12}$ (less than 170 pg/mL). If B$_{12}$ level is equivocal, serum methylmalonic acid and homocysteine should be measured, as they are considered the most reliable indicators of tissue cobalamin deficiency. Treatment is with parenteral B$_{12}$ in cases of pernicious anemia; otherwise, oral B$_{12}$ is adequate.

Folic Acid Deficiency

Folic acid deficiency is another etiology of megaloblastic, or macrocytic, anemia. Macroovalocytes and hypersegmented neutrophils are seen on peripheral smear. The serum vitamin B$_{12}$ concentration has to be normal. The most common etiology of folate deficiency is inadequate dietary intake. Treatment is with oral folic acid supplements.

Hemolytic Anemias

In *hemolytic anemia,* the life span of the RBC is reduced. The bone marrow responds to this reduced survival with an increase in production of RBCs; hence, reticulocytosis is an important clue to the presence of hemolysis. The offending factor may be intrinsic or external to the RBC.

Treatment depends on the specific etiology. In hereditary spherocytosis, there is an autosomal dominant membrane abnormality in the RBC, which causes the RBC to acquire a spherical shape. This abnormal shape leads to lack of RBC strength and RBC deformability, trapping of the RBC in the spleen, and hemolysis. The treatment of choice is splenectomy, which eliminates the site of hemolysis. Uninterrupted supplementation of folic acid is also needed.

In paroxysmal nocturnal hemoglobinuria, the RBC membrane is sensitive to lysis by complement. The best screening test is flow cytometry, which has largely replaced the classic sucrose hemolysis test. Prednisone is helpful in decreasing the hemolysis. In glucose-6-phosphate dehydrogenase (G6PD) deficiency, a hereditary enzyme defect causes hemolytic anemia due to decreased ability of the RBC to deal with oxidative stresses. Oxidized hemoglobin precipitates and forms precipitants called *Heinz bodies*. The RBC is then removed by the spleen. The triggering factor is usually an infection or exposure to a specific drug. Specific G6PD assays are available. Treatment consists of avoiding known oxidant drugs.

Sickle cell disease

In *sickle cell anemia,* an abnormal hemoglobin leads to chronic hemolytic anemia, an autosomal recessive disorder causing an amino acid substitution on the beta chain. The new hemoglobin is called *hemoglobin S.* This in turn damages the RBC membrane and leads to sickling. Parental diagnosis is now available for couples at risk for producing a child with sickle cell anemia. Genetic counseling should be made available for such couples. One out of 400 blacks born in the United States has sickle cell anemia. Chronic hemolytic anemia can produce jaundice, gallstones, splenomegaly, and poorly healing ulcers over the lower tibia.

Sickle cell disease is manifested by acute painful episodes that are caused by the sickling of the RBCs and that can be precipitated by infection, dehydration, and hypoxia. Vascular occlusion can lead to necrosis of bone and to infection. Hematuria can be caused by infarction of the renal papillae. Sickle cell retinopathy can lead to vision loss in severe cases. With improved supportive care, an affected person now has an average life expectancy of between 40 and 50 years. Most clinical laboratories offer a screening test for sickle cell hemoglobin. For patients who have a positive screening test, the diagnosis is confirmed by hemoglobin electrophoresis, which can detect the presence and measure the amount of hemoglobin S. Patients should be given folic acid supplements, pneumococcal vaccination, and, if infections arise, specific treatment for infections. Patients should be kept well hydrated, and they should be given oxygen if they are hypoxic. Allogenic bone marrow transplantation is being studied as a possible curative option for severely affected young patients. See also BCSC Section 12, *Retina and Vitreous.*

Autoimmune hemolytic anemia

In autoimmune hemolytic anemia, an IgG autoantibody is formed and binds to the RBC membrane, leading to formation of a spherocyte and sequestration in the spleen. Half of all cases of autoimmune hemolytic anemia are idiopathic; others are associated with autoimmune diseases such as systemic lupus and chronic leukemia. The Coombs test is positive. Treatment consists of administration of prednisone and, if the disease is recurrent, splenectomy.

Disorders of Hemostasis

Disorders of hemostasis may be due to defects in either platelet number or function or to problems in formation of a fibrin clot (coagulation). A basic understanding of the hemostatic process and the manifestations associated with specific abnormalities helps the ophthalmologist with both medical and surgical management. (See Fig 7-1 for a diagram of blood-clotting pathways.) For the purpose of laboratory test interpretation, the coagulation cascade can be divided into intrinsic and extrinsic pathways. However, it is now understood that this is an oversimplification. For example, factor IX (an intrinsic factor) can be activated by factor VII (an extrinsic factor).

Hemostasis is initiated by damage to a blood vessel wall. This event triggers constriction of the vessel, followed by accumulation and adherence of platelets at the site of injury. Coagulation factors in the blood are activated, leading to formation of a fibrin clot. Slow fibrinolysis ensues, dissolving the clot while the damage is repaired. Circulating inhibitors are also present, modulating the process by inactivating coagulation factors to prevent widespread clotting. Normal endothelium plays a critical role in naturally anticoagulating blood by preventing fibrin accumulation. The following physiologic antithrombotic components can produce this effect:

- antithrombin III
- protein C and protein S

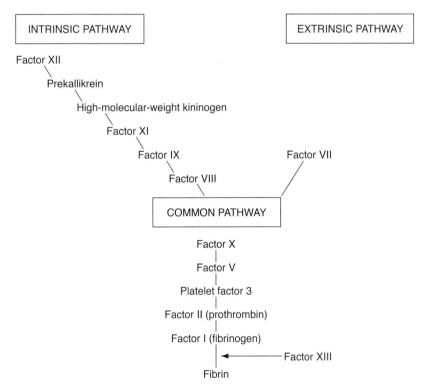

Figure 7-1 Blood-clotting pathways.

- tissue factor pathway inhibitor
- the fibrinolytic system

Antithrombin III (AT III) inactivates thrombin. Activated protein C (APC), with its co-factor protein S, functions as a natural anticoagulant by destroying factors Va and VIIa. Thrombin itself activates protein C. Although inherited deficiencies of AT III, protein C, or protein S are associated with a lifelong thrombotic tendency, tissue factor pathway inhibitor deficiency has not yet been related to the hypercoagulable state (see the discussion of thrombotic disorders later in the chapter).

Laboratory Evaluation of Hemostasis and Blood Coagulation

Various techniques are used to assess the status of a patient's hemostatic mechanisms. Following are some of the most common tests:

- *Platelet count.* Minor bleeding may occur at platelet counts below 50,000/μL. Abnormal bleeding at higher platelet counts suggests abnormal platelet function. Below 20,000/μL, spontaneous bleeding may be serious.
- *Bleeding time.* A small dermal wound is created, and the duration of bleeding is recorded. This is a screening test of the vascular and platelet components of hemostasis. Because disorders of blood vessels are rare, the results essentially reflect platelet number and function. Bleeding time is rarely prolonged when platelet counts are above 50,000/μL.
- *Activated partial thromboplastin time (aPTT).* The aPTT requires all of the coagulation factors involved in the intrinsic and common pathways. The aPTT is most commonly used to measure the effect of heparin therapy. Platelet abnormalities do not affect the result of this test.
- *Prothrombin time (PT).* The PT measures the integrity of the extrinsic and common pathways. It requires a 30% concentration of the vitamin K–dependent factors II, VII, and X (though not factor IX, a part of the intrinsic pathway) and therefore is prolonged in conditions affecting these factors (see Disorders of Blood Coagulation later in this chapter). The PT is most commonly used to monitor anticoagulant therapy. The action of heparin may slightly prolong PT.

Efforts have been made to tailor anticoagulation therapy to the problem being treated. For example, treatment or prevention of deep venous thrombosis is thought to require less oral anticoagulation therapy than treatment of endocardial mural thrombi or cardiac replacement valves. However, because of intralaboratory and interlaboratory variation in test results, it has been difficult to standardize therapeutic dosages. To solve this problem, the international normalized ratio (INR) was developed. The INR modifies the standard PT ratio (patient PT/control PT) to reflect the particular thromboplastin reagent used by a laboratory. The resulting reported INR value is an expression of the ratio of the patient's PT to the laboratory's mean normal PT. Thus, for prevention or treatment of deep venous thrombosis, the recommended INR value (comparable to subsequent values measured over time or across different laboratories) is 2.0–3.0; for tissue replacement valves, 2.0–3.0; for mechanical replacement valves, 2.5–3.5.

Recently, genetic testing in the form of a DNA assay to determine the right warfarin dose for an individual patient has been implemented, especially in cases where resistance to the drug is suspected. This knowledge has substantially reduced the risk of bleeding or clotting events.

Clinical Manifestations of Hemostatic Abnormalities

Hemorrhage resulting from hemostatic derangement must be differentiated from hemorrhage caused by localized processes. The presence of generalized or recurrent bleeding suggests abnormal hemostasis. *Petechiae* (small capillary hemorrhages of the skin and mucous membranes) and *purpura* (ecchymoses) are typical of platelet disorders and vasculitis. Subcutaneous hematomas and hemarthroses characterize coagulation abnormalities. Bleeding due to trauma may be massive and life threatening in coagulation disorders, whereas bleeding is more likely to be slow and prolonged when platelet function is impaired.

Vascular Disorders

A number of inherited and acquired disorders of blood vessels and their supporting connective tissues result in pathologic bleeding. *Hereditary hemorrhagic telangiectasia* (Osler-Weber-Rendu disease) is an autosomal dominant condition characterized by localized dilation of capillaries and venules of the skin and mucous membranes. The lesions increase over a period of decades, often leading to profuse bleeding.

Several inherited connective tissue disorders are associated with hemorrhage. *Ehlers-Danlos syndrome* is characterized by hyperplastic fragile skin and hyperextensible joints; it is dominantly inherited. In *osteogenesis imperfecta,* also a dominant trait, bone fractures and otosclerosis (leading to deafness) are common. In both of these conditions, easy bruising and hematomas are common. *Pseudoxanthoma elasticum,* a recessive disorder, is much rarer but is often complicated by gastrointestinal hemorrhage. *Marfan syndrome* is sometimes associated with mild bleeding as well as with aortic dissection.

Scurvy, the result of severe ascorbic acid deficiency, is associated with marked vascular fragility and hemorrhagic manifestations resulting from abnormal synthesis of collagen. In addition to the classic findings of perifollicular petechiae and gingival bleeding, intradermal, intramuscular, and subperiosteal hemorrhages are common. *Amyloidosis* is another acquired disorder in which petechiae and purpura are common.

All of the inherited vascular disorders have associated ocular findings. Conjunctival telangiectasias occur in hereditary hemorrhagic telangiectasia. Blue sclerae are typical of osteogenesis imperfecta. Ocular manifestations of Ehlers-Danlos syndrome include microcornea, myopia, and angioid streaks; retinal detachment and ectopia lentis have also been reported. Angioid streaks also occur in patients with pseudoxanthoma elasticum. Fifty percent of patients with Marfan syndrome have ectopia lentis; severe myopia and retinal detachment are common.

Platelet Disorders

By far the most common cause of abnormal bleeding, platelet disorders may result from an insufficient number of platelets, inadequate function, or both. Mild derangement of platelet function may be asymptomatic or may cause minor bruising, menorrhagia, or bleeding after surgery. More severe dysfunction leads to petechiae, purpura, and gastrointestinal bleeding and other types of serious bleeding.

Thrombocytopenia

The number of platelets may be reduced by decreased production, increased destruction, or abnormal distribution. Production may be suppressed by many factors, including radiation, chemotherapy, alcohol use, malignant invasion of the bone marrow, aplastic anemia, and vitamin B_{12} or folic acid deficiency.

Accelerated destruction may occur through immunologic or nonimmunologic causes. *Idiopathic thrombocytopenic purpura (ITP)* is the result of platelet injury by antiplatelet antibodies. The acute form of ITP usually occurs in children and young adults, often following a viral illness, and commonly undergoes spontaneous remission. Chronic ITP is more common in adults and is characterized by mild manifestations; spontaneous remission is uncommon. Treatment consists of corticosteroid therapy or splenectomy. Danazol is also effective in treating ITP, and when combined therapy is necessary, danazol allows the use of lower doses of corticosteroids. New forms of treatment are based on the use of Rituximab, which is a monoclonal antibody against lymphocytes. A neonatal form occurs in babies born to women with ITP; this form results from transplacental passage of antiplatelet antibodies. Recovery follows physiologic clearance of the antibodies from the child's circulation.

Many drugs, including quinine, quinidine, digitalis, procainamide, thiazide diuretics, sulfonamides, phenytoin, aspirin, penicillin, heparin, and gold, have been implicated as causes of immunologic platelet destruction. Drug-induced thrombocytopenia is common. Another important cause is *posttransfusion isoantibody production,* which occurs predictably after transfusions containing platelets, unless human leukocyte antigen typing is undertaken, and leads to decreasing efficacy of later platelet transfusions.

Nonimmune causes of thrombocytopenia include *thrombotic thrombocytopenic purpura* and the syndromes of intravascular coagulation and fibrinolysis (see "Disseminated intravascular coagulation" later in the chapter). In addition to the symptoms of thrombocytopenia, thrombotic thrombocytopenic purpura is characterized by thrombotic occlusions of the microcirculation and hemolytic anemia. Fever, neurologic symptoms, anemia, and renal dysfunction occur with abrupt onset, with death occurring in days to weeks in the majority of untreated cases. Early treatment with exchange plasmapheresis has improved the survival rate to over 80%. Additional treatment includes antiplatelet drugs, corticosteroids, and splenectomy.

Abnormal distribution of platelets is most commonly caused by splenic sequestration. The usual clinical setting is hepatic cirrhosis, and the level of thrombocytopenia is mild. Patients with severely depressed platelet counts probably also have accelerated platelet destruction in the spleen.

Platelet dysfunction

Patients with platelet dysfunction usually come to the physician's attention because of easy bruising, epistaxis, menorrhagia, or excessive bleeding after surgery or dental work.

Unlike patients with marked thrombocytopenia, patients with platelet dysfunction rarely have petechiae.

Hereditary disorders of platelet function are rare. Much more important clinically are the acquired forms, of which drug ingestion is the most common cause. As with drugs causing antiplatelet antibodies, the list of causative agents is very long. A single aspirin tablet taken orally irreversibly inhibits platelet aggregation for the life span of the circulating platelets present, causing a modest prolongation of the bleeding time for at least 48–72 hours following ingestion. This reaction has remarkably little effect in otherwise healthy individuals, although intraoperative blood loss may be slightly increased. However, in patients with hemophilia, severe thrombocytopenia, or uremia and in those on warfarin or heparin therapy, bleeding may be significant.

Nonsteroidal anti-inflammatory drugs cause reversible inhibition of platelet function in the presence of the drug; the effect disappears as the drug is cleared from the blood. Other commonly used drugs that may affect platelet function include ethanol, tricyclic antidepressants, and antihistamines.

In addition to uremia, clinical conditions associated with abnormal platelet function include liver disease, multiple myeloma, systemic lupus erythematosus, chronic lymphocytic leukemia, and Hermansky-Pudlak syndrome (an autosomal recessive form of oculocutaneous albinism).

Disorders of Blood Coagulation

Hereditary coagulation disorders

Inherited coagulation abnormalities involve all of the coagulation factors except factors III and IV. The most common and most severe is factor VIII deficiency, called *hemophilia A,* or *classic hemophilia.* Typical manifestations of this X-linked disease include severe and protracted bleeding, after even minor trauma, and spontaneous bleeding into joints (hemarthroses), the central nervous system, and the abdominal cavity.

Treatment involves infusion of coagulation factor VIII. In the past, transfusion of pooled human factor VIII always carried a significant risk of hepatitis B virus transmission; in the 1980s, transmission of the human immunodeficiency virus became a major problem as well. With the availability of recombinant factor VIII, however, those risks have now been mostly eliminated. Up to 10% of patients with hemophilia A develop antibodies, presumably due to sensitization following administration of factor VIII. These anticoagulants can also develop in healthy older patients, in nonhemophilic patients after drug reactions, and in those with collagen vascular diseases. Clinical manifestations range from mild bleeding to full-blown hemophilia. The result of the aPTT is prolonged, and the result of the PT is normal. Treatment involves various regimens of coagulation factor replacement and immunosuppression to try to eliminate the inhibitor. Gene therapy is currently in the developmental phase but could further transform the outlook for these patients.

Von Willebrand disease, another relatively common hereditary disorder, is caused by deficiency or abnormality of a portion of the factor VIII molecule called von Willebrand factor. This deficiency causes platelet adhesion abnormalities, leading to bleeding symptoms that are mild in most cases and may escape detection until adult years.

Acquired coagulation disorders

Vitamin K deficiency   Vitamin K is required for the production of factors II (prothrombin), VII, IX, and X in the liver. Normal diets contain large amounts of vitamin K, which is also synthesized by gut flora. Causes of vitamin K deficiency include biliary obstruction and various malabsorption syndromes (including sprue, cystic fibrosis, and celiac disease), in which intestinal absorption of vitamin K is reduced. Suppression of endogenous gastrointestinal flora, seen commonly in hospitalized patients on prolonged broad-spectrum antibiotic therapy, decreases intestinal production of vitamin K. However, clinical deficiency occurs only if dietary intake is also diminished. Nutritional deficiency is unusual but may occur with prolonged parenteral nutrition. Laboratory evaluation reveals prolongation of both PT and aPTT. Most forms of vitamin K deficiency respond to subcutaneous or intramuscular administration of 20 mg of vitamin K_1, with normalization of coagulation defects within 24 hours. Vitamin K_1 should not be given intravenously because of the risk of sudden death from an anaphylactoid reaction. One special form of vitamin K deficiency is *hemorrhagic disease of the newborn,* which is the result of a normal mild deficiency of vitamin K–dependent factors during the first 5 days of life and the absence of the vitamin in maternal milk. This condition is now rare in developed countries because of the routine administration of vitamin K to newborns. See also Antiphospholipid Antibody Syndrome in Chapter 8, Rheumatic Disorders.

Liver disease   Hemostatic abnormalities of all types may be associated with disease of the liver, the site of production of all the coagulation factors except factor VIII. As liver dysfunction develops, levels of the vitamin K–dependent factors decrease first, followed by those of factors V, XI, and XII; both PT and aPTT are prolonged. Thrombocytopenia, primarily the result of hypersplenism, and a prolonged bleeding time due to platelet dysfunction are common. In addition, intravascular coagulation and fibrinolysis (see "Disseminated intravascular coagulation," next) are common, further complicating the clinical picture.

Mild hemorrhagic symptoms are common in patients with significant liver disease. Severe bleeding is usually gastrointestinal in origin, arising from peptic ulcers, gastritis, and esophageal varices. Treatment is difficult at best and consists of blood and coagulation factor replacement. Local measures, such as vasopressin infusion or balloon tamponade of bleeding varices, can sometimes control potentially catastrophic bleeding.

Disseminated intravascular coagulation   *Disseminated intravascular coagulation (DIC)* is a complex syndrome involving widespread activation of the coagulation and fibrinolytic systems within the general circulation. Utilization and consumption of coagulation factors and platelets produce bleeding; formation of fibrin and fibrin degradation products (fibrin split products) leads to occlusion of the microcirculation, various forms of organ failure, and occasionally thrombosis of larger vessels. Laboratory findings may vary but usually include thrombocytopenia, hypofibrinogenemia, and elevated levels of fibrin split products. PT and aPTT are usually, though not invariably, prolonged.

Clinically, 2 forms of DIC are recognized. *Acute DIC* is characterized by the abrupt onset of severe, generalized bleeding. The most common causes are obstetric complications (most notably abruptio placentae and amniotic fluid embolism), septicemia, shock, massive trauma, and major surgical procedures. Treatment, other than specific measures aimed at the underlying disease, is controversial. Among the modalities used are heparinization and replacement of blood, platelets, and fibrinogen.

Chronic DIC is associated with disseminated neoplasms, some acute leukemias, and autoimmune diseases. Laboratory values range from normal to moderately abnormal; levels of coagulation factors may even be elevated. Bleeding and thrombosis (especially leg vein thrombosis and pulmonary embolism) may occur, but in most patients the syndrome remains undiagnosed unless renal failure results from intravascular coagulation in the kidney. In these patients, the disease has been demonstrated via biopsy to detect fibrin in renal tissue. On occasion, chronic DIC may convert to the acute form.

Thrombotic disorders

The hypercoagulable states encompass a group of inherited or acquired thrombotic disorders *(thrombophilia)* that increase the risk of thrombosis. The primary hypercoagulable states are caused by abnormalities of specific coagulation proteins involving inherited mutations in one of the antithrombotic factors. The trigger for a thrombotic event is often the development of one of the acquired secondary hypercoagulable states superimposed on an inherited state of hypercoagulability. The secondary hypercoagulable states cause a thrombotic tendency by complex and often multifactorial mechanisms.

Primary Hypercoagulable States

Antithrombin III deficiency

Antithrombin III deficiency leads to increased fibrin accumulation and a lifelong propensity for thrombosis.

Protein C deficiency

Protein C deficiency leads to unregulated fibrin generation because of impaired inactivation of factors VIIIa and Va, 2 essential cofactors in the coagulation cascade.

Protein S deficiency

Protein S is the principal cofactor of APC, and therefore its deficiency mimics that of protein C.

Activated protein C resistance

Inherited APC resistance causing thrombophilia was originally detected by the finding that the activated aPTT of the plasma of affected persons could not be appropriately prolonged by the addition of exogenous APC in vitro. The great majority of these subjects are now recognized to harbor a single specific point mutation in the factor V gene, termed *factor V Leiden*. This mutation is remarkably frequent (3%–7%) in healthy white populations but appears to be far less prevalent or even absent in certain black and Asian populations.

Prothrombin gene mutation

The prothrombin gene mutation has been associated with elevated plasma levels of prothrombin; it is second only to factor V Leiden as a genetic risk factor for venous thrombosis.

Hyperhomocysteinemia

Hyperhomocysteinemia, which is due to elevated blood levels of homocysteine, leads to severe neurologic developmental abnormalities in the homozygous state. Adults with the heterozygous deficiency state may have only thrombotic tendencies. Acquired causes of hyperhomocysteinemia in adults commonly involve nutritional deficiencies of pyridoxine, vitamin B_{12}, and folate, all cofactors in homocysteine metabolism. High blood concentrations of homocysteine constitute an independent risk factor for both venous and arterial thrombosis; in contrast, all of the other primary hypercoagulable states are associated only with venous thromboembolic complications, usually involving the lower extremities. The initial treatment of acute venous thrombosis in these patients is not different from treatment in those without genetic defects.

Secondary Hypercoagulable States

Malignancy may stimulate thrombosis directly by elaborating procoagulant substances that initiate chronic DIC. This appears to be most prominent in patients with pancreatic cancer, adenocarcinoma of the gastrointestinal tract or lung, and ovarian cancer. *Myeloproliferative disorders* (polycythemia vera, essential thrombocythemia, chronic myelogenous leukemia, and myelofibrosis) are major causes of thrombosis and paradoxical bleeding, as is the related stem cell disorder *paroxysmal nocturnal hemoglobinuria*. The *phospholipid antibody syndrome* is characterized by both venous and arterial thrombosis, including recurrent spontaneous abortions, deep venous thrombosis, and cerebrovascular arterial thrombotic events. Ophthalmic complications include retinal vein and artery occlusion, retinal vasculitis, choroidal infarction, and anterior ischemic optic neuropathy. Tests for patients with this syndrome include anticardiolipin antibodies and lupus anticoagulants. The hypercoagulability associated with *pregnancy* involves a progressive state of DIC throughout the course of pregnancy, activated in the uteroplacental circulation. *Oral contraceptives* induce similar changes. The *postoperative state* and *trauma* are significant causes of venous thrombosis. Detailed discussion of treatment of these various and complex disorders is beyond the scope of this text.

Therapeutic anticoagulation

Many clinical situations require intentional disruption of the hemostatic process. The effect of aspirin on platelet function has already been discussed.

Unfractionated *heparin* is a mucopolysaccharide that binds antithrombin III, inhibiting the formation of thrombin. It is given intravenously or subcutaneously, and therapy is assessed by measuring the aPTT. Aspirin should not be given to patients on heparin because the resultant platelet dysfunction may provoke bleeding. Additional parenteral anticoagulants are low-molecular-weight heparins, which usually don't require dosage monitoring, and direct antithrombinic agents like lepirudin and argatroban.

The orally administered warfarin derivatives, of which warfarin sodium (Coumadin) is the most widely used, inhibit the production of normal vitamin K–dependent coagulation factors (II, VII, IX, and X). Therapeutic effect is assessed by measuring the patient's INR. One critical issue is the long list of commonly used drugs that interact with warfarin. These interactions may cause an unintended increase or decrease in the INR, depending on the drug.

Heparin and the warfarin derivatives are used to prevent the formation of new thrombi and the propagation of existing thrombi, but neither affects the original clot. Thrombolytic agents such as *streptokinase, urokinase,* and *tissue plasminogen activator (tPA)* are used to dissolve existing thrombi, most notably in the very early stages of myocardial infarction resulting from coronary artery thrombosis. These agents are also currently being used for early treatment of thrombotic stroke; this form of treatment increases the risk of converting a thrombotic stroke into a hemorrhagic stroke.

Hall CJ, Richards S, Hillmen P. Primary prophylaxis with warfarin prevents thrombosis in paroxysmal nocturnal hemoglobinuria (PNH). *Blood.* 2003;102(10):3587–3591.

Means RT Jr. Recent developments in the anemia of chronic disease. *Curr Hematol Rep.* 2003; 2(2):116–121.

Provan D, O'Shaughnessy DF. Recent advances in haematology. *BMJ.* 1999;318(7189): 991–994.

Schafer AI. Approach to the patient with bleeding and thrombosis. In: Goldman L, Ausiello DA, eds. *Cecil Medicine.* 23rd ed. Philadelphia: Elsevier/Saunders; 2008:chap 178.

Schafer AI. Thrombotic disorders: hypercoagulable states. In: Goldman L, Ausiello DA, eds. *Cecil Medicine.* 23rd ed. Philadelphia: Elsevier/Saunders; 2008:chap 182.

The authors would like to thank Liborio Tranchida, MD, for his contributions to this chapter.

CHAPTER 8

Rheumatic Disorders

Recent Developments

- A number of new biologic agents are either in use or being developed for treating rheumatologic diseases. These include drugs that interfere with tumor necrosis factor α (TNF-α), interleukin-1, interleukin-6, and T-cell receptor CD28. Biologic agents that were initially released as chemotherapeutic agents are also being used.
- Anti–TNF-α agents such as etanercept (Enbrel) and infliximab (Remicade) may cause uncommon but significant adverse effects, such as lymphoma, opportunistic infections, and demyelinating disease that can include optic neuritis. Etanercept has also been implicated as a possible cause of uveitis.
- Many rheumatologic diseases, such as the spondyloarthropathies and juvenile arthritides, are undergoing reclassification to allow a more uniform approach to defining treatment and prognosis.

Introduction

The rheumatic disorders are a heterogeneous collection of diseases that include rheumatoid arthritis; the spondyloarthropathies; juvenile idiopathic (rheumatoid) arthritis; systemic lupus erythematosus; antiphospholipid antibody syndrome; scleroderma; Sjögren syndrome; polymyositis and dermatomyositis; relapsing polychondritis; the vasculitides, including giant cell arteritis, polyarteritis nodosa, and Wegener granulomatosis; and Behçet syndrome. Ocular involvement is common in the rheumatic diseases but varies among the different disorders.

Rheumatoid Arthritis

Rheumatoid arthritis (RA) is the most common rheumatic disorder, affecting approximately 1% of adults. RA is classically an additive, symmetric, deforming, peripheral polyarthritis characterized by synovial membrane inflammation. All joints may be involved, but this disorder affects primarily the small joints of the hands and feet. Like all inflammatory arthritides, RA is associated with the *gel phenomenon,* a stiffness at rest that improves with use; patients often complain of morning stiffness, which is a hallmark of inflammatory joint disease.

Approximately 80% of patients with RA are positive for a rheumatoid factor, which is an autoantibody directed against immunoglobulin G (IgG). Seropositive RA aggregates in families. Human leukocyte antigen DR4 (HLA-DR4) is found in 70% of white seropositive patients. A more recent test involves identification of anticyclic citrullinated peptide (anti-CCP) antibodies, which are antibodies directed toward certain peptides in the skin that contain the amino acid citrulline. Testing for both anti-CCP antibodies and rheumatoid factor increases the sensitivity for detecting early RA; patients with anti-CCP antibodies may tend to have more erosive disease.

Extra-articular disease in RA may affect a wide variety of nonarticular tissues. Rheumatoid nodules, located subcutaneously on extensor surfaces, occur in approximately 25% of patients with RA. The lungs may be affected with rheumatoid pleural effusions, pleural nodules, pulmonary nodules, and, occasionally, interstitial fibrosis. Cardiac disease includes pericarditis and rheumatoid nodules involving the conducting system, heart valves, or both. Mild anemia of chronic disease is the rule. *Felty syndrome* is a triad of RA, splenomegaly, and neutropenia. Patients with Felty syndrome can also have hyperpigmentation, chronic leg ulcers, and recurrent infections. Rheumatoid vasculitis affects less than 1% of patients with RA. It generally presents either as peripheral polyneuropathy or as refractory skin ulcers. Patients may develop digital gangrene or, occasionally, visceral ischemia. The most common neuropathy is median nerve compression caused by synovitis of the wrist. Ocular manifestations of RA include Sjögren syndrome, scleritis, episcleritis, and marginal corneal ulcers. The ocular manifestations of RA are discussed in BCSC Section 8, *External Disease and Cornea,* and Section 9, *Intraocular Inflammation and Uveitis.*

Therapy

We now know that significant joint damage occurs early in the course of the disease. Thus, the goal is to identify and aggressively treat even subtle evidence of disease activity. A patient's physician can determine disease activity by analyzing a combination of symptoms, clinical findings, laboratory testing, and imaging. Treatment of RA is then approached in a stepwise additive fashion. Nonpharmacologic and preventive measures, such as physical therapy and actions ensuring bone health, form the basis of treatment.

Analgesics and nonsteroidal anti-inflammatory drugs (NSAIDs) are used to control acute symptoms but do not alter disease outcome. Most patients with active disease require at least 1 *disease-modifying antirheumatic drug (DMARD),* also known as *slow-acting antirheumatic drugs (SAARDs).* These drugs, which include hydroxychloroquine (Plaquenil), methotrexate, and sulfasalazine (Azulfidine), are capable of reducing or preventing joint damage. Methotrexate is perhaps the most commonly used DMARD. Depending on disease response and severity, patients may need more aggressive medications such as cyclosporine (Neoral, Sandimmune), cyclophosphamide (Cytoxan), or the various anticytokine drugs. (All of these medications are reviewed at the end of this chapter.) Combination therapy is often used to minimize the toxicity of any one class of medication. Prednisone is often used, ideally at low doses, to increase the patient's mobility and functional capacity. Joint surgery for pain and impaired function may also be necessary.

Spondyloarthropathies

The spondyloarthropathies are a group of diseases that have been referred to as the *sero-negative spondyloarthropathies*, with the term *seronegative* referring to a negative rheumatoid factor test. As newer and more specific clinical definitions are created, however, that term has become redundant and is less commonly used. The defining clinical term is *spondyloarthropathy* (or *spondyloarthritis*), which refers to a spectrum of diseases that share certain clinical features. There is a predilection for axial (spinal and sacroiliac joint) inflammation, with a hallmark being inflammatory spinal pain. Inflammatory spinal pain is distinguished from more typical low back pain symptoms by the tendency to be worse after rest (morning stiffness) and to improve with activity. Other distinctive features of the various spondyloarthropathies include asymmetric arthritis, genital and skin lesions, eye and bowel inflammation, and an association with previous or ongoing infectious disorders. The presence of these other features is used to distinguish between the various types of spondyloarthropathies, although there may be a great deal of overlap. These diseases are also linked by their statistical association with the antigen type HLA-B27 and by a tendency to have a specific type of joint inflammation known as *enthesitis*. (The enthesis is a complex structure that extends into bone at the point where ligaments and tendons are attached; the most common observable clinical manifestation of enthesitis is swelling at the heels, where the Achilles tendon inserts, or the insertion of the plantar fascia ligament into the calcaneus.)

The spondyloarthropathy family consists of undifferentiated spondyloarthropathy, both the juvenile and adult forms of ankylosing spondylitis, reactive arthritis, and Reiter syndrome. The spondyloarthropathies associated with psoriasis and inflammatory bowel disease (ulcerative colitis and Crohn disease) are also included.

Undifferentiated spondyloarthropathy is a newer category created for patients who do not fall into one of the other categories. It was formed with the recognition that for the majority of patients with spondyloarthropathy, there is no apparent antecedent cause. Most patients present primarily with arthritis. Undifferentiated spondyloarthropathy is probably the most common of the spondyloarthropathies, followed by ankylosing spondylitis, with reactive arthritis and Reiter syndrome being much less common. It is hoped that the addition of this new category will eventually lead to better understanding and management of this subset of rheumatologic diseases.

Awareness of these various entities is important for the ophthalmologist because they all share the potential to develop acute HLA-B27–associated anterior uveitis. At times, the characteristic uveitis may be the presenting feature of a spondyloarthropathy, and the ophthalmologist may therefore be crucial in suggesting the diagnosis. See BCSC Section 9, *Intraocular Inflammation and Uveitis,* for further discussion of the ophthalmic manifestations.

Ankylosing Spondylitis

Ankylosing spondylitis (AS) is characterized by involvement of the axial skeleton and by bony fusion (ankylosis). The cause is unknown, but the strong association with HLA-B27

(90% of patients) suggests a genetic predisposition. Men are affected 3 times more often than women are, and the radiographic features seem to evolve more slowly in women.

The classic features of ankylosing spondylitis are inflammatory low back pain, fusion of the axial skeleton (spinal ankylosis), and sacroiliitis on x-ray examination. The last stage of this process is a completely fused and immobilized spine, also known as a *bamboo* or *poker spine*. In addition to the spinal arthritis that is the hallmark of the disease, patients may develop arthritis of peripheral joints, limited chest expansion, and restrictive lung disease. Other extra-articular features include apical pulmonary fibrosis, ascending aortitis, aortic valvular incompetence, and heart block. Ankylosing spondylitis is surprisingly resistant to the usual rheumatologic therapeutics. The most effective agents seem to be sulfasalazine and TNF-α inhibitors such as infliximab (Remicade). Therapeutic agents for rheumatologic diseases are discussed at the end of this chapter.

The primary ocular manifestation of ankylosing spondylitis is recurrent, acute, nongranulomatous iridocyclitis, which occurs in approximately 25% of these patients and does not seem to be correlated with the activity of the joint disease. Conversely, a study of patients presenting with HLA-B27 uveitis showed that approximately 45% either were known to have or ultimately developed AS. A rheumatologic evaluation of patients with HLA-B27 uveitis should be considered, because early diagnosis and treatment of AS with physical therapy may slow disease progression.

Reactive Arthritis

In the broadest sense, the term *reactive arthritis* implies an autoimmune response to some sort of antecedent infection that usually involves the genitourinary or gastrointestinal system. Reiter syndrome, which features the classic triad of arthritis, urethritis, and conjunctivitis, can be considered to be a subset of reactive arthritis, although different authors may use the 2 terms interchangeably because the classification of the various spondyloarthropathies is in flux. Like ankylosing spondylitis, reactive arthritis has a clear genetic predisposition in that 63%–95% of patients are positive for HLA-B27. The male–female ratio is at least 5:1. Precipitating agents include *Chlamydia trachomatis* in the genitourinary tract and *Salmonella, Shigella, Yersinia,* or *Campylobacter* organisms in the gastrointestinal tract. Fragments of *Yersinia, Salmonella,* and *Chlamydia* organisms have been identified in the synovial tissues of patients with reactive arthritis, but intact organisms have not been cultured—hence the designation "reactive" and not "infective."

The arthritis of reactive arthritis typically appears within 1–3 weeks of the inciting urethritis or diarrhea. It is an asymmetric, episodic oligoarthritis affecting primarily the lower extremities, in particular the large joints such as the knees or ankles. Other features include inflammatory spinal pain; enthesitis; interphalangeal arthritis of the toes and fingers, which produces "sausage digits"; and sacroiliitis. Mucocutaneous lesions include urethritis in men and cervicitis in women, shallow ulcers on the glans penis (circinate balanitis), painless oral ulcers, nail lesions, and skin lesions on the soles and palms (keratoderma blennorrhagicum). Patients may also have systemic symptoms, including fever and weight loss. The disease tends to follow an episodic course, and most patients go into remission within 2 years, although some may develop long-term disease. Systemic treatment includes use of NSAIDs and sulfasalazine in addition to appropriate antibiotic therapy if an active infection is still present after initial treatment.

⊙ Ophthalmic considerations   Conjunctivitis is one of the most common manifestations of reactive arthritis. It tends to be mild and bilateral with a mucopurulent discharge. There may be follicular or papillary changes. Cultures are negative, and the conjunctivitis typically resolves within 10 days without treatment. A more serious ocular manifestation is uveitis, which occurs in 15%–25% of patients with reactive arthritis. It is often the acute, nongranulomatous, recurrent iridocyclitis that is characteristic of HLA-B27 disease. The uveitis may also be chronic, and some patients may even require long-term immunosuppressive therapy.

The conjunctivitis and urethritis of reactive arthritis are, by definition, sterile autoimmune phenomena that can occur after either gastrointestinal tract or genital infections. Confusion occurs because *Chlamydia trachomatis* can cause both conjunctivitis and urethritis, and a *Chlamydia* infection can stimulate a genetically predisposed individual to develop reactive arthritis. It is important to rule out an infectious cause in a patient with presumed reactive arthritis, especially because chlamydial urethritis may be asymptomatic. Most of the time, however, the precipitating infection will have resolved by the time the reactive autoimmune response supervenes. See BCSC Section 9, *Intraocular Inflammation and Uveitis,* for additional information on Reiter syndrome.

Other Spondyloarthropathies

Spondyloarthropathy may also occur in association with ulcerative colitis or with Crohn disease. *Ulcerative colitis* is an inflammatory disorder of the gastrointestinal mucosa with diffuse involvement of the colon. *Crohn disease* is a focal granulomatous disease involving all areas of the bowel and affecting both the large and the small intestine. Crohn disease is also known as *regional enteritis, granulomatous ileocolitis,* and *granulomatous colitis.* Symptoms of inflammatory bowel disease include diarrhea, bloody diarrhea, and cramping abdominal pain.

Extraintestinal manifestations of inflammatory bowel disease include dermatitis, mucous membrane disease, ocular inflammation, and arthritis. Arthritis associated with inflammatory bowel disease is referred to as *enteropathic arthritis* and may include a peripheral arthritis or a spondyloarthropathy or both. Multiple series have shown that 50%–75% of patients with inflammatory bowel disease–associated spondyloarthropathy are positive for HLA-B27, which also predisposes them to iridocyclitis. The activity of the spondyloarthropathy is unrelated to the activity of the bowel disease. Enteropathic arthritis that involves the peripheral joints is not associated with HLA-B27, and disease activity tends to parallel the activity of the bowel disease.

Psoriasis is another systemic disease that may be associated with spondyloarthropathy. Psoriatic arthritis may have multiple presentations, including an oligoarthritis, a distal polyarthritis, and a destructive arthritis known as *arthritis mutilans*. Spondyloarthropathy is often seen in psoriatic arthritis, and there is an increased frequency of HLA-B27 in these patients, although the frequency of HLA-B27 in psoriatic arthritis is not as high as it is in ankylosing spondylitis or Reiter syndrome. Uveitis in patients with psoriatic arthritis tends to be more insidious in onset, smoldering, posterior, and bilateral compared with the more typical HLA-B27–associated anterior uveitis.

Spondyloarthropathies may occur in childhood, although their occurrence is rare before the second decade. The diagnosis may be difficult to make because the recurrent arthritis may be initially misdiagnosed as being caused by multiple injuries. Patients may develop all the features of ankylosing spondylitis (juvenile ankylosing spondylitis), or they may have systemic diseases similar to those of the adults (eg, inflammatory bowel disease, reactive arthritis, or psoriasis). Many patients may not meet the criteria for any particular type of spondyloarthropathy and are therefore considered to have undifferentiated disease. As in adults, the majority of young patients are HLA-B27 positive. There tends to be a preponderance of males, and these patients may develop acute uveitis characteristic of HLA-B27–associated uveitis. The juvenile-onset spondyloarthropathies are considered to be a separate category of juvenile idiopathic (rheumatoid) arthritis referred to as enthesitis-related arthritis.

Kiss S, Letko E, Qamruddin S, Baltatzis S, Foster CS. Long-term progression, prognosis, and treatment of patients with recurrent ocular manifestations of Reiter's syndrome. *Ophthalmology.* 2003;110(9):1764–1769.

Monnet D, Breban M, Hudry C, Dougados M, Brézin AP. Ophthalmic findings and frequency of extraocular manifestations in patients with HLA-B27 uveitis: a study of 175 cases. *Ophthalmology.* 2004;111(4):802–809.

Paiva ES, Macaluso DC, Edwards A, Rosenbaum JT. Characterisation of uveitis in patients with psoriatic arthritis. *Ann Rheum Dis.* 2000;59(1):67–70.

Juvenile Idiopathic Arthritis

The older term *juvenile rheumatoid arthritis (JRA)* is being replaced by the term *juvenile idiopathic arthritis (JIA),* or *juvenile chronic arthritis.* The term *rheumatoid* is not considered accurate because for most children, these entities have no relationship to adult-onset RA. The juvenile arthritides have, classically, been divided into 3 subsets based on associated symptoms and the number of joints involved. (Juvenile spondyloarthropathies are included as a fourth category but are discussed separately in the previous section.)

Pauciarticular- (or *oligoarticular-*) *onset JIA* includes patients with involvement of fewer than 5 joints after 6 months of illness. It accounts for approximately 50% of JIA cases. The antinuclear antibody (ANA) test is positive in many of these patients, and there is a strong predilection for females. The arthritis tends to remit, but 10%–50% of patients may develop chronic iridocyclitis. Thus, periodic eye examinations are important in order to detect occult ocular inflammation. (See BCSC Section 6, *Pediatric Ophthalmology and Strabismus,* and Section 9, *Intraocular Inflammation and Uveitis.*)

Responsible for 30%–40% of JIA cases, *polyarticular-onset arthritis* is defined by the involvement of more than 4 joints after 6 months of illness. As with pauciarticular-onset JIA, there is a female preponderance. The arthritis tends to be severe, but uveitis is rare.

Responsible for approximately 10%–15% of JIA cases, *systemic-onset arthritis* (formerly called *Still disease*) refers to patients with fever, rash, and arthritis of any number of joints. Patients may also have hepatosplenomegaly and lymphadenopathy. The male–female ratio for systemic-onset arthritis is approximately 1:1, in contrast with that of the other variants. Ocular disease is generally not associated with this variant.

This classification is now considered insufficient to reflect the many subgroups that exist within each category. Recently proposed criteria for classification of the idiopathic arthritides of childhood attempt to define these diseases in a way that will allow differentiation of etiologic mechanisms, prognostication, and response to therapy. This newer classification system includes systemic arthritis, polyarthritis, pauciarthritis, psoriatic arthritis, and enthesitis-related arthritis (the last category includes spondyloarthropathies). Each category then has various subcategories, such as ANA positivity and the presence of uveitis. However, because there is currently no universal agreement regarding this approach, several different classification systems are still in use. It is therefore likely that the older terminology will persist at the interface of pediatric rheumatology and ophthalmology, at least for now, because the screening and treatment guidelines for uveitis are based on the classic categories.

Systemic Lupus Erythematosus

Systemic lupus erythematosus (SLE) is generally regarded as the prototypical autoimmune disease. The cause of SLE is unknown, but familial aggregation of autoimmune diseases and association with the HLA types DR2 and DR3 suggest a genetic predisposition. Pathogenically, SLE is characterized by B-cell hyperreactivity, polyclonal B-cell activation, hypergammaglobulinemia, and a plethora of autoantibodies. These autoantibodies include antinuclear antibodies, antibodies to DNA, and antibodies to cytoplasmic components. SLE classically has been considered an immune complex disease in which immune complexes incite an inflammatory response and lead to tissue damage.

Women, especially in their 20s and 30s, are affected more frequently than men. Patients with SLE are subject to myriad symptoms and to inflammation that can affect virtually every organ. Although multiple system involvement is typical, patients may also present with single organ involvement such as nephritis or cytopenia. Cutaneous disease, which occurs in approximately 70%–80% of patients, is most often manifested by the characteristic butterfly rash across the nose and cheeks, also known as a *malar rash*. Other cutaneous manifestations include discoid lesions, vasculitic skin lesions such as cutaneous ulcers or splinter hemorrhages, purpuric skin lesions, and alopecia. Mucosal lesions, characteristically painless oral ulcers, occur in 30%–40% of patients. Photosensitivity occurs in many patients with SLE.

Approximately 80%–85% of patients with SLE experience articular disease at some point, either a polyarthralgia or a nondeforming, migratory polyarthritis. Systemic features—including fatigue, fever, and weight loss—occur in more than 80% of patients with lupus. Renal disease is present in approximately 50%–75% of patients, presenting clinically as either proteinuria with nephrotic characteristics or glomerulonephritis with an active urinary sediment. Lupus nephritis is a major cause of the morbidity and mortality of SLE.

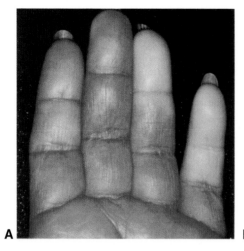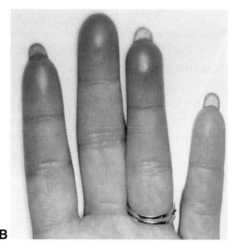

A   **B**

Figure 8-1 Raynaud phenomenon. **A,** Sharply demarcated pallor resulting from the closure of digital arteries. **B,** Digital cyanosis of the fingertips in a patient with primary Raynaud phenomenon. *(Reproduced with permission from Wigley FM. Clinical Practice. Raynaud's phenomenon. N Engl J Med. 2002;347(13):1001. Copyright ©2002 Massachusetts Medical Society.)*

Raynaud phenomenon occurs in 30%–50% of SLE patients (Fig 8-1), and hepatosplenomegaly and adenopathy occur in more than 50%. Cardiac disease includes pericarditis, occasionally myocarditis, and Libman-Sacks endocarditis. Pleuropulmonary lesions cause pleuritic chest pain and, less commonly, pneumonitis.

Central nervous system (CNS) involvement occurs in more than 35% of patients with SLE, and manifestations are typically transient. The most common manifestations of CNS lupus are headache, seizures, an organic brain syndrome, and psychosis. Transverse myelitis is an uncommon manifestation in patients with SLE, but it can occur in association with optic neuritis in active disease. Pseudotumor cerebri also can be associated with SLE.

SLE frequently affects the hematologic system. Patients often have an anemia of chronic disease but may also develop an autoimmune hemolytic anemia. Leukopenia, in particular lymphopenia, is a characteristic feature. Thrombocytopenia occurs in approximately one third of patients.

Diagnosis

Because of the protean manifestations of SLE, a list of diagnostic criteria has been established (Table 8-1). Four or more of these criteria must be met for a diagnosis of definite SLE; patients with fewer criteria may be labeled *probable* or *possible SLE*.

The ANA test is the best diagnostic test for SLE and should be performed whenever SLE is suspected. The result of the ANA test is positive in significant titer (usually 1:160 or higher) in virtually all patients with SLE. A positive test at lower titers is not as specific because many diseases other than SLE may be ANA-positive. However, if the ANA test result is negative, it is very unlikely that a patient has SLE.

In the past, diagnostic significance was assigned to the pattern of antibody staining demonstrated by the ANA test (ie, homogeneous, peripheral, speckled, nucleolar).

Table 8-1 ARA Criteria for Diagnosis of Systemic Lupus Erythematosus

Criterion	Definition
Malar rash	Fixed erythema, flat or raised, over the malar eminences, tending to spare the nasolabial folds
Discoid rash	Erythematosus raised patches with adherent keratotic scaling and follicular plugging; atrophic scarring may occur in older lesions
Photosensitivity	Skin rash as a result of unusual reaction to sunlight, by patient history or physician observation
Oral ulcers	Oral or nasopharyngeal ulceration, usually painless, observed by a physician
Arthritis	Nonerosive arthritis involving 2 or more peripheral joints, characterized by tenderness, swelling, or effusion
Serositis	Pleuritis—convincing history of pleuritic pain or rub heard by a physician or evidence of pleural effusion **OR** pericarditis—documented by EKG, rub, or evidence of pericardial effusion
Renal disorder	Persistent proteinuria greater than 0.5 gram per day or greater than 3+ if quantitation not performed **OR** cellular casts—may be red cell, hemoglobin, granular, tubular, or mixed
Neurologic disorder	Seizures **OR** psychosis—in the absence of offending drugs or known metabolic derangements (uremia, ketoacidosis, or electrolyte imbalance)
Hematologic disorder	Hemolytic anemia—with reticulocytosis **OR** leukopenia—less than 4000/mm^3 total on 2 or more occasions **OR** lymphopenia—less than 1500/mm^3 on 2 or more occasions **OR** thrombocytopenia—less than 100,000/mm^3 in the absence of offending drugs
Immunologic disorders	Positive antiphospholipid antibody **OR** anti-DNA—antibody to native DNA in abnormal titer **OR** anti-Sm—presence of antibody to Sm nuclear antigen **OR** false-positive serologic test for syphilis known to be positive for at least 6 months and confirmed by *Treponema pallidum* immobilization or fluorescent treponemal antibody absorption test
Antinuclear antibody	An abnormal titer of antinuclear antibody by immunofluorescence or an equivalent assay at any point in time and in the absence of drugs known to be associated with "drug-induced lupus" syndrome

SM = Smith.

From Schur PH, Wallace DJ. Diagnosis and differential diagnosis of systemic lupus erythematosus in adults. In: *UpToDate*, Rose BD (ed), Waltham, MA. Available at www.uptodate.com. Accessed September 14, 2009.

Because the interpretation of these patterns may be subjective, greater emphasis is now placed on assays that look for the specific type of autoantibody that is causing the staining. Two such autoantibodies that are highly specific for SLE are anti–double-stranded DNA (anti-dsDNA) antibodies and anti-Smith (anti-Sm) antibodies. There is also a host of additional specific antinuclear and cytoplasmic antibodies (anti-Ro, or anti–SS-A; anti-La, or anti–SS-B; anti-RNP; and anti-RA33, to name a few) that may indicate a predisposition to specific SLE manifestations or suggest the presence of another autoimmune disease (for instance, Sjögren syndrome is associated with anti–SS-A and anti–SS-B).

Unfortunately, ANA testing is often done to screen for disease in patients with little likelihood of having SLE (such as uveitis patients with no systemic symptoms). The test is very nonspecific under these circumstances. False-positive ANAs are commonly found in the normal population; one study found that 32% of individuals without SLE had an ANA titer above 1:40. The combination of very low titers of antibody (<1:80) and no signs or symptoms of disease suggests that the patient should simply be monitored.

SLE can run a varied clinical course, ranging from a relatively benign illness to fulminant organ failure and death. Most patients have a relapsing and remitting course that requires frequent titration of medications. Treatment depends on disease severity and may include NSAIDs, hydroxychloroquine (Plaquenil), glucocorticoids, and immunosuppressive drugs. Refractory cases may require high-dose pulse therapy with glucocorticoids and cyclophosphamide (Cytoxan). Experimental treatments include immunoablation, with or without hematopoetic stem cell transplantation, and anti–B-cell antibodies. Such treatments are reserved for life-threatening disease that is unresponsive to standard measures.

Reichlin M. Measurement and clinical significance of antinuclear antibodies. In: *UpToDate*, Rose BD (ed), Waltham, MA. Available at www.uptodate.com. Accessed September 14, 2009.

◉ **Ophthalmic considerations**   The major ocular manifestations of SLE include discoid lesions of the skin of the eyelids, keratitis sicca from secondary Sjögren syndrome, and retinal and choroidal microvascular lesions. Retinal lesions include cotton-wool spots, hemorrhages, vascular occlusions, and neovascularization. The prevalence of ocular manifestations varies from 3% of outpatients to 29% of hospitalized patients. The inflammatory vasculopathy of SLE should be distinguished from vascular damage due to secondary problems such as hypertension from renal disease or occlusions due to embolic disease or antiphospholipid antibodies. Typical anterior or intermediate uveitis is not a common feature of SLE. Neuro-ophthalmic involvement in SLE includes cranial nerve palsies, lupus optic neuropathy, and central retrochiasmal disorders of vision. The cerebral disorders of vision include hallucinations, visual field defects, and cortical blindness. (See also BCSC Section 9, *Intraocular Inflammation and Uveitis,* and Section 12, *Retina and Vitreous.*)

Antiphospholipid Antibody Syndrome

The *antiphospholipid antibody syndrome (APS)* is a potential cause of vascular thrombosis. The diagnosis of APS requires the presence of both clinical and laboratory findings, specifically, by fulfilling 1 of the clinical and 1 of the laboratory criteria. The clinical features include one or more episodes of arterial and/or venous thrombosis or complications of pregnancy such as fetal death, spontaneous abortions without a maternal cause, and premature births. Laboratory criteria include anticardiolipin IgG or IgM antibodies present at moderate to high levels and/or lupus anticoagulant activity. Abnormalities in laboratory tests must be detected on at least 2 different occasions at least 12 weeks apart.

Antiphospholipid antibody syndrome can occur in association with SLE and other rheumatic diseases, and it can be caused by certain infections and drugs. When it occurs alone, it is referred to as the *primary APS*. The main clinical manifestation is venous and arterial thrombosis. Deep venous thrombosis is the most common type of thrombosis, occurring in approximately one third of patients. Patients may also have pulmonary embolism and superficial thrombophlebitis. Central nervous system disease can include strokes, transient ischemic attacks, dementia, and even psychosis. APS should be considered when cerebrovascular disease occurs in a young patient without other risk factors for stroke.

Episodes of thrombosis can be recurrent; this recurrence may be more likely in patients with high antiphospholipid antibody titers. Additional manifestations of APS include thrombocytopenia, hemolytic anemia, and livedo reticularis. Cardiac manifestations include valvular thickening and vegetations, both of which are caused by thrombotic endocardial deposits. This syndrome can also cause significant problems with pregnancy. Patients may have multiple first-trimester abortions and premature births due to preeclampsia or placental insufficiency, and fetal death may occur after 10 weeks. In rare instances, a severe form of APS can occur with multiple vessel occlusion and multiorgan failure. This is referred to as *catastrophic antiphospholipid syndrome* and carries a mortality rate of 48%.

Diagnosis

Testing for antiphospholipid antibodies can be divided into 2 broad categories: tests for anticardiolipin antibodies and tests for lupus anticoagulants. Anticardiolipin antibodies are 1 type of antiphospholipid antibody; in testing, researchers usually look for both IgG and IgM antibodies, with medium to high levels being more clinically significant. Among blood donors without APS, 5%–10% may have some level of positive anticardiolipin antibodies, and this percentage can be higher among older donors. However, repeatedly positive results are required for a diagnosis of APS, and, in one study, less than 2% of the normal population remained positive for a period of 9 months. Antiphospholipid antibodies also occur in association with other conditions, such as infections or cancer, and with the use of some drugs. In these cases, the antibodies are present at low levels and are not usually associated with thrombotic events.

In addition to tests for anticardiolipin antibodies, other tests for antiphospholipid antibodies include a false-positive serology for syphilis, tests for antiphosphatidylserine antibodies, and tests for antibodies to the plasma protein β2-glycoprotein I, which is a phospholipid-binding inhibitor of coagulation. The risk of thrombosis may increase with both the absolute level of antiphospholipid antibodies and the number of different antibodies. There is an ongoing effort to standardize the various assays between laboratories and to identify the most clinically relevant types of antiphospholipid antibodies.

Testing for lupus anticoagulant activity involves looking for evidence of a functional inhibition of clotting. Whereas testing for antiphospholipid antibodies simply indicates whether such antibodies are present, testing for lupus anticoagulant activity determines if the antibodies have an identifiable effect on phospholipid-dependent clotting pathways. With lupus anticoagulant positivity, there seems to be a somewhat greater risk for thrombosis than with isolated antiphospholipid positivity. Lupus anticoagulants prolong in vitro clotting assays such as the activated partial thromboplastin time (aPTT), the dilute Russell viper venom time (dRVVT), the kaolin plasma clotting time (KCT), and, in rare cases, the prothrombin time. More than 1 test for lupus anticoagulant is often needed because patients with negative test results for 1 test may have positive results for another.

The antibodies detected by assays for antiphospholipid antibodies may or may not be the same antibodies responsible for lupus anticoagulant activity—hence, the need to perform both types of testing when the disease is suspected. The remarkable complexity of the coagulation system is demonstrated by the apparent paradox of lupus anticoagulants. The in vitro effect of these substances results in inhibition of clotting, yet in vivo the effect is to enhance thrombosis. A number of mechanisms have been postulated for the procoagulant effect. One possibility is that antiphospholipid antibodies may interfere with the normal anticoagulant effect of β2-glycoprotein I and lead to spontaneous thrombosis.

Ophthalmic considerations   Ophthalmic manifestations of APS include amaurosis fugax, ischemic optic neuropathy, and retinal and choroidal vascular occlusion. Visual field loss, diplopia, and even proliferative retinopathy have also been reported. Some studies have suggested that the prevalence of antiphospholipid antibodies is increased in patients with retinal vaso-occlusive disease, but it is difficult to assign a definite causative etiology, given the prevalence of antiphospholipid antibodies in the population without APS. Furthermore, in a study looking for ophthalmic findings in a population of patients with known APS, no patients had definite vaso-occlusive disease, and only 13% of patients had identifiable changes, which largely consisted of mild retinopathy. Patients in this series were more likely to have visual symptoms from neurologic disease.

Although a high index of suspicion for APS should be maintained, testing for this entity may lead to false-positive results, and determining if a cause-and-effect relationship truly exists may be difficult. This is important because treatment of APS may include long-term anticoagulation, which carries a significant risk, and it may be very difficult for a consulting specialist to determine if an isolated ophthalmic vascular occlusion represents the type of thrombotic episode that warrants such treatment. In such cases, it has been proposed that repeatedly positive levels of antiphospholipid antibodies suggest the presence of APS. More studies are needed to determine the prevalence of ophthalmic disease in APS, as well as the significance of positive laboratory test results in patients with ocular vaso-occlusive disease without systemic features of APS.

Treatment

Therapy for thrombosis usually consists of heparin, followed by warfarin (Coumadin). The optimal duration of treatment is not known. Some experts feel that anticoagulation can be discontinued if the antiphospholipid antibody titers decrease, but lifelong treatment is recommended for patients with recurrent disease. Treatment of the pregnant patient remains controversial and may include some combination of heparin or low-molecular-weight heparin and aspirin (warfarin is teratogenic). Patients with antiphospholipid anti-bodies but no prior history of thrombosis may benefit from prophylactic aspirin.

Behbehani R, Sergott RC, Savino PJ. The antiphospholipid antibody syndrome: diagnostic aspects. *Curr Opin Ophthalmol.* 2004;15(6):483–485.

Scleroderma

Scleroderma, also known as *progressive systemic sclerosis,* is a rheumatic disease character-ized by fibrous and degenerative changes in the viscera, skin, or both. The disease seems to be mediated by the activation of fibroblasts that produce excessive fibrosis, but the mechanism by which this occurs is not understood. Scleroderma is much more common in women and rare in childhood. The disorder may be localized (confined to the skin, subcutaneous tissue, and muscle) or systemic (which may be diffuse or limited). Localized scleroderma is not a severe illness and may allow a normal life span. The limited form of systemic scleroderma, known as *CREST* (calcinosis, Raynaud phenomenon, esophageal involvement, sclerodactyly, and telangiectasias), involves internal organs less frequently than does the diffuse form and therefore carries a better prognosis.

In addition to the thickening and fibrous replacement of the dermis, scleroderma is characterized by vascular insufficiency and vasospasm. The hallmark of scleroderma is the skin change, which consists of thickening, tightening, and induration, with sub-sequent loss of mobility and contracture. The disease most characteristically begins pe-ripherally and involves the fingers and hands, with a subsequent centripetal spread up the arms to involve the face and body. Telangiectasia and calcinosis (calcium phosphate nodules under the skin) are common. More than 95% of scleroderma patients experience Raynaud phenomenon (see Fig 8-1). Although Raynaud phenomenon usually represents reversible vasospasm, in scleroderma, episodes may be prolonged, and the structure of vessels is permanently altered, possibly leading to digital ulcers or infarcts.

Organ involvement is common and includes esophageal dysmotility with gastro-esophageal reflux in more than 90% of patients. The small and large intestines may be involved, with decreased motility, malabsorption, and diverticulosis. Cardiopulmonary disease is manifested primarily by pulmonary fibrosis, which results in restrictive lung disease with a decreased diffusing capacity. The consequences of the interstitial fibrosis include pulmonary hypertension and right-sided heart failure. Conduction abnormali-ties and arrhythmias result from cardiac fibrosis. Musculoskeletal features include polyar-thralgias, tendon friction rubs, and, occasionally, myositis. There is no known cure for the disease, and treatment is largely directed toward controlling problems related to the organ systems involved.

Most patients with scleroderma have positive ANA test results. It was thought that certain antinuclear staining patterns were fairly specific for scleroderma (such as the nucleolar pattern), but it is now recognized that these are not especially sensitive or spe-cific. Instead, testing is done looking for specific ANAs such as anti-centromere, anti-topoisomerase I (anti–Scl-70), and anti-RNA polymerase. These tests can help with the diagnosis and may help identify various syndromes that overlap with scleroderma. The best-known overlap syndrome is *mixed connective tissue disease,* which has features of SLE, systemic sclerosis, and myositis. This syndrome is characterized by autoantibodies directed at U1-ribonucleoprotein complex.

Renal disease is a major cause of mortality and is often associated with the onset of malignant hypertension and a rapid progression to renal failure *(scleroderma renal crisis).* This complication was uniformly fatal until the late 1970s, when aggressive antihypertensive therapy was found to be able to sometimes reverse the scleroderma renal crisis.

Ophthalmic considerations   Ocular manifestations of scleroderma include eyelid involvement resulting in tightness and blepharophimosis (but only rarely corneal exposure); conjunctival vascular abnormalities, including telangiectasia and vascular sludging; and keratoconjunctivitis sicca. Patchy choroidal nonperfusion can be seen on fluorescein angiography as part of the diffuse microvascular damage caused by scleroderma. Occasionally, as a result of scleroderma renal crisis, a patient develops retinopathy of malignant hypertension, with cotton-wool spots, intraretinal hemorrhages, and optic disc edema.

Sjögren Syndrome

Sjögren syndrome was originally described as a triad of dry eyes, dry mouth, and RA. Subsequently, it became apparent that Sjögren syndrome could coexist with a variety of other connective tissue diseases, including SLE and scleroderma (secondary Sjögren syndrome), or without a definable connective tissue disease (primary Sjögren syndrome). The ophthalmologist is often the first physician to see these patients once they become symptomatic.

The dry eyes and dry mouth in patients with Sjögren syndrome are the result of an inflammatory mononuclear infiltrate involving the lacrimal and salivary glands that causes glandular destruction and dysfunction. Several studies have demonstrated the usefulness of minor salivary gland biopsy in documenting the presence of such an inflammatory infiltrate. Patients with Sjögren syndrome often have autoantibodies known as anti–SS-A and anti–SS-B. Criteria for the diagnosis of Sjögren syndrome have been published, including parameters referring to oral and ocular symptoms, ocular signs, salivary gland involvement, histopathologic features, and the presence of autoantibodies anti–SS-A and anti–SS-B. The presence of 4 of 6 items confers high sensitivity and specificity. Patients with primary Sjögren syndrome may have a number of possible systemic manifestations that extend far beyond dry eyes and mouth, including upper-airway dryness and mucous plugs, purpuric vasculitis, hyperglobulinemia, CNS inflammation that may mimic multiple sclerosis, psychiatric problems, and an increased risk of lymphoma. Treatment is aimed at symptomatic relief and substitution of the missing secretions, although immunosuppression may be necessary for patients with systemic manifestations. (Sjögren syndrome is discussed in detail in BCSC Section 8, *External Disease and Cornea.*)

Polymyositis and Dermatomyositis

Polymyositis and *dermatomyositis* are inflammatory diseases of skeletal muscle characterized by pain and weakness in the involved muscular groups. Typically, weakness begins insidiously and involves the proximal muscle groups, particularly those of the shoulders and hips. Dermatomyositis is distinguished from polymyositis by the presence of cutaneous lesions. These skin lesions are an erythematous to violaceous rash variably affecting the eyelids (heliotrope rash), cheeks, nose, chest (V-neck sign), and extensor surfaces (Gottron sign). Pathogenically, dermatomyositis is associated with immune complex deposition in the vessels, whereas polymyositis appears to reflect direct T-cell–mediated muscle injury. Laboratory findings include elevated serum levels of skeletal muscle enzymes and abnormal electromyography results; also, muscle damage and inflammation may be revealed by muscle biopsy. These entities may be primary, or they may arise in association with a malignancy. They may also overlap with other connective tissue diseases, such as in mixed connective tissue disease, which has features of scleroderma, SLE, and myositis.

Ocular involvement is relatively uncommon in inflammatory myositis, other than the heliotrope rash of dermatomyositis, which is very specific but not often present (Fig 8-2). Occasionally, ophthalmoplegia may occur because of involvement of the extraocular muscles, which myositis can provoke.

Relapsing Polychondritis

Relapsing polychondritis is an episodic autoimmune disorder characterized by recurrent, widespread, potentially destructive inflammation of cartilage, the cardiovascular system, and the organs of special sense. The most common clinical features are auricular inflammation, arthropathy, and nasal cartilage inflammation. Auricular chondritis and nasal chondritis are the features that most often suggest the diagnosis. Laryngotracheobronchial disease may lead to a fatal complication from laryngeal collapse. Involvement of the internal ear, cardiovascular system, and skin is less common. Cardiovascular lesions include aortic insufficiency (due to progressive dilation of the aortic root) and vasculitis. Skin lesions are most often due to cutaneous vasculitis.

This disease can be associated with other autoimmune diseases such as SLE or RA or with any of the systemic vasculitides, such as Wegener granulomatosis, polyarteritis

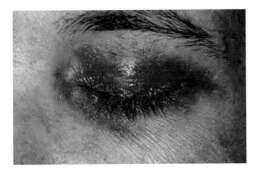

Figure 8-2 Heliotrope rash in dermatomyositis. A reddish purple eruption on the upper eyelid (the heliotrope rash), accompanied by swelling of the eyelid in a patient with dermatomyositis. This is the most specific rash in DM, although it is present only in a minority of patients. *(Reproduced with permission from Miller ML, MD. Clinical manifestations and diagnosis of adult dermatomyositis and polymyositis. In: UpToDate, Rose BD (ed), Waltham, MA. Available at www.uptodate.com.)*

nodosa, and Behçet disease. Other associations include Sjögren syndrome, Graves disease, and myelodysplastic syndromes (dysplastic and ineffective blood cell production due to malignant stem cells). Ocular manifestations occur in approximately 50% of patients with relapsing polychondritis. The most common ocular conditions are conjunctivitis, scleritis, uveitis, and retinal vasculitis.

Vasculitis

The primary systemic vasculitides are a group of diseases whose principal pathology involves autoimmune damage to blood vessels. The classification of these entities is largely based on the size of the vessel involved and the various clinical features. Table 8-2 outlines the definitions created by the Chapel Hill Consensus Conference on these diseases. Recently, an algorithm was developed to allow more specific classification of patients with Wegener granulomatosis, microscopic polyangiitis, Churg-Strauss syndrome, and polyarteritis nodosa. The algorithm expands on the Chapel Hill classification by using features such as the clinical presentation, the presence of antineutrophil cytoplasmic antibodies (ANCA), and histology to distinguish these often overlapping diseases.

A number of other diseases are capable of causing vasculitis as part of their clinical spectrum; these are considered to be secondary vasculitides. Secondary causes of vasculitis include exogenous factors such as infections, neoplasia, or use of certain drugs. Secondary vasculitis can also occur as part of other autoimmune disorders such as SLE or Behçet disease. This section emphasizes the primary vasculitides that are more likely to have ophthalmic involvement.

Watts R, Lane S, Hanslik T, et al. Development and validation of a consensus methodology for the classification of the ANCA-associated vasculitides and polyarteritis nodosa for epidemiological studies. *Ann Rheum Dis.* 2007;66(2):222–227.

Large-Vessel Vasculitis

Giant cell (temporal) arteritis
Giant cell arteritis is of particular concern to ophthalmologists and is discussed thoroughly in BCSC Section 5, *Neuro-Ophthalmology.*

Takayasu arteritis
Takayasu arteritis affects large arteries, particularly branches of the aorta. It occurs primarily in children and young women. The disease is rare in the West but common in the Far East, particularly Japan. Other names for Takayasu arteritis include *aortic arch arteritis, aortitis syndrome,* and *pulseless disease.*

The disease may involve the entire aorta or be localized to any segment of the aorta or its primary branches. The inflammatory process is characterized by a panarteritis with a granulomatous inflammation. The involved vessels may ultimately become narrowed or obliterated, resulting in ischemia to the supplied tissues. Areas of weakened vascular wall may develop dissections or aneurysms.

Systemic features such as fatigue, weight loss, or low-grade fever are common. Evidence of vascular insufficiency due to large-artery narrowing leads to the characteristic

Table 8-2 Names and Definitions of Vasculitides Adopted by the Chapel Hill Consensus Conference on the Nomenclature of Systemic Vasculitis

Name	Definition
Large-vessel vasculitis*	
Giant cell (temporal) arteritis	Granulomatous arteritis of the aorta and its major branches, with a predilection for the extracranial branches of the carotid artery. *Often involves the temporal artery. Usually occurs in patients older than 50 and often is associated with polymyalgia rheumatica.*
Takayasu arteritis	Granulomatous inflammation of the aorta and its major branches. *Usually occurs in patients younger than 50.*
Medium-sized–vessel vasculitis	
Polyarteritis nodosa†	Necrotizing inflammation of medium-sized or small arteries without glomerulonephritis or vasculitis in arterioles, capillaries, or venules.
Kawasaki disease	Arteritis involving large, medium-sized, and small arteries and associated with mucocutaneous lymph node syndrome. *Coronary arteries are often involved. Aorta and veins may be involved. Usually occurs in children.*
Small-vessel vasculitis	
Wegener granulomatosis‡	Granulomatous inflammation involving the respiratory tract, and necrotizing vasculitis, affecting small to medium-sized vessels. *Necrotizing glomerulonephritis is common.*
Churg-Strauss syndrome‡	Eosinophil-rich and granulomatous inflammation involving the respiratory tract, and necrotizing vasculitis affecting small to medium-sized vessels, and associated with asthma and eosinophilia.
Microscopic polyangiitis† (microscopic polyarteritis)‡	Necrotizing vasculitis, with few or no immune deposits, affecting small vessels (ie, capillaries, venules, arterioles). *Necrotizing arteritis involving small and medium-sized arteries may be present. Necrotizing glomerulonephritis is very common. Pulmonary capillaritis often occurs.*
Henoch-Schönlein purpura	Vasculitis, with IgA-dominant immune deposits, affecting small vessels (ie, capillaries, venules, arterioles). *Typically involves skin, gut, and glomeruli and is associated with arthralgias or arthritis.*
Essential cryoglobulinemic vasculitis	Vasculitis, with cryoglobulin immune deposits, affecting small vessels (ie, capillaries, venules, arterioles), and associated with cryoglobulins in serum. *Skin and glomeruli are often involved.*
Cutaneous leukocytoclastic angiitis	Isolated cutaneous leukocytoclastic angiitis without systemic vasculitis or glomerulonephritis.

*"Large vessel" refers to the aorta and the largest branches directed toward major body regions (eg, to the extremities and the head and neck); "medium-sized vessel" refers to the main visceral arteries (eg, renal, hepatic, coronary, and mesenteric arteries); "small vessel" refers to venules, capillaries, arterioles, and the intraparenchymal distal arterial radicals that connect the arterioles. Some small- and large-vessel vasculitides may involve medium-sized arteries, but large- and medium-sized–vessel vasculitides do not involve vessels smaller than arteries. Essential components are represented by normal type; italicized type represents usual, but not essential, components.

†Preferred term.

‡Strongly associated with antineutrophil cytoplasmic autoantibodies.

Reprinted with permission from Jennette JC, Falk RJ, Andrassy K, et al. Nomenclature of systemic vasculitides. Proposal of an international consensus conference. *Arthritis Rheum.* 1994;37(2):187–192.

pulseless phase. The disease is most often diagnosed via arteriography. Treatment is generally with systemic corticosteroids, which may successfully suppress the disease. Cyclophosphamide or methotrexate is added in resistant cases. Surgical reconstruction of damaged vessels may be necessary.

Ophthalmic considerations   Patients with Takayasu arteritis may report transient visual disturbances and blindness due to decreased perfusion. The most characteristic ocular findings are retinal arteriovenous anastomoses, best demonstrated by fluorescein angiography. Milder changes found earlier in the course of the disease include small-vessel dilation and microaneurysm formation; more severe ischemia may result in peripheral retinal nonperfusion, iris and retinal neovascularization, and vitreous hemorrhage.

Medium-sized–Vessel Vasculitis

Polyarteritis nodosa

Classic *polyarteritis nodosa (PAN)* is characterized by necrotizing vasculitis of the medium-sized and small muscular arteries. The lesions are segmental, and aneurysms may develop, which can be detected by angiography. One of the most common presenting symptoms is mononeuritis multiplex, which is simultaneous or sequential ischemic damage to anatomically unrelated peripheral nerves. CNS lesions can also occur. Renal involvement is common, and hypertension develops as a consequence of the renal disease. Gastrointestinal disease with infarction of the viscera is also common. Polyarteritis nodosa may be limited to a single organ, such as the appendix, uterus, or testes. It may be triggered by hepatitis B.

The mean age of onset of PAN is 40–50 years; men are affected more often than women. Survival in patients with untreated PAN is poor. However, most patients are now treated with a combination of corticosteroids and an immunosuppressive drug such as cyclophosphamide, and this therapy appears to improve disease control and long-term outcome.

Ophthalmic considerations   Ocular manifestations occur in approximately 10%–20% of patients with PAN and include hypertensive retinopathy, retinal vasculitis, and visual field loss from CNS lesions. Cranial nerve palsies can occur, as well as scleritis and marginal corneal ulceration. Choroidal vasculitis is often overlooked in PAN and may cause transient visual symptoms, exudative retinal detachments, and pigment changes. Fluorescein angiography may be necessary to identify choroidal involvement. *Cogan syndrome,* manifested by interstitial keratitis, hearing loss, tinnitus, and vertigo, may be associated with PAN (see also BCSC Section 8, *External Disease and Cornea*). There is no specific test to diagnose PAN. Rather, the diagnosis depends on characteristic clinical features, angiographic findings, and biopsy results. Results of hepatitis B studies may be positive in a subset of patients.

Small-Vessel Vasculitis

Wegener granulomatosis

Wegener granulomatosis (also known as ANCA-associated granulomatosis vasculitis) was originally described as the classic triad of necrotizing granulomatous vasculitis of both the upper and lower respiratory tract and focal segmental glomerulonephritis. The clinical features of Wegener granulomatosis include granulomatous inflammation of the paranasal sinuses in 90% of cases, nasopharyngeal disease in 63%, cutaneous vasculitis in 45%, and vasculitis affecting the nervous system in 25%. Ocular disease occurs in up to 60% of patients and may be the presenting feature. Ocular findings include scleritis with or without peripheral keratitis, orbital pseudotumor, and vasculitis-mediated retinal vascular or neuro-ophthalmic lesions. Limited forms of the disease may occur without significant systemic involvement and may be difficult to diagnose. Approximately 80% of patients with Wegener granulomatosis are serum-positive for a cytoplasmic pattern of ANCA (c-ANCA). As this cytoplasmic pattern is usually caused by the presence of autoantibodies to proteinase 3, the specificity of positive findings for c-ANCA may be enhanced by testing for these antibodies. (See also BCSC Section 7, *Orbit, Eyelids, and Lacrimal System,* and BCSC Section 9, *Intraocular Inflammation and Uveitis.*)

Before immunosuppressive drugs were used to treat Wegener granulomatosis, the disease was uniformly fatal, with a mean untreated survival rate of 5 months. With corticosteroid treatment, the mean survival time increased to 12.5 months; long-term survival occurred only in patients with limited disease. However, the use of cytotoxic drugs, especially cyclophosphamide (Cytoxan), has dramatically improved the outcome for patients with Wegener granulomatosis. Once the disease is controlled, it may be possible to switch to safer immunosuppressive agents such as methotrexate. Trimethoprim-sulfamethoxazole (Bactrim, Septra) may also be helpful in preventing relapses.

Microscopic polyangiitis is a systemic necrotizing vasculitis affecting small vessels and associated with necrotizing glomerulonephritis. It is felt by some investigators to be part of a spectrum of Wegener granulomatosis. Characteristic features include constitutional symptoms, renal disease, pulmonary involvement, arthralgias, rash, and neuropathy. Patients with microscopic polyangiitis often have positive findings for ANCA, with peripheral staining around the nucleus (p-ANCA). This particular staining pattern is nonspecific and needs to be confirmed by testing for autoantibodies to myeloperoxidase (MPO-ANCA). Peripheral ulcerative keratitis may be a presenting feature of this entity.

Churg-Strauss syndrome

An allergic diathesis, particularly asthma, is present in Churg-Strauss syndrome (CSS) (allergic granulomatosis and angiitis). Eosinophilia is generally present, often before the disease manifests, and pathologic examination often shows granulomas with eosinophilic tissue infiltration of smaller vessels. The disease tends to overlap both PAN and Wegener granulomatosis. Asthma is the principal feature of the disease, and the systemic vasculitis may, in addition, involve the heart, skin, kidneys, and gastrointestinal tract. CNS disease may also occur, and mononeuritis multiplex is common. Ophthalmic manifestations include conjunctival granulomas, retinal vasculitis and occlusion, uveitis, and cranial nerve palsies. The diagnosis depends on the presence of several criteria, including asthma, eosinophilia, eosinophilic vasculitis, transient pulmonary infiltrates, and neuropathy. Patients with CSS may also have positive p-ANCA titers.

Behçet Syndrome

Behçet syndrome was initially described as a triad of oral ulcers, genital ulcers, and uveitis with hypopyon. It is now recognized as a multisystem vasculitis of unknown etiology with various clinical manifestations. The disease is most common in the Middle East and Far East, particularly Japan. Oral ulcers are the most common clinical feature, affecting 98%–99% of patients. Genital ulcers occur in 80%–87%; skin disease occurs in 69%–90% and includes erythema nodosum, superficial thrombophlebitis, and pyoderma. Pathergy (pustular response to skin injury) and dermatographism (firmly stroking the skin causes a urticarial wheal) can also be seen. Some 44%–59% of patients have asymmetric, nondeforming, large-joint polyarthritis that frequently responds to corticosteroids.

Vascular disease, which occurs in 10%–35% of patients, can present as migratory superficial thrombophlebitis, major-vessel thrombosis, arterial aneurysms, or even peripheral gangrene. CNS disease, found in 10%–30% of patients, has classically been divided into 3 types: brainstem syndrome, meningoencephalitis, and confusional states. Most often, patients present with combinations of the three. The major cause of mortality in Behçet syndrome is CNS involvement or large-vessel disease.

A number of nonspecific abnormalities in laboratory findings may be seen in these patients, including an elevated ESR, C-reactive protein, and circulating immune complexes. Patients may also have serologic evidence of a hypercoagulable state and elevated levels of intracellular adhesion molecule-1. The prevalence of HLA-B51 is also greater in some populations with Behçet syndrome. However, no specific laboratory tests define Behçet disease. The diagnosis is based on the patient's meeting clinical criteria that include oral ulcers and any 2 of the following: uveitis, genital ulcers, skin involvement, or pathergy. Other criteria may be used, depending on regional differences in disease presentation.

Treatment

The use of corticosteroids alone may control acute exacerbations but does not seem to alter the ultimate outcome of this disease. As a result, one or more immunosuppressive agents is usually added as therapy. Unfortunately, many small studies suggest, but do not prove, the effectiveness of various agents, and there is a paucity of large well-controlled trials to guide the choice of therapy. Common treatments include use of drugs such as azathioprine (Imuran) and cyclosporine (Neoral, Sandimmune), although there may be an increased risk of inducing CNS disease with use of cyclosporine. Alkylating agents such as cyclophosphamide (Cytoxan) and chlorambucil (Leukeran) may be used in refractory cases, although these drugs may have significant toxicity. Newer agents that may hold promise include infliximab (Remicade) and interferon alfa-2a (Roferon-A), especially for treatment of ophthalmic disease.

👁 **Ophthalmic considerations**   Ophthalmic disease is a significant cause of morbidity in Behçet syndrome, with the most common ocular manifestations being iridocyclitis, with or without hypopyon, and retinal vasculitis. The natural history of retinal vasculitis in Behçet syndrome is poor. The majority of untreated patients lose all or part of their vision within 5 years of onset. See also BCSC Section 9, *Intraocular Inflammation and Uveitis.*

Medical Therapy for Rheumatic Disorders

Medications are used in rheumatology for a number of purposes, including analgesia, an anti-inflammatory effect, and immunosuppression. These drugs and their use in treating ocular inflammatory diseases are also discussed in BCSC Section 9, *Intraocular Inflammation and Uveitis.*

Corticosteroids

Although the overall anti-inflammatory effect of glucocorticoids is the result of a number of mechanisms, one important action involves the inhibition of prostaglandin synthesis. This inhibition results from preventing the release of the prostaglandin precursor arachidonic acid from membrane phospholipids. In addition to their anti-inflammatory activity, glucocorticoids have a variety of other effects. Gluconeogenesis is promoted, with a concomitant negative nitrogen balance and reduction in protein production. Fat oxidation, synthesis, storage, and mobilization are also affected. The number of circulating neutrophils increases because mature neutrophils are released from bone marrow and their movement from blood to other tissues decreases, whereas the number of other circulating leukocytes decreases after glucocorticoid administration. Associated mineralocorticoid activity increases sodium retention and potassium excretion.

Table 8-3 lists the relative potency of commonly used glucocorticoid preparations. The molecular structure of the corticosteroid nucleus can be modified to dissociate glucocorticoid from mineralocorticoid activity. Unfortunately, the goal of dissociating beneficial

Table 8-3 Comparison of Commonly Used Glucocorticoid Preparations

	Approximate Equivalent Dose, mg	Relative Potency	Mineralocorticoid Activity
Cortisol	20	1.0	Yes
Cortisone	25	0.8	Yes
Prednisone	5	4.0	No
Prednisolone	5	4.0	No
Triamcinolone	4	5.0	No
Dexamethasone	0.75	30–150	No

From Kovacs WJ. Structure-function relationships of synthetic glucocorticoids. In: *UpToDate*, Rose BD (ed), Waltham MA. Available at www.uptodate.com. Accessed October 2008.

anti-inflammatory effects from the harmful side effects of glucocorticoid activity has not been achieved. The ophthalmologist must be aware of both ocular and systemic toxicity in patients who are receiving systemic corticosteroids. Adverse ocular effects of systemic corticosteroids include posterior subcapsular cataracts, glaucoma, mydriasis, ptosis, papilledema associated with pseudotumor cerebri, reactivation or aggravation of ocular infection, and delay of wound healing. Systemic complications may include peptic ulceration, osteoporosis, aseptic necrosis of the femoral head, and muscle and skin atrophy. Hyperglycemia, hypertension, edema, weight gain, and changes in body fat distribution resulting in cushingoid habitus can occur. Other adverse effects include hyperosmolar nonketotic coma, hypokalemia, and growth retardation in children. Mental changes are a common problem and may range from mild mood alterations to severe psychological reactions. Psychological dependence may also occur with use of glucocorticoids, particularly in patients who have been given repeated courses of therapy for recurring problems, such as asthma or certain dermatologic conditions.

Osteoporosis is a particularly insidious problem that may increase the risk of fractures as early as a few months after beginning treatment with corticosteroids. In the past, little could be done to prevent this, but today several approaches can help minimize the risk, including bone mineral density testing to assess the degree of osteoporosis. Patients can be treated with calcium and vitamin D supplementation. More sophisticated interventions include hormone replacement therapy or the use of nasal calcitonin supplements or bisphosphonates. Specialty consultation should be obtained to optimize the identification and management of this disease.

Another frequently overlooked complication of systemic corticosteroid therapy is rapid withdrawal. The rate of corticosteroid withdrawal should be determined by the degree of hypothalamic-pituitary-adrenal (HPA) suppression, which, in turn, is related to dose and duration of therapy, as well as by the response of the underlying disease to the corticosteroid withdrawal. A variety of schedules have been suggested. Glucocorticoids given in large doses for 1–3 weeks probably suppress HPA function only temporarily, so they can be withdrawn suddenly or gradually over 1 week. After 1 or more months of treatment, a dosage-reduction protocol is usually followed. Otherwise, sudden withdrawal of corticosteroid therapy may result in adrenal insufficiency, with symptoms such as fatigue, weakness, arthralgias, nausea, orthostatic hypotension, and hypoglycemia. In severe cases, adrenal suppression may be fatal. After corticosteroid therapy has been discontinued, adrenal function may not return to normal for 1 year or more; thus, supplementary corticosteroids may be needed if the patient has a serious illness or undergoes surgery during this recovery period. Because of the likelihood of withdrawal symptoms, even physiologic doses of long-term corticosteroids (eg, 5 mg of prednisone a day) should be gradually reduced.

Ophthalmologists may occasionally initiate corticosteroid therapy for ophthalmic diseases, ideally with the assistance of their patients' general medical doctors, given the need to monitor patients for these potential problems. Physicians may become complacent with the use of corticosteroids because of their effectiveness and relative ease of use to control symptoms. However, studies have shown that a dosage as low as 5 mg a day is associated with increased adverse events over time. For patients who seem to require high or extended doses of corticosteroids, clinicians should strongly consider early use of other immunosuppressive medications, which can decrease patient dependency on corticosteroids. The ophthalmologist may need to be responsible for initiating this discussion if the cortico-steroids are being used to treat localized ocular disease. The other physicians involved in the patient's care may be unaware of or uninterested in making relatively onerous changes in the management of a disease viewed as being a part of the ophthalmologist's "turf."

> Cervantes RA, Kump LI, Neer RM, Foster CS. Glucocorticoid-induced osteoporosis: consider-ations in ophthalmology. *Ophthalmology.* 2004;111(8):1437–1438.

Nonsteroidal Anti-inflammatory Drugs

A wide variety of NSAIDs have been developed in recent years to treat RA and other rheumatic diseases. The names of and starting dosages for some of these agents are listed in Table 8-4. All of these agents decrease synthesis of inflammatory mediators such as the

Table 8-4 The Nonsteroidal Anti-inflammatory Drugs

NSAID	Trade Name	Usual Dose
Carboxylic acids		
Aspirin (acetylsalicylic acid)		2.4–6 g/24 h in 4–5 divided doses
Buffered aspirin	Multiple	Same
Enteric-coated salicylates	Multiple	Same
Salsalate	Disalcid	1.5–3.0 g/24 h bid
Diflunisal	Dolobid	0.5–1.5 g/24 h bid
Choline magnesium trisalicylate	Trilisate	1.5–3 g/24 h bid-tid
Proprionic acids		
Ibuprofen	Motrin, Rufen, OTC	OTC: 200–400 mg qid Rx: 400–800 mg; max 3200 mg/24 h
Naproxen (enteric-coated)	Naprosyn, Anaprox OTC: Alleve	250, 375, 500 mg bid 225 mg bid
Fenoprofen	Nalfon	300–600 mg qid
Ketoprofen	Orudis; Oruvail	75 mg tid; q day
Flurbiprofen	Ansaid	100 mg bid-tid
Oxaprozin	Daypro	600 mg; 2 tabs/day
Acetic acid derivatives		
Indomethacin	Indocin, Indocin SR	25, 50 mg tid-qid; SR: 75 mg bid; rarely >150 mg/24 h
Tolmetin	Tolectin	400, 600, 800 mg; 800–2400 mg/24 h
Sulindac	Clinoril	150, 200 mg bid; some increase to tid
Diclofenac	Voltaren; Cataflam;	50, 75 mg bid-qid
(plus misoprostol)	(Arthrotec)	(50 mg bid)
Etodolac	Lodine	200, 300 mg bid-qid Max: 1200 mg/24 h
Fenamates		
Meclofenamate	Meclomen	50–100 mg tid-qid
Mefenamic acid	Ponstel	250 mg qid
Enolic acids		
Piroxicam	Feldene	10, 20 mg q day
Phenylbutazone	Butazolidin	100 mg tid up to 600 mg/24 h
Naphthylkanones		
Nabumetone	Relafen	500 mg bid up to 1500 mg/24 h
Selective COX-2 inhibitors		
Celecoxib	Celebrex	100, 200 mg q day-bid

Modified with permission from Solomon DH. NSAIDs: overview of adverse effects. In: *UpToDate,* Rose BD (ed), Waltham, MA. Available at www.uptodate.com. Accessed September 7, 2009.

prostaglandins by inhibiting the enzyme cyclooxygenase (COX), and all of them are analgesic, antipyretic, and anti-inflammatory. Their relative efficacy remains largely untested, and the response of individual patients to these drugs varies.

Complications from NSAID use result in approximately 100,000 hospitalizations and 10,000–20,000 deaths per year. The most significant adverse effects from use of oral NSAIDs are gastrointestinal bleeding, renal failure, worsening hypertension, and heart failure, as well as onset of asthma in aspirin-sensitive individuals. Oral NSAIDs can interfere with platelet function and clotting and can cause bone marrow suppression, hepatic toxicity, and CNS symptoms, including headache, dizziness, and confusion. In rare cases, NSAIDs have been associated with ocular adverse effects such as nonspecific blurred vision and diplopia. There have also been reports of possible optic neuropathy and macular edema, especially with use of ibuprofen (Motrin).

There are 2 isoforms of the COX enzyme. COX-1 is present in most cells and appears to be involved in various aspects of cellular metabolism, such as gastric cytoprotection, platelet aggregation, and renal function. COX-2 is present in some tissues, such as brain and bone, but it also is expressed in other sites in response to inflammation. The traditional NSAIDs inhibit both forms, but in 1999 selective COX-2 inhibitors were introduced that reduced the risk of gastrointestinal damage and had less effect on platelet function. Unfortunately, 2 of these drugs (rofecoxib [Vioxx] and valdecoxib [Bextra]) have been removed from the market because of adverse cardiovascular events identified in various studies. Similar concerns have been raised about celecoxib (Celebrex), and although it is still available, this drug now carries significant warnings. It has been proposed that the selective blocking of COX-2 decreases the production of prostacyclins, which cause vasodilation and inhibit platelet aggregation, leading to increased prothrombotic activity. Ophthalmologists should be aware that conjunctivitis, temporary blindness, and vague visual blurring have been reported with use of COX-2 inhibitors.

The exact role of oral NSAIDs in treating ocular inflammation remains uncertain. For instance, systemic NSAIDs may be useful in partially controlling uveitis or scleritis in some patients. In general, however, these drugs are not as effective as corticosteroids. Several topical NSAIDs have been approved for ocular use, and these are discussed in BCSC Section 8, *External Disease and Cornea*, and Section 9, *Intraocular Inflammation and Uveitis*.

Methotrexate

Methotrexate, a structural analogue of folic acid, interferes both with folate-dependent metabolic pathways such as purine and with pyrimidine metabolism. Its disease-modifying effect may in part be mediated via increased extracellular adenosine, which has intrinsic anti-inflammatory activity. Methotrexate is given weekly, usually beginning at a dose of 7.5–10 mg, and gradually increasing to a maximum dose of 25 mg, depending on disease response. All patients are supplemented with folic acid. Major adverse effects include hepatic fibrosis, interstitial lung disease, marrow toxicity, and sterility. Minor problems include gastric upset, stomatitis, and rash.

Hydroxychloroquine

Hydroxychloroquine (Plaquenil) is an antimalarial compound commonly used to treat rheumatologic diseases (chloroquine [Aralen] is a related drug that has an increased risk of retinal toxicity and is rarely used). The drug seems to work by slightly raising the pH of various cellular compartments. This has multiple subtle effects that include decreased cytokine production and decreased lymphocyte proliferation. The response to treatment may take weeks to months, in part because of the drug's half-life (1–2 months) and the time required to achieve steady-state levels.

Hydroxychloroquine is one of the safest immunomodulating drugs. Gastrointestinal symptoms may occur and, in rare cases, a myopathy. When the drug is first started, patients may complain of a self-limited decrease in accommodation, which is probably mediated by transient effects on ciliary muscle function. Retinopathy (bull's-eye maculopathy) due to use of hydroxychloroquine is relatively unusual. A screening protocol has been developed that assigns a patient's level of risk for retinopathy based on factors such as duration of drug use, age, the presence of preexisting retinal disease, and the presence of renal or liver disease. Dosing greater than 6.5 mg/kg/day also increases the risk. This drug is not retained in fatty tissues, so the dosage limit refers to lean body weight—not the patient's actual weight. That is, a short obese patient may actually be at greater risk for toxicity than a taller, leaner patient of similar weight. Higher-risk patients should have annual examinations that include, at a minimum, Amsler grid testing and/or central visual field tests. Patients should be given an Amsler grid for self-monitoring at home because subtle paracentral changes may be the earliest sign of toxicity. Retinopathy is discussed more fully in BCSC Section 12, *Retina and Vitreous*.

> Marmor MF, Carr RE, Easterbrook M, et al. Recommendations on screening for chloroquine and hydroxychloroquine retinopathy: a report by the American Academy of Ophthalmology. *Ophthalmology*. 2002;109(7):1377–1382.

Sulfasalazine

Sulfasalazine (Azulfidine) is effective in treating RA, although the exact mechanism of action is unclear. As they are with other sulfa drugs, side effects may be due to idiosyncratic hypersensitivity (skin reactions, aplastic anemia) or may be dose-related (gastrointestinal tract symptoms, headache). Sulfasalazine is often used in combination with other drugs such as hydroxychloroquine and methotrexate.

Gold Salts

Gold salts are rarely used because of modest efficacy and a high side-effect profile involving hematologic, renal, and dermatologic reactions.

Anticytokine Therapy and Other Immunosuppressive Agents

More detailed understanding of the immune response has allowed the development of drugs targeting specific mediators. Cytokines, which are compounds generated by activated immune cells, can enhance or inhibit the immune response. Tumor necrosis factor α

(TNF-α) is a major proinflammatory cytokine involved in the pathogenesis of RA and other inflammatory diseases. Three TNF-α antagonists are in common use. *Etanercept* (Enbrel) is a recombinant TNF-α receptor protein fused to the Fc portion of an IgG molecule. It works by binding free TNF-α and preventing it from attaching to cell membrane receptors. *Infliximab* (Remicade) and *adalimumab* (Humira) are different types of antibodies that directly target TNF-α. Etanercept and adalimumab are given approximately once a week as subcutaneous injections. Infliximab is given as an IV infusion every 4–8 weeks. Newer TNF-α antagonists include *certolizumab pegol* (Cimzia), which has recently been released, and *golimumab* (Simponi), which has recently been approved by the FDA.

The drugs are usually well tolerated, but there is a potential for severe side effects. These include the development of opportunistic infections such as tuberculosis or atypical mycobacteria; a possible association with demyelinating disease; and a possible association with lymphoma, especially in the pediatric population. Other associations include cytopenias, heart failure, shingles, antibodies to the drugs, and a lupuslike syndrome. Ophthalmologists should be aware that these drugs have been reported to cause optic neuritis due to demyelinization. Also, etanercept has been implicated in causing or exacerbating uveitis and does not seem to be very effective as a treatment for the disease (unlike the other drugs in this class, which can be very effective in uveitis). The drugs are also very expensive; the cost of infliximab, for example, is approximately $12,000 per year based on an average of 8 treatments. In spite of these problems, these drugs can be very effective medications in the treatment of autoimmune diseases, and they herald the onset of immunomodulatory therapies that target specific aspects of the immune response.

Biologic agents used to treat autoimmune disease can affect pathways other than TNF-α. Anakinra (Kineret) is an anticytokine drug that inhibits interleukin 1 (IL-1) by binding to IL-1 receptors on the cell surface. Daclizumab (Zenapax) is an antibody that binds to the IL-2 receptor. Tocilizumab (Actemra) is an anti–IL-6 receptor antibody that is in advanced clinical testing and appears promising for both RA and JIA. It works best when combined with other disease-modifying agents such as methotrexate. Abatacept (Orencia) has recently been approved for the treatment of rheumatoid arthritis that is poorly responsive to other therapies. This drug blocks the T-cell receptor CD28, which is involved in T-cell activation and can be very effective in refractory disease. Rituximab (Rituxan) is a B-cell–depleting monoclonal antibody used for chemotherapy that is also being used in rheumatoid arthritis unresponsive to other agents. Alemtuzumab (Campath) is another monoclonal antibody used to treat chronic lymphocytic leukemia that has shown promise in autoimmune diseases.

There are also traditional immunosuppressive drugs that work by interfering with lymphocyte proliferation. *Leflunomide* (Arava) inhibits pyrimidine synthesis, targeting rapidly dividing cell populations such as activated lymphocytes. Potential adverse effects include liver toxicity, neuropathy, and birth defects. This drug is approximately as effective as methotrexate, and the two are often combined when methotrexate is ineffective alone.

Cyclophosphamide (Cytoxan) and *chlorambucil* (Leukeran) are alkylating agents that are very potent immunosuppressive agents. Their primary mechanism of action involves the cross-linking of DNA molecules, which halts cellular processes. They also have potentially severe adverse effects, including infertility, bone marrow suppression, increased risk of infection, and late malignancy (particularly bladder cancer with use of cyclophosphamide). Consequently, these drugs are saved for very resistant or life-threatening diseases such as Wegener granulomatosis, for which the benefits are worth the substantial risk. Cyclophosphamide is the most commonly used drug, and it may be given as a daily oral dose or as intermittent IV pulse therapy.

Azathioprine (Imuran) is an antimetabolite that ultimately interferes with purine metabolism. The most common adverse effects are gastrointestinal tract symptoms, infection, and bone marrow suppression. Up to 10% of the population may have decreased levels of the enzyme thiopurine methyltransferase (TPMT), which is important in the metabolism of this drug. Because decreased levels of TPMT may lead to more pronounced bone marrow suppression and toxicity, measuring the levels of this enzyme may help identify patients at risk.

Cyclosporine (Neoral, Sandimmune) and *tacrolimus* (Prograf) are drugs that inhibit the transcription of interleukin-2 and other cytokines, primarily in helper T cells. They are used primarily in transplant patients to prevent rejection, but there is increasing recognition of their usefulness in treating autoimmune diseases. The chief adverse effects of both drugs are nephrotoxicity and hypertension. Other potential problems include neurologic symptoms, infections, and malignancy. Because of such risks, these agents are reserved for recalcitrant cases that do not respond to standard therapies. Although rare, ophthalmic adverse effects have been reported with use of systemic cyclosporine, including disc edema, hallucinations, and unexplained eye pain.

Mycophenolate mofetil (CellCept) inhibits the production of guanosine in lymphocytes and thereby decreases cellular proliferation and antibody production. It is another drug that was initially used in transplant patients and is increasingly used in patients with immunologic diseases. Primary adverse effects include gastrointestinal symptoms, bone marrow suppression, and increased risk of infection. Overall, the drug seems to be well tolerated by patients and may serve as an adjunct to other medications.

Cush JJ, Kavanaugh A, Stein CM. *Rheumatology: Diagnosis and Therapeutics.* 2nd ed. Philadelphia: Lippincott Williams & Wilkins; 2005.

Firestein GS, Budd RC, Harris ED, McInnes IB, Ruddy S, Sergent JS. *Kelley's Textbook of Rheumatology.* 8th ed. 2 vols. Philadelphia: Elsevier/Saunders; 2008.

Foster CS, Tufail F, Waheed NK, et al. Efficacy of etanercept in preventing relapse of uveitis controlled by methotrexate. *Arch Ophthalmol.* 2003;121(4):437–440.

Fraunfelder FT, Fraunfelder FW, Chambers WA. *Clinical Ocular Toxicology: Drug-Induced Ocular Side Effects.* Philadelphia: Elsevier/Saunders; 2008.

UpToDate. www.uptodate.com.

The authors would like to thank Karen Ringwald, MD, and Susan Ballinger, MD, for their contributions to this chapter.

CHAPTER 9

Endocrine Disorders

Recent Developments

- Simple measures such as moderate exercise and weight loss can prevent the onset of type 2 diabetes in patients at risk for developing the disease.
- Although careful glucose control is the mainstay of diabetic therapy, newer treatments are being developed that target downstream mechanisms of diabetic pathophysiology in order to help prevent complications. Examples of these treatments include protein kinase C inhibitors, drugs that decrease advanced glycosylation end products, and inhibitors of growth factors such as vascular endothelial growth factor (VEGF).
- There is heightened recognition that poor glucose control is only 1 of several risk factors contributing to the complications of diabetes and that equal attention must be paid to other factors, such as hypertension and lipid abnormalities.
- A brief period (2–4 weeks) of intensive insulin treatment at the onset of type 2 diabetes can result in remission of diabetes for 1 year or longer compared to initiating treatment with standard oral agents.

Diabetes Mellitus

The prevalence of diabetes in the United States is estimated to be as high as 8% of the population. Obesity is a major contributing factor and continues to increase in prevalence yearly. In 2007, the total economic impact of diabetes in the United States was $174 billion, due to both direct medical costs and costs related to work loss, disability, and early mortality. New diabetes is diagnosed in more than 1 million people each year, a number expected to increase 165% by 2050. Annual spending is increasing by 14.5% for diabetes treatment and is now the fastest growing therapeutic category. As diabetes is still the leading cause of new cases of blindness among adults 20–74 years old, the ophthalmologist plays a crucial role as part of a multidisciplinary team involved in prevention, treatment, and management of this disease.

Basics of Glucose Metabolism

The plasma glucose level is reduced by a single hormone, insulin. In contrast, 6 hormones increase the plasma glucose level: somatotropin, adrenocorticotropin, cortisol, epinephrine, glucagon, and thyroxine. All of these hormones are secreted as needed to maintain normal serum glucose levels in the face of extremely variable degrees of glucose intake and utilization. In the fed state, *anabolism* is initiated by increased secretion of insulin and growth hormone. This leads to conversion of glucose to glycogen for storage in the liver and muscles, synthesis of protein from amino acids, and combining of fatty acid and glucose in adipose tissue to form triglycerides.

In the fasting state, *catabolism* results from the increased secretion of hormones that are antagonistic to insulin. In this setting, glycogen is reduced to glucose in the liver and muscles; proteins are broken down into amino acids in muscles and other tissues and transported to the liver for conversion to glucose or ketoacids; and triglycerides are degraded into fatty acids and glycerol in adipose tissue for transport to the liver for conversion to ketoacids and glucose (or for transport to muscle for use as an energy source).

The normal lean adult secretes approximately 33 units of insulin per day. If the pancreatic β-cell mass is reduced (as it is in type 1 diabetes), then insulin production falls. The relative excess of catabolic hormones results in fasting hyperglycemia, and persistent catabolism may lead to fatal diabetic ketoacidosis if insulin therapy is not started. This disastrous chain of events explains why type 1 diabetes was uniformly fatal before the development of insulin. It also explains why insulin-dependent diabetic patients require a continuous baseline dose of insulin, even in the fasting state: some level of insulin is needed to offset the effect of all the other hormones.

In the obese overfed adult, insulin secretion can increase almost 4-fold to approximately 120 units per day. In this state, the plasma glucose level may rise only slightly, but pancreatic β-cell mass increases. When serum insulin levels are elevated, the number of insulin receptors on the surface of insulin-responsive cells actually decreases, and formerly insulin-sensitive tissues become resistant to the glucose-lowering effects of both endogenous and exogenous insulin. This condition may progress to fasting hyperglycemia and type 2 diabetes. The risk of hyperglycemia is 2 times as great in persons who are 20% above ideal body weight, compared with persons at ideal body weight; 4 times as great at 40% above; 8 times as great at 60% above; 16 times as great at 80% above; and 32 times as great at 100% above.

Definition

The definition of diabetes mellitus has changed considerably in recent years. *Diabetes mellitus* is now defined as a group of metabolic diseases characterized by hyperglycemia resulting from defects in insulin secretion, insulin action, or both. The American Diabetes Association Expert Panel recommends a diagnosis of diabetes when 1 of the 3 criteria shown in Table 9-1 is met (and confirmed with retesting by any of the 3 methods on a subsequent day).

Classification

Diabetes can be caused by a number of different mechanisms. Although this chapter emphasizes types 1 and 2, which are most frequently seen in clinical practice, many diseases and drugs can be associated with diabetes. For instance, diabetes can be seen with pancreatitis, endocrinopathies such as Addison disease, and genetic diseases such as Down

Table 9-1 American Diabetes Association Plasma Glucose Diagnostic Criteria for Diabetes Mellitus

Diagnosis	Test Condition Plasma Glucose, mg/dL	
	Fasting ≥8 hr	2 hr after 75 g oral glucose
Normal	<110	<140
Impaired glucose tolerance (IGT)	<126	≥140–<200
Impaired fasting glucose (IFG)	≥110–<126	<200
Diabetes mellitus	≥126	—
Diabetes mellitus	<126	≥200
Diabetes mellitus (classic symptoms + casual plasma glucose, ≥200 mg/dL)	—	—

	Plasma Glucose, mg/dL	
Gestational diabetes mellitus (GDM)	Fasting	After 100 g oral glucose
	>105*	1 hr ≥190*
	>105*	2 hr ≥165*
	>105*	3 hr ≥145*

Note: The Fourth International Workshop–Conference on Gestational Diabetes Mellitus has proposed lower criteria, which would increase the percentage of cases from 4% to 7% in white women. These criteria are fasting, 95; 1 hour, 180; 2 hours, 155; and 3 hours, 140, after 100 g oral glucose.
*Two of these 4 criteria must be met for diagnosis of GDM.

Reproduced with permission from Genuth S. Diabetes mellitus. May 2004 Update. ACP Medicine website, available at www.acpmedicine.com. Accessed March 1, 2005.

syndrome. Drugs that can cause diabetes include synthetic glucocorticoids, thiazide diuretics, and the atypical antipsychotic medications.

Type 1 diabetes

Type 1 diabetes was previously called *insulin-dependent diabetes mellitus* or *juvenile-onset diabetes.* Although it does have a peak incidence around the time of puberty, approximately 25% of cases present after 35 years of age. This form of diabetes is due to a deficiency in endogenous insulin secretion secondary to destruction of insulin-producing β cells in the pancreas.

Most type 1 diabetes is due to immune-mediated destruction characterized by the presence of various autoantibodies. The rate of destruction varies, but it is usually rapid in children and slow in adults. One or more autoantibodies are present in 90% of patients at initial presentation of fasting hyperglycemia. Studies have shown that patients newly diagnosed with type 1 diabetes can avoid the use of insulin if they are placed on systemic immunosuppressive agents to prevent further β-cell destruction. Unfortunately, this treatment is too toxic to be practical. There are strong human leukocyte antigen (HLA) associations with and multiple genetic predispositions related to type 1 diabetes. These patients are also prone to other autoimmune disorders, such as Graves disease, Hashimoto thyroiditis, Addison disease, vitiligo, and pernicious anemia. However, environmental factors may also play a role, as studies of monozygotic twins have shown that both twins develop diabetes only 30%–50% of the time.

Type 2 diabetes

Type 2 diabetes was formerly known as *non–insulin-dependent* or *adult-onset diabetes mellitus*. This type, which accounts for 90% of Americans with diabetes, has a strong genetic predisposition. Type 2 patients are usually, but not always, older than age 40 at presentation. Obesity is a frequent finding and, in the United States, is present in 80%–90% of these patients. Other risk factors for type 2 diabetes include hypertension, gestational diabetes, physical inactivity, and low socioeconomic status. This form of diabetes is frequently undiagnosed for years because the hyperglycemia develops slowly and symptoms are not severe enough to warrant attention. Although symptoms may initially be minimal, these patients are at increased risk for microvascular and macrovascular complications.

Although there is a strong genetic tendency for developing type 2 diabetes, no specific genetic locus has been uniquely associated with the disease. Type 2 diabetes is likely a function of a variable number of abnormal genes that combine to create a tendency for obesity and abnormal glucose metabolism, as well as a predisposition to complications of the disease.

Autoimmune destruction of β cells does not usually occur in type 2 diabetes. The β cells continue to function at first, but their ability to control hyperglycemia gradually diminishes, in part owing to a process known as *glucose toxicity*, which is basically a positive feedback loop involving glucose metabolism. Glucose toxicity occurs when elevated glucose levels result in increasing insulin resistance in target tissues and a gradual loss of compensatory insulin production by the β cells. The result is a vicious cycle, as elevated glucose levels lead to even higher glucose levels. It is therefore crucial to encourage the patient to try to break this cycle by decreasing the glucose level. In a significant number of these patients, the elevated plasma glucose level can revert to normal simply with caloric restriction and weight loss.

Although gestational diabetes is a separate entity (see Table 9-1), it is metabolically similar to type 2 disease. In 30%–50% of affected women, type 2 diabetes develops within 10 years of initial diagnosis. Defined as any degree of glucose intolerance with onset or first recognition during pregnancy, gestational diabetes complicates approximately 4% of all pregnancies in the United States. It is also significant for the risk it poses to the fetus, including intrauterine mortality, neonatal mortality, metabolic problems, and large birth weight.

Approximately 10% of patients presenting with type 2 diabetes may also have serum islet cell autoantibodies typical of type 1 diabetes. This combination of disease types is referred to as *latent autoimmune diabetes in adults (LADA)*. These patients are more likely to need insulin therapy than are the more typical type 2 diabetic patients.

Prediabetic disorders: impaired glucose tolerance and impaired fasting glucose

Impaired glucose tolerance (IGT) is defined as a standard 75-g oral glucose tolerance test yielding a 2-hour plasma glucose level of ≥140 mg/dL to <200 mg/dL. A new category, *impaired fasting glucose (IFG)*, requires a fasting plasma glucose level of ≥110 mg/dL to <126 mg/dL (see Table 9-1). Both conditions can be considered early stages of type 2 diabetes and are often referred to as *prediabetic states*. For instance, 30%–50% of patients with IGT develop type 2 diabetes within 10 years of diagnosis. Although there is a great deal of overlap, IGT and IFG are not identical states.

Patients with these conditions do not yet appear to be at risk for nephropathy or significant retinopathy, although recent studies suggest that, occasionally, patients may have mild background retinopathy. These patients do, however, have an elevated risk of macrovascular disease compared with persons who have normal glucose tolerance.

Metabolic syndrome

Closely associated with type 2 diabetes, *metabolic syndrome* (formerly known as *metabolic syndrome X* or the *insulin resistance syndrome*) is not a disease but a collection of disorders. The definition of this syndrome includes obesity, lipid abnormalities, hypertension, and some type of glucose intolerance (see Chapter 5, Hypercholesterolemia)—risk factors for both diabetes and cardiovascular disease. Thus, awareness of this syndrome is becoming increasingly important. There is a significant prevalence in the United States, with metabolic syndrome being present in 44% of those older than 50 years. Men with a majority of the features of the syndrome have roughly 4 times the risk of coronary heart disease and 25 times the risk of diabetes as those without these abnormalities. Metabolic syndrome represents a profound public health risk, and treatment of the syndrome may have a significant impact on preventing diabetes and cardiovascular diseases.

Clinical Presentation of Diabetes

The classic findings of diabetes mellitus are polyuria, polydipsia, and polyphagia. Type 1 diabetes tends to present more acutely than type 2, and the diagnosis is usually made based on the presence of these classic symptoms, in association with an elevated plasma glucose level. The diagnosis of type 2 diabetes often depends more on laboratory testing, because patients may have abnormal glucose metabolism long before overt symptoms develop. Other important historical findings that suggest the diagnosis of diabetes include complications during pregnancy or giving birth to large babies, reactive hypoglycemia, family history, advanced vascular disease, impotence, leg claudication, and neuropathy symptoms.

Physical findings, particularly in type 2 diabetes, may include obesity, hypertension, arteriopathy, neuropathy, genitourinary tract abnormalities (especially recurrent *Candida* infections or bacterial bladder or kidney infections), periodontal disease, foot abnormalities, skin abnormalities, and unusual susceptibility to infections.

Diagnosis and Screening

Table 9-1 lists the criteria for diagnosing diabetes mellitus. The preferred test for type 2 diabetes is a fasting plasma glucose test (FPG). Although the oral glucose tolerance test (OGTT) is more sensitive than the FPG, it is not recommended for routine use because it is more costly, inconvenient, and difficult to reproduce. Note that newly revised American Diabetes Association guidelines now recommend the use of hemoglobin A_{1c} as a screening test. Criteria for diabetes testing in asymptomatic persons are given in Table 9-2.

Prevention of Diabetes

Several clinical trials have recently demonstrated that the risk of progression from IGT to type 2 diabetes can be markedly reduced—approximately 50% over several years—with

Table 9-2 Criteria for Testing for Diabetes Mellitus in Asymptomatic Patients in Whom Diabetes Has Not Been Diagnosed

1. Testing for diabetes should be considered in all persons at age 45 years and older; if results are normal, testing should be repeated at 3-yr intervals.
2. Testing should be considered at younger ages or performed more frequently in persons who
   - are obese (≥120% desirable body weight or a BMI ≥25 kg/m²)*
   - have a first-degree relative with diabetes
   - are members of a high-risk ethnic population (eg, African American, Hispanic American, Native American, Asian American, Pacific Islander)
   - have delivered a baby weighing >9 lb or have a diagnosis of gestational diabetes mellitus
   - are hypertensive (≥140/90 mm Hg)
   - have an HDL cholesterol level ≤35 mg/dL (0.90 mmol/L) and/or a triglyceride level ≥250 mg/dL (2.82 mmol/L)
   - were shown to have impaired glucose tolerance or impaired fasting glucose
   - have polycystic ovary syndrome
   - have history of vascular disease
   - are habitually physically inactive

*May not be correct for all ethnic groups.

Modified from American Diabetes Association. Screening for type 2 diabetes. *Diabetes Care.* 2004; 27(suppl 1):S12.

relatively simple lifestyle modifications such as a combination of diet and exercise therapy. The amount of weight loss and exercise required to achieve this result is surprisingly modest. For instance, in the Diabetes Prevention Program, patients who were asked to perform only 150 minutes of brisk walking a week (a little over 20 minutes a day) on average lost only about 12 pounds of weight but reduced their risk by 50%. Other studies have suggested that early pharmacologic intervention with oral hypoglycemic agents also decreases the risk of progression to diabetes. There are, as yet, no known ways to prevent type 1 diabetes, although trials looking at potential interventions for high-risk individuals such as first-degree relatives of type 1 diabetic patients are under way.

Jeon CY, Lokken Rp, Hu FB, van Dam RM. Physical activity of moderate intensity and risk of type 2 diabetes: a systematic review. *Diabetes Care.* 2007;30(3):744–752.

Knowler WC, Barrett-Connor E, Fowler SF, et al; Diabetes Prevention Program Research Group. Reduction in the incidence of type 2 diabetes with lifestyle intervention or metformin. *N Eng J Med.* 2002;346(6):393–403.

Management

Diet and exercise

Adherence to nutrition and meal-planning principles is a challenging but essential component of successful diabetes management. Diet planning should include lifestyle and nutrition goals as well as specific biochemical and other physiologic parameters for the individual. Insulin requirements are then matched to the patient's diet, not vice versa. Although the "one-type-fits-all" diabetic diet is no longer recommended, meals should be consistent, regularly spaced, and low in cholesterol, with less than 10% of calories coming from saturated fat and 10%–20% of calories derived from protein (some studies, however, suggest better control can be obtained with a low-carbohydrate diet, assuming good renal function). If type 2 diabetes is diagnosed and the patient is overweight, a diet that is prudently low fat and low cholesterol should be started and an exercise routine initiated, with the goal of approaching ideal weight. This goal is often not realized, but even a modest weight loss of 10–20 pounds may ameliorate the diabetes or cause its remission. Extensive and continuing counseling on weight reduction may be necessary. A good exercise program helps the weight-loss program and improves fitness. Before an exercise program is prescribed for anyone older than age 35, a determination must be made that the heart is normal and that there are no contraindications. Anyone who has been sedentary or who is out of shape should start slowly and work up to more demanding activities.

Unfortunately, it may be difficult for patients with type 2 diabetes to maintain these lifestyle changes, especially those involving weight loss. This difficulty should not simply be attributed to a lack of willpower on the part of the patient, as it may well represent a CNS manifestation of the multifactorial genetics of this disease. Psychiatric counseling also seems to be an important part of treating patients with type 2 diabetes. Studies suggest that efforts directed toward treating the stress and depression often associated with this disease may help improve glucose control.

Bariatric surgery—surgery that promotes weight loss—is a popular option for very obese individuals who are unresponsive to other forms of therapy. The National Institutes of Health recommends considering bariatric surgery for well-informed and motivated patients with severe obesity for whom conventional treatment modalities have failed or for those who have multiple comorbidities or severe lifestyle limitations. There are 3 general techniques for bariatric surgery: restrictive surgery, which restricts stomach volume; malabsorptive surgery, which minimizes the ability of the gastrointestinal tract to absorb nutrients; and a combination of restrictive and malabsorptive approaches.

Bariatric surgery may be advertised as the only "cure" for type 2 diabetes, but there is potential for both morbidity and mortality. Morbidity can include venous thrombosis, infection, nutritional complications, and complications related to the surgery itself; the risk of mortality is approximately 0.1%–1.0%, depending on the procedure. In addition, the surgery is not universally effective, with perhaps 50%–70% of patients actually losing about half of their weight and maintaining the weight loss. Significant counseling and lifestyle changes are still required, and patients can undermine the eating limitations imposed by the surgery by eating small amounts of food very frequently—especially high-carbohydrate liquids such as milk shakes.

Thomas D, Elliott EJ. Low glycaemic index, or low glycaemic load, diets for diabetes mellitus. *Cochrane Database Syst Rev.* 2009;(1):CD006296.

Insulin therapy

Approximately 1 million North Americans require insulin therapy. Such therapy is indicated for diabetic patients who are pregnant or are at or below ideal body weight with sustained hyperglycemia, ketoacidosis, or a hyperosmotic state. The use of insulin in type 2 diabetes actually decreases the number of target-cell insulin receptors, increases food intake, and promotes weight gain. Therefore, patients who are above ideal body weight, who have not experienced ketoacidosis, and who are not pregnant should not be treated with insulin initially. However, a brief period (2–4 weeks) of intensive insulin treatment at the onset of type 2 diabetes can result in remission of diabetes for 1 year or longer compared to initial treatment with standard oral agents. This approach is not commonly used, though, and most patients with type 2 diabetes are treated with oral therapy initially.

The goal of therapy is to simulate the physiologic changes in insulin levels that would normally occur in response to food intake and activity level. This therapy usually involves use of a longer-acting insulin to maintain a baseline level and then use of a rapid-acting insulin to cover meals. As insulins can be created with different rates of absorption by substituting amino acids or complexing with zinc, patients can fine-tune glucose control (Table 9-3). In the past, most insulin was derived from animals, but currently, recombinant human insulin is used almost exclusively.

Regular insulin is the traditional rapid-acting agent used for short-term coverage; however, the development of very rapid-acting insulins allows diabetic patients the convenience of timing injections just a few minutes before meals. Very rapid-acting insulins include insulin lispro (Humalog), insulin aspart (NovoLog), and insulin glulisine (Apidra). Isophane insulin suspension (NPH insulin) is an intermediate-acting insulin. Glargine (Lantus) and detemir (Levemir) are newer long-acting insulins with very stable absorption characteristics that result in a constant level of basal insulin. Insulin zinc suspension (Lente insulin) and extended insulin zinc (Ultralente insulin) are no longer available.

Sophisticated patients can adjust each injection using formulas that depend on preprandial glucose level, activity level, and amount of food to be ingested, provided they have extensive knowledge of the carbohydrate types and overall nutritional value of each meal. Intensive insulin therapy requires that patients become very involved with their own management and, ideally, almost as familiar as their health care professionals with the disease pathophysiology. Premixed combinations of various insulins are also available for patients less able to work with all these variables.

In addition to exercise and intake, 2 physiologic phenomena may need to be accounted for with insulin therapy. The *Somogyi phenomenon* is the occurrence of posthypoglycemic rebound hyperglycemia. Hypoglycemia as mild as 50–60 mg/dL of plasma glucose (which may be asymptomatic) can activate counterregulation. Current evidence indicates that catecholamines and growth hormone are the major factors involved. Recognition of

Table 9-3 Pharmacokinetics of Most Commonly Used Insulin Preparations

Insulin Type	Onset of Action	Time to Peak Effect	Duration of Action
Lispro (Humalog), aspart (Novolog), glulisine (Apidra)	5–15 min	45–75 min	2–4 h
Regular	About 30 min	2–4 h	5–8 h
NPH	About 2 h	6–10 h	18–28 h
Insulin glargine (Lantus)	About 2 h	No discernible peak	20–>24 h
Insulin detemir (Levemir)	About 2 h	No discernible peak	10–24 h

Modified with permission from McCulloch DK. Insulin therapy in type 1 diabetes mellitus. In: *UpToDate*, Rose BD (ed), Waltham, MA. Available at www.uptodate.com. Accessed August 1, 2007.

this process is important because patients may incorrectly decide to increase their longer-acting insulin dose to treat the hyperglycemia and thereby increase the hypoglycemia that precipitated the problem. The incidence of the Somogyi phenomenon is not known, but it is probably not frequent.

The second phenomenon is the *dawn phenomenon,* which occurs when a normal physiologic process is exaggerated, resulting in substantial hyperglycemia. Characterized by early morning hyperglycemia not preceded by hypoglycemia or waning of insulin, this phenomenon is thought to be caused by a surge of growth hormone secretion shortly after the patient falls asleep. It can occur with equal frequency in type 1 and type 2 diabetes, but its severity varies, making this condition difficult to treat. Management consists of increasing a patient's before-supper intermediate-acting insulin or delaying insulin administration until just before bedtime.

Continuous subcutaneous insulin infusion (CSII) pumps allow even more physiologic levels of insulin than do traditional injections. For instance, CSII pumps can be programmed to increase the basal insulin level during the latter half of the night in anticipation of the dawn effect. CSII is not a simple treatment, however, as patients must be able to understand the more sophisticated demands of using a pump, and improvement in glucose control is not automatic. In the Diabetes Control and Complications Trial (DCCT), the overall rate of control was not better in patients using the pump than in patients using multiple injections, although more recent studies using very rapid-acting insulins do demonstrate slightly better control with a pump compared with multiple injections.

The pump tends to be used when multiple-injection therapy fails, although some endocrinologists will consider using it with motivated patients who understand the nuances of living with the pump because it can provide greater lifestyle flexibility. Disadvantages include a higher cost, infection at the infusion site, and infusion failure. Infusion failure is significant, because patients can develop diabetic ketoacidosis if the pump fails for as little as 4–6 hours. The pump delivers a low dose of rapid-acting insulin that quickly disappears if the infusion is stopped. The patient may be unaware of a failure at first (unlike with a multiple-injection regimen, in which the patient is absolutely aware of giving a dose). A state of hypoinsulinemia develops, with resulting hyperglycemia and possible ketoacidosis if pump failure is not recognized. Finally, because patients need to wear the pump on an almost constant basis, some patients discontinue use simply because it interferes with activities such as bathing or sex. CSII technology is continually improving, however, and for many patients the pump is becoming a preferred option over multiple injections.

A surgically implanted programmable insulin pump is available in the European Union and under investigation in the United States. This pump has the advantage of a lower incidence of severe hypoglycemia and less day-to-day fluctuation in blood glucose concentrations, compared with intensive regimens using injections or external pumps. These advantages may occur, in part, because implantable pumps deliver insulin into the peritoneal cavity or intravascularly, where rapid absorption provides more physiologic insulin profiles. However, implantable insulin pumps are more prone to catheter blockage, and anti-insulin antibodies occur more commonly with continuous intraperitoneal insulin infusion than with CSII.

Complications of insulin therapy   *Hypoglycemia* is the most significant complication of insulin therapy. Stimulation of the adrenal medulla with resulting hyperepinephrinemia may result in anxiety, palpitations, perspiration, pallor, tachycardia, hypertension, and dilated pupils. Neurologic dysfunction is manifested as headache, paresthesia, blurred vision, drowsiness, irritability, bizarre behavior, mental confusion, combativeness, and a variety of other symptoms. Short-term hypoglycemia can lead to accidental injury and even criminal behavior. Prolonged hypoglycemia can result in irreversible brain damage or death. Unfortunately, the epinephrine response to hypoglycemia can diminish over time, often in association with the global autonomic neuropathy that occurs in diabetes. As a result, patients have fewer warning symptoms of hypoglycemia, as well as a decreased ability to metabolically respond to the hypoglycemia. Thus, the first clinical manifestation of a hypoglycemic episode is CNS dysfunction, and by then it may be too late for the patient to recognize and self-treat the episode. This is the clinical syndrome of *hypoglycemia unawareness*. The result may be a very rapid deterioration from normal functioning to dangerous hypoglycemia in patients with long-standing diabetes.

Hypoglycemia is usually caused by inadequate carbohydrate intake secondary to a missed or delayed meal, vigorous exercise, decreased hepatic gluconeogenesis, or an excessive dose of insulin. The condition needs to be promptly verified by testing for a venous plasma glucose level of lower than 50 mg/dL. Patients who are still able to swallow should be given candy, soft drinks, orange juice, food, or glucose. For those unable to swallow, 25 g of intravenous glucose or 1 mg of subcutaneous or intramuscular glucagon is administered. The patient needs to be observed until recovery is complete, and the plasma glucose test is repeated with additional food given.

Other complications of insulin include lipoatrophy (loss of fat) or lipohypertrophy (accumulation of fat) at sites of insulin injection. Local insulin allergy can occur and usually clears as therapy continues. Generalized anaphylaxis, hives, and angioedema may also develop and may need to be treated with desensitization techniques. Immunologic insulin resistance may occur because of production of insulin-neutralizing antibodies. All of these immunologic phenomena have become much less frequent with the use of human insulins.

Oral agents

See Table 9-4 and Figure 9-1. Figure 9-1 shows an algorithm for treating hyperglycemia in type 2 diabetes.

Sulfonylureas   The sulfonylureas have been widely used in the United States and Canada since 1967 for treatment of type 2 diabetes. Their major mechanism of action is stimulation of pancreatic insulin secretion, although some studies have suggested a peripheral augmentation of insulin action.

The major problem with sulfonylurea therapy is that approximately one third of patients who begin therapy do not become normoglycemic (they are considered "primary failures"). Furthermore, during a 5-year period, 85% of those who initially respond to the drug experience secondary failure to control blood glucose. The sulfonylureas are

Table 9-4 **Pharmacokinetics of Oral Hypoglycemic Drugs**

Drug	Usual Daily Dose, mg	Dosing per Day
First-generation sulfonylureas		
Acetohexamide	500–750	Once or divided
Chlorpropamide (Diabinese)	250–500	Once
Tolbutamide (Orinase)	1000–2000	Once or divided
Second-generation sulfonylureas		
Glipizide (Glucotrol)	2.5–10	Once or divided
(Glucotrol XL)	5–10	Once
Glyburide (DiaBeta, Micronase, Glynase)	2.5–10	Once or divided
Glimepiride (Amaryl)	2–4	Once
Biguanides		
Metformin (Glucophage, Glucophage XR)	1500–2550	Twice to 3 times
α-Glucosidase inhibitors		
Acarbose (Precose)	150–300	3 times
Miglitol (Glyset)	150–300	3 times
Thiazolidinediones		
Rosiglitazone (Avandia)	4–8	Once or divided
Pioglitazone (Actos)	15–45	Once
Meglitinides		
Repaglinide (Prandin)	2–16	3 times w/meals
Nateglinide (Starlix)	360	3 times w/meals
Other		
Sitagliptin (Januvia)	100	Once

Modified with permission from McCulloch DK. Treatment of blood glucose in type 2 diabetes mellitus. In: *UpToDate*, Rose BD (ed), Waltham, MA. Available at www.uptodate.com. Accessed March 1, 2005.

also contraindicated in diabetic patients who are pregnant and in those who have had ketoacidosis.

The most significant adverse effect of the sulfonylureas is hypoglycemia, which, though infrequent, may be severe and prolonged, depending on the half-life of the specific drug. First-generation sulfonylureas compete for carrier protein–binding sites with many other drugs, including sulfonamides, salicylates, and thiazides. Because the pharmacologic effect of the sulfonylureas may be increased when they are displaced from their albumin-combining sites, combination drug therapy may have unforeseen toxic consequences.

Second-generation sulfonylurea agents *glipizide* (Glucotrol, Glucotrol XL), *glyburide* (DiaBeta, Micronase, Glynase), and *glimepiride* (Amaryl) differ from the first-generation agents in structure and potency. On a weight-for-weight basis, the newer sulfonylureas are approximately 50–100 times more potent than first-generation agents, and these drugs generally need to be given only once daily. Complications are less frequent with the second-generation agents because of their nonionic binding to albumin, and patients may be less susceptible to drug interactions. Although these newer agents are more potent than the first-generation sulfonylureas in facilitating insulin release, this enhanced β-cytotrophic effect is not associated with better control of hyperglycemia. As a result, in

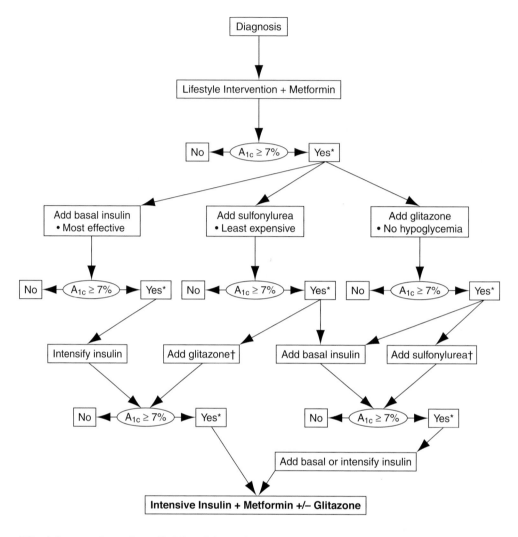

Figure 9-1 Management of hyperglycemia in type 2 diabetes. *(Modified with permission from Nathan DM, Buse JB, Davidson MB, et al. Management of hyperglycemia in type 2 diabetes: a consensus algorithm for the initiation and adjustment of therapy. A consensus statement from the American Diabetes Association and the European Association for the Study of Diabetes.* Diabetes Care. *2006;29:1963. Copyright © 2006 The American Diabetes Association.)*

most cases the choice of initial sulfonylurea depends on cost and availability; the efficacy of the various agents tends to be similar.

Biguanides   A major advance occurred with the development of *metformin* (Glucophage, Glucophage XR), currently the only available biguanide. Metformin improves insulin sensitivity, unlike the sulfonylureas and meglitinides (discussed later in the chapter). Metformin may also lead to modest weight loss or at least stabilization (in contrast to the weight gain that may occur with use of insulin or sulfonylureas). In addition, it is less likely to cause hypoglycemia and can be used in nonobese patients. Metformin is generally the first agent used in patients whose hyperglycemia cannot be controlled with lifestyle changes alone (see Fig 9-1).

Although metformin is generally very safe, patients may complain of gastrointestinal tract symptoms, including a metallic taste, nausea, and diarrhea. A more severe potential problem is lactic acidosis. Although rare, this problem is more likely to occur in patients with renal insufficiency. Metformin should therefore not be prescribed to patients with elevated serum creatinine levels, and the drug should be discontinued before patients take part in any studies involving iodinated contrast materials, given the risk of renal failure. The same precaution should be taken before major surgery when there is a possibility of circulatory compromise and secondary renal insufficiency. Metformin is also available as a combination pill with glyburide (Glucovance), with glipizide (Metaglip), and with rosiglitazone maleate (Avandamet).

α-Glucosidase inhibitors   *Acarbose* (Precose) and *miglitol* (Glyset) are administered with meals to delay digestion and absorption of carbohydrates by inhibiting the enzymes that convert complex carbohydrates into monosaccharides. Although relatively safe, these agents often cause flatulence, which limits patient compliance, and they are to be avoided in patients with intestinal disorders.

Thiazolidinediones   This new class of orally active drugs, represented by *rosiglitazone* (Avandia) and *pioglitazone* (Actos), is thought to increase insulin sensitivity in muscle and adipose tissue and to inhibit hepatic gluconeogenesis, thereby increasing glycemic control while reducing circulating insulin levels. These drugs also act to increase insulin secretion. The first available agent of this class, *troglitazone* (Rezulin), was withdrawn from the market in 2000, when the FDA noted that this drug had a higher rate of liver toxicity than did the other drugs. In 2010, the FDA significantly restricted the use of rosiglitazone because of an increased risk of cardiovascular complications in patients using this drug. Both rosiglitazone and pioglitazone can cause weight gain, in part owing to the proliferation of new adipocytes. Another problem is fluid retention, which has been associated with cases of macular edema.

The general approach to treating type 2 diabetes begins with diet and exercise modifications. If this does not work, the patient is given an oral agent, usually metformin or a sulfonylurea. If this is insufficient, a second agent with a different mechanism is usually added. If even better control is required, then insulin is usually added to the current 1- or 2-drug oral therapy. This regimen is less expensive and more effective than 3-drug oral therapy. If patients are underweight or ketotic at any point, or if they are losing weight, insulin may need to be started earlier in the course.

Meglitinides   *Repaglinide* (Prandin) and *nateglinide* (Starlix) are meglitinides, whose mechanism of action and side effect profile are similar to those of the sulfonylureas. However, they are more expensive and generally no more efficacious than the sulfonylureas. Because of their rapid onset of action and short duration, these agents are taken daily with meals. They can be used as single agents or in combination therapy with other oral hypoglycemic agents.

Other therapies

An inhaled form of rapid-acting insulin was available for a short time but was discontinued in 2007.

Incretins are gut-derived factors that are released when nutrients enter the stomach; they help to stimulate postprandial insulin release. *Incretin mimetics* improve glycemic control by enhancing pancreatic secretion of insulin in response to nutrient intake, inhibiting glucagon secretion and promoting early satiety. Two recently approved injectable incretin mimetics are *exenatide* (Byetta), used as adjunctive therapy for patients with type 2 diabetes who are inadequately controlled by oral agents, and *pramlintide* (Symlin), a synthetic analogue of amylin, used in patients treated with mealtime insulin.

Dipeptidyl peptidase IV (DPP-IV) is an enzyme that deactivates bioactive peptides, including incretins; therefore, inhibiting this enzyme can enhance glucose regulation. Sitagliptin (Januvia) is an oral DPP-IV inhibitor that requires only once a day dosing, but it is expensive, only modestly effective, and not commonly used.

Glucose transport inhibitors are a new class of drugs in phase 3 studies. Glucose is filtered in the renal glomerulus and reabsorbed in the proximal tubule. Beyond a certain threshold (usually 160–180 mg/dL), it is excreted in the urine. Glucose transport inhibitors prevent the reabsorption, and thereby increase the loss, of glucose in the urine. The lost calories then cause weight loss and improved blood glucose values.

Pancreatic transplantation

For type 1 diabetic patients, pancreas transplantation can be performed in conjunction with renal transplantation. With modern techniques and immunosuppression, there is a high transplant survival rate, and the majority of patients become euglycemic without the need for insulin. Although quality of life is usually improved, the patient faces the risks of both surgery and long-term immunosuppression. Pancreas transplantation alone is therefore used only in certain situations, such as in patients with frequent metabolic complications or patients for whom standard insulin therapy consistently fails to control disease. When combined with renal transplantation in a patient with end-stage renal disease, however, the benefits of pancreas transplantation far outweigh the risks.

Islet cells can be injected directly into the liver without the need for formal transplantation. This procedure has been attempted in humans, but rejection leads to a high failure rate. Studies are under way to identify effective immunosuppressive regimens as well as other sites for cell placement. Islet cell–producing stem cell research is still at a basic stage.

The Importance of Glucose Control

The Diabetes Control and Complications Trial showed that intensive therapy aimed at maintaining near-normal glucose levels had a large and beneficial effect on delaying the development and retarding the progression of long-term complications for type 1 diabetic patients. These levels were obtained either by 3 or more daily self-administered insulin injections or via a battery-powered insulin pump. Intensive therapy decreased the risk of the development and progression of retinopathy, nephropathy, and neuropathy by 40%–76%. The beneficial effects increased over time but came with a 3-fold increased risk of hypoglycemia. Thus, intensive therapy is recommended for most patients with type 1 disease, but with careful self-monitoring of blood glucose levels to prevent hypoglycemic episodes. A related study, the United Kingdom Prospective Diabetes Study (UKPDS), was designed to assess the effect of intensive control on patients with type 2 diabetes. The UKPDS used a combination of diet, sulfonylureas, and insulin to achieve a median HbA_{1c} of 7.0 in the intensive care group and also showed a reduction in complications. See also BCSC Section 12, *Retina and Vitreous.*

Tight control has a tremendous effect on the development of complications. As Figure 9-2 shows, the risk of retinopathy progression rises almost exponentially as the HbA_{1c} increases. However, patients who decrease their HbA_{1c} by 1 percentage point (eg, from 8% to 7%) decrease the risk of retinopathy approximately 30%, and this benefit holds for other diabetic complications, such as nephropathy and neuropathy. Health care providers involved with diabetic patients need to emphasize the importance of tight control and encourage patients to achieve it.

For patients with type 1 diabetes, intensive control also provides protection against macrovascular complications, such as cardiovascular disease. For patients with type 2 diabetes, however, the role of glycemic control in reducing cardiovascular risk has not been established. In this group, macrovascular disease may be affected more by other risk factors, such as smoking, obesity, and lipid abnormalities. A recent study, the Action to Control Cardiovascular Risk in Diabetes (ACCORD) trial, even suggested that intensive glycemic control in patients with type 2 diabetes might actually increase the risk of cardiovascular mortality. Although this result received wide coverage in the lay press, the finding may be related more to the study's methodology; the result has not been confirmed in other trials. Nevertheless, based on this, some experts suggest that a target HbA_{1c} of 7.0%–7.9% may be safer for patients with long-standing type 2 diabetes who are at high risk for cardiovascular disease.

Gerstein HC, Miller ME, Byington RP, et al; Action to Control Cardiovascular Risk in Diabetes Study Group. Effects of intensive glucose lowering in type 2 diabetes. *N Engl J Med.* 2008;358(24):2545–2559.

Kravetz JD, Federman DG. Implications of new diabetes treatment trials: should current clinical practice be altered? *Postgrad Med.* 2009;121(3):67–72.

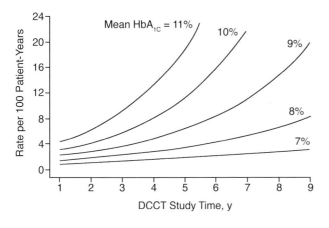

Figure 9-2 Rate of retinopathy progression relative to mean hemoglobin A_{1c}. *(Redrawn with permission from the DCCT Research Group. The relationship of glycemic exposure (HbA_{1c}) to the risk of development and progression of retinopathy in the Diabetes Control and Complications Trial. Diabetes. 1995;44(8):968–983.)*

Glucose Surveillance

Probably the most important advance in glycemic control is self-monitoring of blood glucose using finger sticks. Newer blood-testing devices require smaller amounts of blood than do older units; they are also less painful. The glucose values are stored in memory and downloaded to give an accurate assessment of glucose control without depending on the patient to recall or reconstruct the data. Having patients maintain a glucose log is still useful, however, because it can serve as an important reminder of their progress.

Continuous blood glucose–monitoring systems, which measure the glucose content of interstitial fluid either using a needle sensor inserted subcutaneously or implanting the whole device subcutaneously are also available. This approach offers the promise of continuous control of insulin infusion based on real-time glucose levels. However, the efficacy of these systems compared with that of finger-stick monitoring is uncertain, leading to the need for continuing the latter. The greatest potential of continuous blood glucose monitoring is for patients with hypoglycemic unawareness; unfortunately, currently available meters are most inaccurate in the low range of glucose. The technology is also expensive.

In recent decades, the ability to measure *glycosylated hemoglobin levels* has significantly improved long-term glucose-control surveillance. All serum-bound and membrane-bound proteins are exposed to glucose and undergo a nonenzymatic postsynthetic modification that results in the attachment of glucose to the protein (glycosylation). Higher concentrations of glucose and longer periods of exposure result in a higher concentration of glycosylated proteins. The time period reflected by the glycosylated protein concentration depends on the particular protein's turnover rate. Red blood cells and hemoglobin have a half-life of 60 days; thus, the glycosylated hemoglobin level reflects the mean blood glucose concentration during the preceding 2 months. The amount of glycosylated hemoglobin is expressed as a percentage of total hemoglobin.

Hemoglobin A_{1c}, the most abundant of the glycosylated hemoglobins, is the assay most commonly performed. The HbA_{1c} assay is used to monitor the level of long-term glucose control in both type 1 and type 2 disease and is especially useful in uncooperative or unreliable patients. Glucose levels less than 6 indicate nondiabetic individuals, those generally less than 7 are goal values for patients with diabetes, and those greater than 8 indicate that further interventions are warranted. The American Diabetes Association recommends measuring levels at least twice a year for well-controlled diabetic patients and quarterly for those with less-optimal control.

Acute Complications of Diabetes

The acute complications of diabetes are *nonketotic hyperglycemic-hyperosmolar coma* and diabetic *ketoacidosis.* Either of these, if not recognized promptly and treated aggressively, can lead to death. These complications should be considered part of a continuum of hyperglycemia rather than separate entities; the main difference between the 2 is whether ketoacids accumulate. Both are often precipitated by some sort of stress, such as infection, that results in the increased production of glucagon, catecholamines, and cortisol, which in turn enhances gluconeogenesis. If insufficient amounts of insulin or oral hypoglycemic agents are used, the resulting elevated glucose level will lead to osmotic diuresis and volume depletion. If insulin levels are extremely low or absent (such as in a type 1 diabetic patient), then catabolic processes prevail (such as the conversion of lipids to ketones), and ketoacids are produced, superimposing severe metabolic acidosis on the hyperosmotic volume-depleted state.

The treatment of both these entities involves correcting any precipitating factors, such as infection, and addressing metabolic abnormalities, which includes reversing the hypovolemia, hyperglycemia, or metabolic acidosis and correcting electrolyte abnormalities such as hypokalemia. The treatment is complex and usually involves admission to an intensive care unit and careful monitoring of all metabolic parameters.

Long-term Complications of Diabetes

The long-term complications of diabetes are usually secondary to vascular disease. Nephropathy, neuropathy, peripheral vascular disease, coronary atherosclerosis, secondary cerebral thrombosis, cardiac infarction, and retinopathy are all important causes of morbidity and mortality. (Diabetic retinopathy is discussed in BCSC Section 12, *Retina and Vitreous*.)

The precise mechanism for the development of diabetic complications is elusive, but hyperglycemia plays some central role by triggering a number of different mechanisms. These mechanisms include toxicity from elevated sorbitol due to activation of the enzyme aldose reductase by hyperglycemia. An elevated glucose level also results in increased activity of the enzyme protein kinase C (PKC), which in turn results in phosphorylation of various proteins (reversible phosphorylation of proteins is the principal means of governing protein activity within cells). The resultant imbalance of enzymatic activity ultimately causes vascular damage from processes such as excessive endothelial cell basement membrane formation.

Another mechanism involved in diabetic pathophysiology is the formation of advanced glycosylation end products (eg, HbA_{1c}) due to nonenzymatic attachment of glucose to various proteins. These advanced glycosylation end products interfere with a number of metabolic processes and have been implicated in the development of all major complications of diabetes. In the retina, all of these mechanisms may in turn stimulate production of VEGF, the compound that appears to be associated with the development of vascular leakage and with the proliferation seen in diabetic retinopathy.

Although careful glucose control is the mainstay of diabetic therapy, the recognition of these additional pathways has led to research into treatments targeting these more distal processes. Potential new treatments include aldose reductase inhibitors, protein kinase C inhibitors, drugs that prevent the formation of advanced glycosylation end products, and VEGF inhibitors. Clinical studies of these potential treatments are under way. Studies have also looked at medications for diseases other than diabetes to see if they have any effect on retinopathy. For instance, studies have found that candesartan (Atacand), an angiotensin II receptor antagonist, and fenofibrate (Tricor), a cholesterol-lowering agent, have a possible mild effect on slowing retinopathy progression.

Glucose control is not the only risk factor that can be modified to minimize the development of complications. In particular, hypertension and lipid abnormalities seem to be inextricably intertwined with glucose control. Thus, any attempt to minimize complications must include aggressive control of these other factors. Additional risk factors for diabetic complications include duration of disease, smoking, pregnancy, and a genetic predisposition for the disease and for specific complications. Risk factors that seem to exacerbate diabetic retinopathy in particular include early renal disease and anemia.

Nephropathy

Approximately 40% of patients who have had diabetes mellitus for 20 or more years have nephropathy. Albuminuria greater than 300 mg/24 hours, which is about the level at which a standard urine dipstick test becomes positive, is the hallmark of diabetic nephropathy. The disease can be diagnosed clinically if diabetic retinopathy is also present and there is no other kidney or renal tract disease. Renal failure eventually occurs in approximately 50% of patients who develop diabetes before age 20 and in 6% of those with onset after age 40. Diabetic nephropathy is the leading cause of end-stage renal disease, and the 5-year survival rate of diabetic patients on maintenance dialysis is less than 20%. Almost invariably, nephropathy and retinopathy develop within a short time of each other.

The progression of diabetic nephropathy is as follows: microalbuminuria (urine albumin levels of 30–300 mg/24 hours), macroalbuminuria (urine albumin levels of over 300 mg/24 hours), nephrotic syndrome, and finally end-stage renal disease. Tight control of blood glucose can delay and perhaps prevent the development of microalbuminuria. Controlling hypertension (particularly with angiotensin-converting enzyme inhibitors) and adhering to low-protein diets may help decrease the rate of decline in glomerular filtration rate.

Neuropathy

Diabetic neuropathy is a common problem. After 30 years of diabetes mellitus, half of diabetic patients have signs of neuropathy, and 15%–20% have symptoms of distal symmetric polyneuropathy. Changes in nerve metabolism and function are thought to be mediated in part through increased aldose reductase activity; Schwann cell synthesis of myelin is impaired, and axonal degeneration ensues. In addition, microangiopathy of the endoneural capillaries leads to vascular abnormalities and microinfarcts of the nerves, with multifocal fiber loss. Symptoms in the feet and lower legs are most common. Foot pain, paresthesias, and loss of sensation occur frequently and probably result from both ischemic and metabolic nerve abnormalities. Weakness may occur as part of mononeuritis or a mononeuritis multiplex and is usually associated with pain. Cranial neuropathies may also occur (see BCSC Section 5, *Neuro-Ophthalmology*). Significant morbidity affecting the autonomic nervous system can also occur from neuropathy. Problems can include male and female sexual dysfunction, impaired urination, delayed gastric emptying, orthostatic hypotension, and tachycardia due to loss of vagal tone.

There is no specific treatment for diabetic neuropathy. Aldose reductase inhibitors (not yet commercially available) may improve nerve conduction slightly but do not result in major clinical improvement. The pain may respond to tricyclic antidepressants or capsaicin cream (capsaicin, a component of hot peppers, causes analgesia through local depletion of substance P). Anticonvulsant drugs such as carbamazepine (Tegretol) and gabapentin (Neurontin) may also be useful.

Large-vessel disease

In diabetic patients, the risk of coronary artery disease is 2–10 times higher than that of the general population, and the mortality rate in diabetic patients with an anterior myocardial infarction is twice that of nondiabetic patients. Because myocardial infarction in patients with diabetes may present without the classic symptom of chest pain, an increased index of suspicion is required to make the diagnosis. Hypertension adds significantly to the risk of cardiovascular disease for persons with diabetes. Cerebral thrombosis is approximately twice as prevalent in the diabetic population as it is in the nondiabetic population, and peripheral vascular disease is 40 times more prevalent in the diabetic population.

◉ Ophthalmic considerations   Managing diabetic patients can be challenging. Often the ophthalmologist is the physician who identifies and manages what may be the first apparent complication related to a patient's diabetes, whether a transient refractive change due to glucose elevation or actual diabetic retinopathy. Sometimes the ophthalmologist is a patient's only regular health care provider. Thus, it is important that both the patient and the ophthalmologist be aware of the patient's HbA_{1c} level, a specific and objective measure of glucose control.

Patients may need to be educated about the glucose test, the great importance of maintaining good control, and the possible consequences of poor control. In addition, patients should be reminded that other modifiable risk factors for retinopathy progression, including hypertension, lipid abnormalities, early renal failure, and anemia, are also important.

From an ophthalmic perspective, awareness of a patient's control is important because it may affect the rate of retinopathy progression (and thereby affect decisions regarding treatment and frequency of follow-up). Studies have shown that poor control can increase the rate of retinopathy progression after cataract surgery and blunt the treatment response to laser for diabetic macular edema. Educating patients with poorly controlled diabetes about their prognosis prior to surgical intervention may facilitate more realistic expectations. However, attempting to improve glucose control rapidly in a patient with poor control at the same time that cataract surgery is performed may actually contribute to retinopathy progression and a poorer visual outcome.

The importance of all the risk factors for retinopathy progression should be conveyed to the patient's medical doctor as well so that all potential exacerbating factors are controlled as much as possible. The ophthalmologist should strive to be aware of how well these issues are being controlled, because a patient with significant problems in any of these areas is likely to have less-than-optimal results with any ophthalmic surgical intervention. (The management of diabetic patients at the time of surgery is reviewed in Chapter 15.)

Do DV, Shah SM, Sung JU, Haller JA, Nguyen QD. Persistent diabetic macular edema is associated with elevated hemoglobin A_{1c}. *Am J Ophthalmol.* 2005;139(4):620–623.

Hauser D, Katz H, Pokroy R, Bukelman A, Shechtman E, Pollack A. Occurrence and progression of diabetic retinopathy after phacoemulsification cataract surgery. *J Cataract Refract Surg.* 2004;30(2):428–432.

Suto C, Hori S, Kato S, Muraoka K, Kitano S. Effect of perioperative glycemic control in progression of diabetic retinopathy and maculopathy. *Arch Ophthalmol.* 2006;124(1):38–45.

UpToDate. www.uptodate.com.

Thyroid Disease

Physiology

Functionally, the thyroid gland can be thought of as having 2 parts. The *parafollicular* (or C) cells secrete calcitonin and do not play a role in thyroid physiology. Thyroid *follicles* are made up of a single layer of epithelial cells surrounding colloid, which consists mostly of thyroglobulin, the storage form of the thyroid hormones T_4 and T_3.

T_4 (thyroxine), the main secretory product of the thyroid gland, contains 4 iodine atoms. Deiodination of T_4, which occurs mainly in the liver and kidneys, gives rise to T_3 (triiodothyronine), the metabolically active form of thyroid hormone. Eighty percent of serum T_3 is derived through deiodination; the remainder is secreted by the thyroid. Only a small fraction of the hormones circulate freely in the plasma (0.02% of total T_4 and 0.3% of total T_3); the remainder is bound to the proteins thyroxine-binding globulin (TBG), transthyretin, and albumin.

Thyroid function is regulated by the interrelationships of hypothalamic, pituitary, and thyroid activity. Thyrotropin-releasing hormone (TRH) is secreted by the hypothalamus, causing the synthesis and release of thyrotropin (or thyroid-stimulating hormone, TSH) from the anterior pituitary. TSH, in turn, stimulates the thyroid, leading to the release of T_4 and T_3. T_4 and T_3 inhibit the release of TSH and the TSH response to TRH at the level of the pituitary.

The main role of the thyroid hormones is regulation of tissue metabolism through their effects on protein synthesis. Normal development of the CNS requires adequate amounts of thyroid hormone during the first 2 years of life. Congenital hypothyroidism results in irreversible mental retardation (cretinism). Normal growth and bone maturation also depend on sufficient hormone levels.

Testing for Thyroid Disease

Detection of thyroid disease and evaluation of the efficacy of therapy require the use of various combinations of laboratory tests. Increased availability of direct measurement of free T_4 and the "sensitive" TSH test have greatly simplified the testing process.

Measurement of serum T_4

Total serum T_4 is composed of 2 parts: the protein-bound fraction and the free hormone. Total T_4 levels can be affected by changes in serum TBG levels, while euthyroidism is maintained and free T_4 levels remain normal. Levels of TBG and total T_4 are elevated in pregnancy and with use of oral contraceptives, while free T_4 levels remain normal. Low

TBG and total T_4 levels are associated with chronic illness, protein malnutrition, hepatic failure, and use of glucocorticoids.

For many years, laboratory determination of total T_4 by radioimmunoassay was the most commonly used direct measurement of thyroid function. Free T_4 was then calculated indirectly via multiplication of total T_4 by the T_3 resin uptake (itself an indirect determination of the fraction of unbound thyroid hormone in the serum). Direct determination of free T_4 is now widely available, however, improving the accuracy of thyroid function testing.

Measurement of serum T_3

Serum T_3 levels may not accurately reflect thyroid gland function for 2 reasons: first, because T_3 is not the major secretory product of the thyroid; and second, because many factors influence T_3 levels, including nutrition, medications, and mechanisms regulating the enzymes that convert T_4 to T_3. Determining T_3 levels is indicated in patients who may have T_3 thyrotoxicosis, an uncommon condition in which clinically hyperthyroid patients have normal T_4 and free T_4 but elevated T_3 levels.

Measurement of serum TSH

TSH secretion by the pituitary is tightly controlled by negative feedback mechanisms regulated by serum T_4 and T_3 levels. TSH levels begin to rise early in the course of hypothyroidism and fall early in hyperthyroidism, even before free T_4 levels are outside the reference range. Therefore, the serum TSH level is a sensitive indicator of thyroid dysfunction.

The concentration of TSH is very low and, until recently, available tests were not sensitive enough to differentiate between normal TSH levels and the reduced TSH levels seen in hyperthyroidism. In recent years, extremely sensitive assays of TSH have been developed that can detect levels down to 0.005 mU/L, making it possible to differentiate low normal values from abnormally low values. The TSH test is useful for (1) screening for thyroid disease, (2) monitoring replacement therapy in hypothyroid patients (TSH levels respond 6–8 weeks after changes in hormone replacement dosage), and (3) monitoring suppressive therapy for thyroid nodules or cancer. In screening for thyroid disease, the combination of free T_4 and sensitive TSH assays has a sensitivity of 99.5% and a specificity of 98%. As a result, the combination of both TSH and free T_4 is used for screening in most situations. There is presently some controversy about the upper limit of normal for TSH, and endocrinologic consultation is indicated in borderline cases.

Serum thyroid hormone–binding protein tests

TBG concentrations can be measured directly by immunoassay. However, it is rarely necessary to determine the levels of circulating TBG and transthyretin in the clinical setting. The T_3 resin uptake test can be used to estimate thyroid hormone binding.

Radioactive iodine uptake

A 24-hour test of the thyroid's ability to concentrate a dose of radioactive iodine, radioactive iodine uptake (RAIU) is not always accurate enough to assess thyroid metabolic status. The RAIU test is used mainly to determine whether a patient's hyperthyroidism is due to Graves disease (elevated RAIU, >30%–40%), toxic nodular goiter (normal to elevated), or subacute thyroiditis (low to undetectable, <2%–4%).

Testing for antithyroid antibodies

Several antibodies related to thyroid disease can be detected in the blood. The most common is *thyroid microsomal antibody,* found in about 95% of patients with Hashimoto thyroiditis, 55% of those with Graves disease, and 10% of adults with no apparent thyroid disease. Antibodies to thyroglobulin are also found in thyroid disease of various causes, including Hashimoto thyroiditis, Graves disease, and thyroid carcinoma. Patients with Graves disease usually have antibodies directed at TSH receptors. These antibodies generally stimulate the release of thyroid hormone, although rare patients may have antibodies that block thyroid hormone release. High serum levels of thyroid-stimulating immunoglobulin and the absence of antithyroperoxidase antibody are both risk factors for ophthalmopathy in Graves disease. Assays are available to detect antibodies against antigens present on extraocular muscles in Graves ophthalmopathy, but it is not clear if such antibodies contribute to the disease or if they are simply secondary to extraocular muscle inflammation and damage.

Thyroid scanning

Scanning with iodine 123 reveals concentration and binding, whereas using technetium 99m demonstrates iodide-concentrating capacity. Thyroid scanning is useful in distinguishing functioning (hot) from nonfunctioning (cold) thyroid nodules and in evaluating chest and neck masses for metastatic thyroid cancer.

Thyroid ultrasonography

Ultrasonography is used to establish the presence of cystic or solid thyroid nodules when palpation is inconclusive in suspicious cases. This modality detects nodules as small as 1 mm, although nodules of this size are not of clinical significance. Thyroid ultrasonography is also useful in assessing the effectiveness of suppressive therapy for reduction of thyroid nodule size.

Biopsy or fine-needle aspiration biopsy

Biopsy or fine-needle aspiration techniques are used to obtain tissue samples for the evaluation of thyroid nodules. Fine-needle aspiration specimens require interpretation by an experienced cytopathologist. Needle aspiration is also used to drain fluid from cystic thyroid nodules.

Hyperthyroidism

Hypermetabolism caused by excessive quantities of circulating thyroid hormones results in the clinical syndrome of *hyperthyroidism (thyrotoxicosis).* This syndrome can be caused by a number of diseases. Graves hyperthyroidism accounts for approximately 85% of cases of thyrotoxicosis. Toxic nodular goiter and thyroiditis account for most of the remaining cases. *Thyroid storm,* a potentially fatal complication seen in some patients with hyperthyroidism, is a medical emergency. It is often precipitated by stress or infection in a patient with otherwise mild hyperthyroidism; modern treatments aimed at controlling the process have dramatically reduced mortality.

Graves hyperthyroidism

Thyroid eye disease (*TED*; also known as *thyroid-associated orbitopathy* or *Graves ophthalmopathy*) is discussed in BCSC Section 5, *Neuro-Ophthalmology,* and Section 7, *Orbit, Eyelids, and Lacrimal System*; this discussion focuses on the thyroid disease.)

Patients with Graves hyperthyroidism (also known as *diffuse toxic goiter*) exhibit various combinations of hypermetabolism, diffuse enlargement of the thyroid gland, TED (ophthalmopathy), and infiltrative dermopathy. Although the exact cause is not known, Graves hyperthyroidism is thought to be an autoimmune disorder: 85%–90% of patients have circulating TSH receptor antibodies.

Graves hyperthyroidism is common, with a 10:1 female preponderance. The incidence peaks in the third and fourth decades of life; there is a strong familial component, and stress may also play a role. Current smoking is associated with an increased incidence of TED that parallels the number of cigarettes smoked per day.

The clinical syndrome is well known; it consists of nervousness, tremor, weight loss, palpitations, heat intolerance, emotional lability, muscle weakness, and gastrointestinal hypermotility. Clinical signs include tachycardia or atrial fibrillation, increased systolic and decreased diastolic blood pressure (widened pulse pressure), and thyroid enlargement. *Infiltrative dermopathy*—brawny, nonpitting swelling of the pretibial area, ankles, or feet—may be present and is almost always associated with TED. Infiltrative dermopathy was known as *pretibial myxedema* in the past. The terminology has changed to avoid confusion with the term *myxedema,* which refers to the diffuse accumulation of glycosaminoglycans and fluid in hypothyroidism. Approximately one third of patients with Graves hyperthyroidism have clinically obvious TED at the time of diagnosis of the hyperthyroidism.

Treatment of Graves hyperthyroidism is aimed at returning thyroid function to normal. A significant proportion of patients (30%–50%) experience remission in association with drug treatment directed at the thyroid. Later in the course of the disease, patients may experience relapse, hypothyroidism, or both.

The first step in treatment is to control symptoms, if necessary, with a β-blocker. In addition, thyroid secretion is suppressed using 1 of the thiourea derivatives, propylthiouracil or methimazole (Tapazole). The drugs inhibit the use of iodine by the gland. Treatment is continued until clinical and laboratory indices show improvement. Adverse effects include rash (common), liver damage (rare), vasculitis (rare), and agranulocytosis (0.02%–0.05% of patients).

There are several options for long-term treatment of Graves hyperthyroidism: the aforementioned antithyroid drugs can be continued for 12–24 months in hopes of a remission; part of the gland can be surgically removed, an option that is frequently successful, although approximately half of such patients eventually become hypothyroid; or radioactive iodine can be used, which is the third and most common choice. Iodine 131 is highly effective, resulting in hypothyroidism in 80% of patients within 6–12 months; some require a second treatment. Side effects are minimal, although use of iodine 131 may be associated with worsening of TED (ophthalmopathy). Corticosteroids may be useful in preventing progression of TED related to this treatment.

Toxic nodular goiter

In toxic nodular goiter, thyroid hormone–producing adenomas (either single or multiple) make enough hormone to cause hyperthyroidism. Hot nodules (those shown to be functioning on thyroid scan) are almost never carcinomatous and often result in hyperthyroidism. Toxic nodules may be treated with radioactive iodine or surgery.

Hypothyroidism

Hypothyroidism is a clinical syndrome resulting from a deficiency of thyroid hormone. *Myxedema* is the nonpitting edema caused by subcutaneous accumulation of mucopolysaccharides in severe cases of hypothyroidism; the term is sometimes used to describe the entire syndrome of severe hypothyroidism.

   Primary hypothyroidism accounts for more than 95% of cases and may be congenital or acquired. Most primary cases are due to Hashimoto thyroiditis (discussed in the following section), "idiopathic" myxedema (thought by many to be end-stage Hashimoto thyroiditis), and iatrogenic causes (after iodine 131 or surgical treatment of hyperthyroidism). *Secondary hypothyroidism,* caused by hypothalamic or pituitary dysfunction (usually after pituitary surgery), is much less common. As in hyperthyroidism, the female preponderance among adults is significant. *Subclinical hypothyroidism* is defined as a normal T_4 concentration and a slightly elevated TSH level. These patients may or may not have symptoms suggestive of hypothyroidism, and there is some controversy about whether such patients should be treated.

   Clinically, the patient with hypothyroidism presents with signs and symptoms of hypometabolism and accumulation of mucopolysaccharides in the tissues of the body. Many of the symptoms are nonspecific—weakness, fatigue, lethargy, decreased memory, dry skin, deepening of the voice, weight gain (despite loss of appetite), cold intolerance, arthralgias, constipation, and muscle cramps—and their relationship to thyroid dysfunction may not be recognized for some time. Clinical signs include bradycardia, reduced pulse pressure, myxedema, loss of body and scalp hair, and menstrual disorders. In severe cases, personality changes ("myxedema madness") and death (following "myxedema coma") may occur.

   Treatment of hypothyroidism is straightforward, consisting of oral thyroid replacement medication to normalize circulating hormone levels. Levothyroxine is the most commonly used preparation. Serum T_4 and TSH levels are monitored at regular intervals to ensure that euthyroidism is maintained.

Thyroiditis

Thyroiditis may be classified as acute, subacute, or chronic. *Acute thyroiditis,* caused by bacterial infection, is extremely rare. *Subacute thyroiditis* occurs in 2 forms: granulomatous and lymphocytic. Hashimoto thyroiditis is the most common type of *chronic thyroiditis.*

   Patients with *subacute granulomatous thyroiditis* present with a painful, enlarged gland associated with fever, chills, and malaise. Thyroid function tests may be helpful because they may reveal the unusual combination of an elevated T_4 level and a low RAIU. Patients may be hyperthyroid because of the release of hormone from areas of thyroid destruction; pathologic examination reveals granulomatous inflammation. The disease is self-limited, and treatment is symptomatic, with use of either analgesics or, in severe cases, oral corticosteroids. After resolution, transient hypothyroidism, which becomes permanent in 5%–10% of patients, may occur.

Patients with *subacute lymphocytic thyroiditis* ("painless" thyroiditis), which commonly occurs 2–4 months postpartum in mothers but may occur in isolation, present with symptoms of hyperthyroidism and a normal or slightly enlarged but nontender thyroid gland. Pathologic investigation shows lymphocytic infiltration resembling Hashimoto thyroiditis, suggesting an autoimmune cause. This disease is also self-limited, generally lasting less than 3 months. Hypothyroidism may ensue. Treatment is symptomatic.

An autoimmune disease that appears to be closely related to Graves hyperthyroidism, Hashimoto thyroiditis is the most common cause of goitrous hypothyroidism in iodine-sufficient areas of the world. Patients have antibodies to 1 or more thyroid antigens and an increased incidence of other autoimmune diseases, such as Sjögren syndrome, systemic lupus erythematosus, idiopathic thrombocytopenic purpura, and pernicious anemia. In rare cases, other endocrine organs—the adrenals, parathyroids, pancreatic islet cells, pituitary, and gonads—may be involved as well.

Patients with Hashimoto thyroiditis may present with hypothyroidism, an enlarged thyroid, or both. Pathologic examination reveals lymphocytic infiltration. Treatment is aimed at normalizing hormone levels with thyroid replacement therapy. Patients with enlarged glands and airway obstruction that do not respond to TSH suppression may require surgery. The risk of primary thyroid lymphoma is slightly increased in patients with Hashimoto thyroiditis.

Postpartum thyroiditis occurs in approximately 5% of women after delivery (often in subsequent pregnancies) and can cause hyperthyroidism or hypothyroidism (or first one problem and then the other). Postpartum thyroiditis is usually painless and self-limited and is often associated with antimicrosomal antibodies.

Thyroid Tumors

Virtually all tumors of the thyroid gland arise from glandular cells and are, therefore, adenomas or carcinomas. Functioning adenomas were discussed previously (in "Toxic nodular goiter").

On thyroid scan, 90%–95% of thyroid adenomas are nonfunctioning ("cold" nodules) and come to attention only if large enough to be physically apparent. Diagnostic testing involves a combination of approaches, including ultrasonography (cysts are benign and simply aspirated), fine-needle aspiration, and surgery, depending on the clinical situation. Treatment options for benign cold nodules are suppressive therapy, in which thyroid hormone replacement is used to suppress TSH secretion and its stimulatory effect on functioning nodules, and surgery.

Carcinomas of the thyroid are of 4 types: papillary, follicular, medullary, and anaplastic (undifferentiated). *Papillary carcinoma* is the most common form of thyroid tumor. Tumors removed prior to extension outside the capsule of the gland appear to have no adverse effect on survival. *Follicular carcinoma* may also be compatible with a normal life span if it is identified before it becomes invasive, although late metastases can occur. *Medullary carcinoma* arises from the C cells and produces calcitonin. The lesion can occur as a solitary malignancy or as part of multiple endocrine neoplasia syndrome type 2 (discussed at the end of the chapter). *Anaplastic carcinoma,* although rare, is the most malignant tumor of the thyroid gland and is found mainly in patients older than age 60. With the giant cell form, the survival time is less than 6 months from time of diagnosis; with the small cell form, the 5-year survival rate is 20%–25%.

The Hypothalamic-Pituitary Axis

The hypothalamus is the coordinating center of the endocrine system. It consolidates signals from higher cortical centers, the autonomic nervous system, the environment, and systemic endocrine feedback. The hypothalamus then delivers precise instructions to the pituitary gland, which releases hormones that influence most endocrine systems in the body. The hypothalamic-pituitary axis directly affects the thyroid gland, the adrenal gland, and the gonads, and it influences growth, milk production, and water balance.

Table 9-5 shows the various hypothalamic and anterior pituitary hormones involved in this system. The hypothalamic hormones are released directly into a primary capillary plexus that empties into the portal venous circulation, travels down the pituitary stalk, and bathes the anterior pituitary gland in a secondary capillary plexus. The hormones released by the hypothalamic neurons, therefore, reach their target cells rapidly and in high concentrations. This proximity allows a rapid, pulsatile response to signals between the hypothalamus and the anterior pituitary. The posterior pituitary is controlled by direct neuronal innervation from the hypothalamus rather than by bloodborne hormones. The main products of the posterior pituitary are vasopressin and oxytocin. Vasopressin (antidiuretic hormone) is primarily involved in controlling water excretion by the kidneys. Oxytocin produces uterine contractions required for delivery.

Pituitary Adenomas

Pituitary tumors constitute 10% of intracranial tumors. They are classified as *microadenomas* (<10 mm in widest diameter) or *macroadenomas* (>10 mm in widest diameter).

Table 9-5 Major Hypothalamic Hormones and Their Effect on Anterior Pituitary Hormones

Corticotropin-releasing hormone releases adrenocorticotropic hormone (ACTH).
Growth hormone–releasing hormone releases growth hormone.
Somatostatin inhibits growth hormone release.
Gonadotropin-releasing hormone releases luteinizing hormone (LH) and follicle-stimulating hormone (FSH).
Thyrotropin-releasing hormone (TRH) releases thyrotropin (TSH).
Prolactin-releasing factors (including serotonin, acetylcholine, opiates, and estrogens) release prolactin.
Prolactin-inhibiting factors (including dopamine) inhibit the release of prolactin.
Melanocyte-stimulating hormone-releasing factor releases melanocyte-stimulating hormone.

Reproduced with permission from Martin KA. Hypothalamic-pituitary axis. In: *UpToDate,* Rose BD (ed), Waltham, MA. Available at www.uptodate.com. Accessed March 1, 2005.

Typically benign, these tumors arise from hormone-producing cells and may be functionally active (ie, producing usually large amounts of hormones) or inactive. The clinical presentation depends on what type of cell the tumor is derived from and whether there is hormone production. Any type of tumor may be clinically nonfunctioning and therefore will become apparent only when it has enlarged enough to cause symptoms, at which time patients may present with headaches, visual symptoms due to chiasmal compression, cranial neuropathies, and/or hypopituitarism from compression of normal pituitary tissue. (The ophthalmic effects of pituitary adenomas and other parasellar lesions are discussed in BCSC Section 5, *Neuro-Ophthalmology*.)

Accounting for approximately 15% of pituitary tumors, *somatotroph adenomas* produce growth hormone and cause acromegaly in adults and gigantism in prepubertal patients. Acromegaly often develops insidiously over several years. Patients may present with headaches and visual symptoms due to enlargement of the adenoma before the diagnosis is recognized. The characteristic findings are an enlarged jaw, coarse facial features, and enlarged and swollen hands and feet. Patients may also have cardiac disease and diabetes mellitus in addition to the typical bone and soft tissue changes.

Lactotroph adenomas (prolactinomas) account for approximately 25% of symptomatic pituitary tumors. Hyperprolactinemia produces amenorrhea and galactorrhea in women and decreased libido and impotence in men. The symptoms tend to be gradual in males, and patients may present with compression symptoms due to tumor enlargement before the hormonal effects are recognized.

Thyrotroph adenomas are rare, accounting for less than 1% of pituitary tumors. They may cause hyperthyroidism, hypothyroidism, or no change in thyroid function, depending on how the TSH subunits are processed in the tumor cells. These tumors tend to be large macroadenomas, and patients may present with compressive symptoms in addition to any thyroid changes.

Corticotroph adenomas account for approximately 15% of pituitary tumors. They are associated with Cushing syndrome, which includes the classic features of centripetal obesity, hirsutism, and plethora. Patients develop fat deposits over the thoracocervical spine (buffalo hump) and temporal regions (moon facies). Psychiatric abnormalities occur in 50% of patients, and long-standing Cushing disease can produce osteoporosis. Patients bruise easily and have violet striae on the abdomen, upper thighs, and arms. Hypertension and glucose intolerance leading to diabetes can also occur. Cushing syndrome can occur as well because of adrenal gland neoplasms and, most commonly, because of iatrogenic administration of glucocorticoids.

Gonadotroph adenomas (approximately 10% of pituitary tumors) may produce serum follicle-stimulating hormone and, in rare cases, luteinizing hormone. Affected patients present with hypogonadism related to gonadal down-regulation. Gonadotropin-producing pituitary tumors may also be clinically nonfunctioning, and patients may present with compression symptoms.

Accounting for approximately 15% of pituitary tumors, *plurihormonal adenomas,* as the name implies, produce more than one type of hormone. Common combinations include elevated growth hormone with prolactin, and growth hormone with TSH.

Null-cell adenomas (approximately 20% of pituitary tumors) do not have any pathologic markers to suggest a certain cell type and do not produce hormone excess. The majority of tumors that present with signs of enlargement and compression are gonado-troph or null-cell adenomas.

Tumors of the pituitary gland are best diagnosed with MRI focused on the pituitary region. Endocrinologic testing is warranted when hypersecretion syndromes are suspected or when the patient has evidence of hypopituitarism due to compression of the normal pituitary by a nonfunctioning adenoma. The treatment approach is complex and depends on a number of factors, including the size of the tumor and the nature of the hormonal activity. Treatment is discussed further in BCSC Section 5, *Neuro-Ophthalmology*.

Pituitary Apoplexy

Pituitary apoplexy results from hemorrhage in a pituitary adenoma that can occur spon-taneously or after head trauma. In its most dramatic presentation, apoplexy causes the sudden onset of excruciating headache, visual field loss, diplopia due to pressure on the oculomotor nerves, and hypopituitarism. All pituitary hormonal deficiencies can occur, but cortisol deficiency is the most serious because it can cause life-threatening hypoten-sion. Imaging of the pituitary reveals intra-adenomal hemorrhage and deviation of the pi-tuitary stalk. Most patients recover but experience long-term pituitary insufficiency. Signs of reduced visual acuity and altered mental status are indications for transsphenoidal sur-gical decompression. Ophthalmologists need to be aware of this entity because of the high incidence of visual symptoms on presentation.

Multiple Endocrine Neoplasia Syndromes

Multiple endocrine neoplasia (MEN) syndromes are rare hereditary syndromes of benign and malignant endocrine neoplasms. There are 2 syndromes, MEN 1 and MEN 2, both of which are inherited in an autosomal dominant fashion. MEN 2 is further divided into types 2A and 2B.

The most common features of MEN 1 are parathyroid, enteropancreatic, and pitu-itary tumors. Hyperparathyroidism is the most common endocrine abnormality. En-teropancreatic tumors include gastrinomas, which cause increased gastric acid output (Zollinger-Ellison syndrome), and insulinomas, which cause fasting hypoglycemia. Pitu-itary adenomas can be present and are usually prolactinomas, though other types can also occur. Carcinoid and adrenal tumors can develop as well.

MEN 2A and 2B are characterized by medullary thyroid cancer, which occurs in 90%–100% of patients and is the main cause of morbidity. Pheochromocytoma occurs with an incidence of approximately 50%. Hyperparathyroidism is seen in approximately 20%–30% of patients with MEN 2A, but is rarely seen in 2B.

MEN 2B is characterized by ganglioneuromas, which occur in 95% of patients. They can occur in the lips, eyelids, and tongue, giving these patients a characteristic phenotype that can be apparent at birth. Patients with MEN 2B may also have marfanoid features but do not have lens subluxation or aortic disease. The eyelid margins may be nodular because of the presence of multiple small tumors (Fig 9-3); neuromas have also been reported subconjunctivally. Perhaps the most striking ophthalmic finding is the presence of promi-nent corneal nerves in a clear stroma; this is reported to occur in 100% of cases (Fig 9-4).

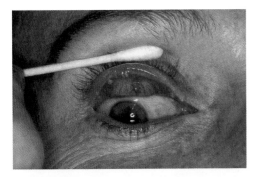

Figure 9-3 Eyelid nodules in MEN 2B. *(Courtesy of Jason M. Jacobs, MD, and Michael J. Hawes, MD.)*

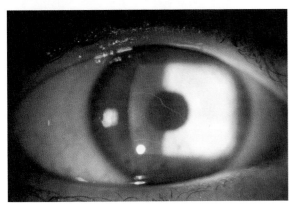

Figure 9-4 Enlarged corneal nerves in MEN 2B. *(Courtesy of Jason M. Jacobs, MD, and Michael J. Hawes, MD.)*

Because the medullary thyroid cancer may not appear until the patient's second or third decade, the ophthalmic manifestations may be the initial indication that a patient has MEN 2B, making ophthalmologists potentially instrumental in diagnosing this disease.

The management of MEN depends on the nature of the tumor and usually involves medical treatment to control hormonal effects and/or surgical excision when possible. The genes that cause all types of MEN have been located, and genetic testing can identify patients at risk. Identification of involved family members is particularly useful in MEN 2 because prophylactic thyroidectomy can decrease the risk of death from medullary thyroid cancer. Screening for pheochromocytoma is also warranted in order to identify problems before complications such as hypertension develop. Ophthalmologists have a critical role to play in recognizing the findings associated with MEN 2B, because early diagnosis of this syndrome may be life-saving.

Jacobs JM, Hawes MJ. From eyelid bumps to thyroid lumps: report of a MEN type IIb family and review of the literature. *Ophthal Plast Reconstr Surg*. 2001;17(3):195–201.

Kronenberg HM, Melmed S, Polonsky KS, Larsen PR, eds. *Williams Textbook of Endocrinology*. 11th ed. Philadelphia: Elsevier/Saunders; 2008.

UpToDate. www.uptodate.com.

Washington University School of Medicine, Department of Medicine; Henderson KE, Baranski TJ, Bickel PE, et al. *The Washington Manual Endocrinology Subspecialty Consult*. 2nd ed. Philadelphia: Lippincott Williams & Wilkins; 2008.

The authors would like to thank David A. Sorg, MD, for his contributions to this chapter.

CHAPTER 10

Geriatrics

The expanding older population in the United States presents a growing challenge to primary care physicians and medical subspecialists. Increasing life expectancies are at a record high of 77.7 years, reported for 2006. The baby boomers will be 65 and older in 2030, accounting for nearly 1 in 5 US residents, and this age group is estimated to increase to 88.5 million by 2050. The 85 and older population is projected to more than triple, from 5.4 million to 19 million between 2008 and 2050.

Ophthalmology is one specialty that will be significantly affected by this demographic shift. Although ophthalmologists already care for older patients, there will be an increasing need for geriatric expertise in all the medical subspecialties, including ophthalmology. In addition, cataracts, age-related macular degeneration (AMD), ischemic optic neuropathy, giant cell arteritis, diabetic retinopathy, and glaucoma are all diseases that disproportionately affect older persons. These eye conditions are discussed elsewhere, but the ophthalmologist needs to consider the impact of visual loss on activities of daily living (ADLs) and functional outcome.

Ophthalmologists may be expert in dealing with ophthalmic problems in the geriatric population, but they may lack experience in identifying and managing geriatric problems in general. In the past, most medical specialties (including ophthalmology) have followed the traditional medical paradigm of diagnosis of illness, treatment of disease, and measurement of objective outcomes (usually vision parameters such as visual acuity or visual field). The relatively new subspecialty of geriatrics emphasizes a different medical paradigm of functional assessment and a more holistic approach to patient care. For example, rather than measuring visual acuity as an independent and isolated outcome, a functional approach might incorporate improvement in ADLs and independence.

Geriatricians have developed validated instruments for assessing ADLs. Practicing ophthalmologists may not use these instruments daily, but they must recognize the potential impact of visual loss on ADLs, as well as the importance of joining the geriatrician or primary care physician in completely evaluating and managing their older patients. The paradigm involves developing a multidisciplinary history and performing a comprehensive physical examination that incorporates measures of physical health (including visual function), psychosocial assessment (including mental health, social support), and functional assessment.

These goals were summarized by the National Institutes of Health Consensus Development Conference on geriatric assessment: "[T]he multiple problems of older persons are uncovered, described, and explained, if possible, and . . . the resources and strengths of the person are catalogued, the need for services assessed, and a coordinated care plan developed to focus interventions on the person's problems" (p 1409).

The ophthalmologist's role in this multidisciplinary evaluation is to communicate the visual limitations and visual needs of the older patient to the geriatrician and to contribute to the integrated goals of the care plan. The role of the ophthalmologist is not to provide a comprehensive geriatric assessment but to screen for and identify particular geriatric conditions (eg, depression, dementia).

Lee and colleagues showed that screening for depression, dementia, and functional impairment in an ophthalmology practice can be accomplished quickly (less than 5 minutes) and easily with a geriatric screening tool they developed. Their investigation selected elements from more comprehensive established tests (clock drawing, instrumental activities of daily living) and from a depression screening. Questions are incorporated into the screening related to using the telephone, traveling, shopping, preparing meals, doing housework, taking medication, and managing money. To screen for depression, the investigators asked, "Do you often feel sad or depressed?" By incorporating questions from accepted geriatric screening tests into their newly devised test, Lee and colleagues were able to screen a selected group of geriatric patients, in a relatively short time, before their eye examination. They demonstrated that 20% of patients studied were depressed or showed early signs of dementia, and 6% of these patients had a functional impairment. Using this tool, the ophthalmologist would be able to identify patients at risk and refer them to appropriate resources.

The psychosocial assessment recognizes the age-related role changes and identifies and coordinates available services. The goals are to increase the level of functioning but maintain patient self-determination. The ophthalmologist should recognize the need for psychosocial assessment when there is a change in the patient's cognitive, affective, or functional abilities (eg, loss of visual function, new signs or symptoms of depression or dementia, inability to drive).

Appropriate referral and coordination of care with the geriatrician or primary care physician should accomplish the following:

- Identify the strengths and weaknesses of patients in their environment.
- Assess cognitive, affective, functional, environmental, and economic issues.
- Include any appropriate changes in social support, and identify caregiver stress.
- Explore possible placement issues and options.

The ophthalmologist should also be able to recognize the effect of vision loss on function. Referral to vision rehabilitation is appropriate for patients with acuity less than 20/40, central scotomata, field loss, or contrast sensitivity loss. The SmartSight patient handout, available on the American Academy of Ophthalmology website, can be given to patients to inform them of how they may be able to access Medicare-funded multidisciplinary vision rehabilitation or other vision rehabilitation services in their community. The Academy's Preferred Practice Pattern *Vision Rehabilitation for Adults* outlines how comprehensive vision rehabilitation addresses reading, ADLs, patient safety, continued community participation, and patient well-being.

Lee AG, Beaver HA, Jogerst G, Daly JM. Screening elderly patients in an outpatient ophthalmology clinic for dementia, depression, and functional impairment. *Ophthalmology.* 2003; 110(4):651–657.

Modules in Clinical Geriatrics. Blue Cross and Blue Shield Association, American Geriatrics Society; 1997.

National Center for Health Statistics (CDC) [online]. Available at www.cdc.gov/nchs.

SmartSight. San Francisco: American Academy of Ophthalmology. Available at http://one.aao.org/CE/EducationalContent/Smartsight.aspx.

Solomon D, Sue Brown A, Brummel-Smith K, et al. Best Paper of the 1980s: National Institutes of Health Consensus Development Conference Statement: geriatric assessment methods for clinical decision-making. *J Am Geriatr Soc.* 2003;51(10):1490–1494.

Vision Rehabilitation Committee. Preferred Practice Patterns. *Vision Rehabilitation for Adults.* San Francisco: American Academy of Ophthalmology; 2007. Available at http://one.aao.org/CE/PracticeGuidelines/PPP.aspx.

Physiologic Aging and Pathologic Findings of the Aging Eye

Changes in the eye due to aging affect everyone, but there are marked differences among individuals. The periorbital and eyelid skin and soft tissues atrophy with age. Dermatochalasis and levator dehiscence may produce secondary ptosis. Lid laxity may cause entropion, ectropion, and trichiasis. Lacrimal gland dysfunction, decreased tear production, meibomian gland disease, and goblet cell dysfunction may cause dry eye symptoms. As a person ages, the conjunctiva undergoes atrophic changes, and corneal sensitivity is reduced. The pupils become progressively miotic and less reactive to light. There is an increasing incidence of presbyopia, cataract, glaucoma, AMD, and diabetic retinopathy. Contrast sensitivity and visual field sensitivity are reduced. In addition, refractive error (of some type) is present in more than 90% of older patients and remains a significant cause of visual disability in the nursing home patient.

The 4 leading causes of visual loss in the older population are AMD, glaucoma, cataract, and diabetic retinopathy. It is estimated that by 2020, 2.95 million will have AMD. Glaucoma becomes more common with increasing age, and screening is recommended for patients older than age 50. It is also estimated that by 2020, 30.1 million Americans will have cataracts, a 50% increase, and 9.5 million will be pseudophakic/aphakic, a 60% increase from the year 2000.

Congdon N, O'Colmain B, Klaver CC, et al; Eye Diseases Prevalence Research Group. Causes and prevalence of visual impairment among adults in the United States. *Arch Ophthalmol.* 2004;122(4):477–485.

Congdon N, Vingerling JR, Klein BE, et al; Eye Diseases Prevalence Research Group. Prevalence of cataract and pseudophakia/aphakia among adults in the United States. *Arch Ophthalmol.* 2004;122(4):487–494.

Friedman DS, O'Colmain BJ, Muñoz B, et al; Eye Diseases Prevalence Research Group. Prevalence of age-related macular degeneration in the United States. *Arch Ophthalmol.* 2004;122(4):564–572.

Pharmacology

Medication use and the number and frequency of medications, adverse reactions to medicines, and drug interactions increase with advancing age. Ophthalmologists need to be aware that ophthalmic medications may have adverse effects in older patients or may interact with other medications. Age-related pharmacokinetic changes include changes in drug absorption, distribution, metabolism, and elimination. Caution is needed when using new agents, which are often less tested and proven in the older population. A complete medication history, including prescription medications, over-the-counter drugs, herbal agents, vitamins and supplements, and topical agents is mandatory in all patients. Because some older patients are unaware of or do not remember their medication allergies, verifying this information with the family or primary care physician would be prudent. See also BCSC Section 2, *Fundamentals and Principles of Ophthalmology.*

The ophthalmologist should regularly review all of a patient's medications (including topical antibiotics, corticosteroids, and antiglaucoma medications). Older patients (especially nursing home patients) often take multiple medications whose indications expired long ago. Review of the indications for current ophthalmic medications and discontinuation of unnecessary medications should reduce ophthalmology's contribution to polypharmacy. In addition, ophthalmologists should be familiar with all the agents they prescribe, including their side effects in older patients and their potential interactions with other medications. For example, the long-term use of systemic corticosteroids in an older patient may cause proximal muscle wasting and may exacerbate osteoporosis. Finally, if medical therapy is needed, the ophthalmologist should recognize that compliance issues are often more complex with older persons. Considerations include dosing frequency, difficulty in applying the medication, remembering complex dosing regimens (because of dementia, arthritis, poor vision), the number of agents, and expense. A list of prescribed eye medications that includes the dose and frequency of administration (preferably printed in large type and color coded to match the caps on the bottles) helps to ensure compliance.

Outpatient Visits

Ophthalmology is largely an outpatient specialty. Access to the ophthalmologist's office can be a major physical barrier to eye care for older patients. The ideal outpatient office should be designed to accommodate geriatric patients with various disabilities. The geriatric-friendly office environment should include the following:

- a safe, well-lit office that is close to drop-off areas and parking
- automatic or assisted doors (doorways with pull levers or handles)
- large-print, legible, and well-placed signs
- wheelchair-accessible entranceways and waiting rooms
- obstacle-free and well-lit, high-contrast walkways, hallways, and waiting areas (free of rugs, electrical cords, and hazards for falls, such as toys)

- accessible bathrooms with elevated toilet seats, grab bars, and a wheelchair-accessible sink
- trained staff to assist the patient with a disability to and from the examination room
- a private area where patients with decreased hearing and vision can receive assistance from staff in completing forms

Elder Abuse

The ophthalmologist may be the first or only physician to see an older patient suffering from maltreatment. The signs of elder abuse may be subtle, and early recognition is key. The national prevalence of elder maltreatment is between 2% and 10% and may affect 1.5–2.0 million older adults each year. The actual numbers are probably significantly higher because of underreporting of cases. Major risk factors for elder abuse include external stresses due to marital, financial, and legal difficulties; dependent relationships (eg, the abuser may be dependent on the older patient for finances or housing); mental illness and substance abuse; social isolation; and misinformation about normal aging or about the patient's medical or nutritional needs. Maltreatment can occur at home, in assisted living, or in nursing homes. It can take the form of physical or psychological abuse, material misappropriation, neglect, or sexual attack.

Physical neglect includes withholding of food or water, medical care, medication, or hygiene. Neglect may be intentional or unintentional and may be fostered by financial constraints or other lack of resources (eg, transportation, supervision). Elder abuse also includes financial abuse or exploitation, deprivation of basic rights (eg, decision making for care, privacy), and abandonment. Actual physical abuse in the form of slapping, restraining, and hitting may cause physical pain or injury.

The ophthalmologist should suspect elder abuse ("red flags") in the following circumstances:

- bruises, black eyes, and fractures
- broken eyeglasses and report by the patient of being slapped or abused
- repeated visits to the emergency room or office
- conflicting or noncredible history from caregiver or patient
- unexplained delay in seeking treatment
- unexplained, inconsistent, vague, or poorly explained injuries
- history of being "accident-prone"
- expressions of ambivalence, anger, hostility, or fear by the patient toward the caregiver
- poor compliance with follow-up or care instructions
- evidence of physical abuse (eg, skin bruises, lacerations, wounds in various stages of healing, unusually shaped bruises, burns, welts, patches of hair loss, or unexplained subconjunctival, retinal, or vitreous hemorrhage)

Sometimes it is necessary to obtain the history with the caregiver absent. Directed questions for the patient include "Has anyone at home tried to harm you?" "Has anyone tried to make you do things that you don't wish to do?" "Has anyone taken anything from you without your consent?"

Any suspected case of elder neglect or abuse should prompt a complete written report. Documentation of any suspicious injuries is mandatory, including type, size, location, and characteristics of injury and stage of healing. Mandatory reporting of elder abuse varies from state to state, and many localities have abuse hotlines for reporting maltreatment. The physician should be aware of local services for adult protection, community social service, and law enforcement agencies.

Lachs MS, Pillemer K. Elder abuse. *Lancet*. 2004;364(9441):1263–1272.

Surgical Considerations

The ophthalmologist should be aware of how preoperative and perioperative evaluation and management differ for the older patient. Loss of visual acuity alone may not be an appropriate sole indication for surgical intervention (eg, cataract surgery). Functional assessment includes determining how visual loss affects IADLs (instrumental activities of daily living; eg, reading, driving, taking medications properly, using telephone independently). Documentation of these functional impairments is important for preoperative assessment. In addition, issues of informed consent are important in patients with mild dementia or in those who have legal guardians or caregivers.

The ophthalmic surgeon should know some general principles regarding the preoperative assessment of older patients. Delirium and confusion affect up to 25% of older patients in the postoperative period. There are numerous causes for confusion in this setting, but many are preventable. Minimization of preoperative sedation or psychotropic medications, appropriate patient and family orientation by nursing or ancillary staff, and careful supervision and reassurance in the postoperative period can decrease postoperative confusion. Often, a confused older patient simply needs a familiar face or reassurance to regain calm. The use of restraints should be minimized.

Confusion may be exacerbated in patients with visual loss or in those who require visual rehabilitation. In monocular older patients, patching of the eye after surgery may aggravate confusion and disorientation. Having a family member in the recovery room can be very helpful. The patch should be removed as soon as possible, and patients should be provided with appropriate eye protection. Topical anesthetic may not be indicated because of comorbidities such as cognitive impairment and inability to cooperate during surgery. In addition, patients with decreased vision following intraocular surgery may experience decreased mobility or be at increased risk for falls. Bed rest and immobilization can lead to disuse of extremities from lying in bed and lack of movement, pressure ulcers, and other problems. Active rehabilitation should be encouraged as soon as possible ("bed is bad").

Although rare in outpatient ophthalmic surgery, surgical or anesthesia complications may produce life-threatening problems. The surgeon must pay careful attention to any preexisting directives (eg, do not resuscitate orders or living wills) prior to any surgical intervention (including laser treatments and periocular injections or anesthetics). By discussing possible treatment decisions early on—preferably before any serious illness arises or, if a serious illness is present, early in its course—the surgeon can avoid emergency decisions.

Some potential issues for discussion include limits of treatment, feeding tubes, antibiotics, and changes in living situation. Candidly and openly discussing these important issues with the patient and the family (especially in cases of dementia) in the preoperative period allows them to consider these matters in the context of their belief systems and without the disorientation and confusion created by an emergency. The content, context, time, and date of such discussions should be well documented in the medical record and communicated to the patient, the family, and the primary care physician or geriatrician.

When difficult decisions do need to be made, the physician should not merely set forth a menu of possible choices but should provide information on probable outcomes (such as survival with cardiopulmonary resuscitation, which patients and family members tend to overestimate). Treatments that are futile need not be offered, but the question of what constitutes medical futility is complex.

Psychology of Aging

The psychology of aging is influenced by a wide range of factors, including physical changes, adaptive mechanisms, and psychopathology. Each older patient has a unique psychological profile and social life history. Deleterious changes are not universal; in fact, in the absence of disease, growth of character and the ability to learn continue throughout life.

As we age, the issue of loss becomes more prevalent. Losses—of status, physical abilities, loved ones, and income—become more frequent. A fear of loss of social and individual power, and with it an attendant loss of independence, is common. In addition, the reality of death has increasing influence on a person's psychological status.

Duthrie EH, Katz PR, Malone M. *Practice of Geriatrics.* 4th ed. Philadelphia: Elsevier/Saunders; 2007.

Geriatric Review Syllabus: A Core Curriculum in Geriatric Medicine. 6th ed (GRS6). New York: American Geriatrics Society; 2009. http://www.americangeriatrics.org.

Katz PR, Grossberg GT, Potter JF, Solomon DH; American Geriatrics Society. *Geriatrics Syllabus for Specialists.* New York: American Geriatrics Society; 2002:chap 11, 19, 36, 39.

Reuben DB, Herr KA, Pacala JT, Pollock BG, Potter JF, Semla TP. *Geriatrics at Your Fingertips.* 11th ed. New York: American Geriatrics Society; 2009.

Normal Aging Changes

Age-related changes in sensation and perception can have great influence, isolating an individual from the surrounding environment and requiring complex psychological reactions. There may be diminution of hearing and vision (see Ophthalmic Considerations, later in this chapter), slowing of intellectual and physical response time, and increasing difficulty with memory.

Many physical and intellectual abilities, however, are retained throughout life, and their loss should not be assumed to be part of the normal aging process. These include the senses of taste and smell, intelligence, the ability to learn, and sexuality. Any change in physical, intellectual, or emotional capabilities may reflect underlying organic or psychological disease.

Psychopathology

Functional disorders

Depression is the most frequent psychiatric problem in the older population. Approximately one quarter of older patients seen in primary care settings are clinically depressed, and the incidence of depression in older patients with other illness is even greater. The suicide rate in white American men older than age 65 is 5 times greater than that of the general population. Loneliness is the main reason cited, along with financial problems and poor health. Successful suicide is much less common in older American women, but older women attempt suicide more often than do men.

Major depressive disorder is characterized by episodes of at least 2 weeks of depressed mood or loss of interest with 4 or more of the following symptoms:

- loss of appetite
- significant weight loss or gain
- sleep disturbance, agitation, or retardation (slowing down)
- loss of energy
- feelings of worthlessness or guilt
- difficulties in concentration and decision making
- recurrent thoughts of suicide or death

The signs and symptoms of depression are similar to those seen in younger age groups, although older depressed patients are *more likely* than younger patients to express somatic or hypochondriacal complaints, minimize depression symptoms (masked depression), and have psychotic delusional disease but *less likely* to report symptoms of guilt. The most frequent presentations of subclinical depression include new medical complaints, fatigue, poor concentration, exacerbation of existing symptoms and medical problems, preoccupation with health, and diminished interest in pleasurable activities.

The ophthalmologist's role is to recognize and refer the patient with depression. In particular, loss of function, such as moderate or severe visual loss, can precipitate depression, as can recent death of a spouse. In addition to the signs of depression listed previously, other red flags may include frequent visits to the ophthalmology office and unexplained visual loss. Early recognition may be crucial because older patients, particularly men older than age 65, are at highest risk for suicide. Further, most older patients who commit suicide have communicated suicidal ideation to family or friends, although there is no evidence that questions about suicide increase the likelihood of suicide attempts.

Another disorder seen in older persons is *paranoia,* which is usually the result of social isolation or reduced cognitive and sensory capabilities rather than the severe personality disorganization seen in younger patients. For example, a hearing-impaired person may have difficulty understanding what is being said and may imagine hostile motivations on the part of others. Although it may begin in adolescence, *hypochondriasis* more often begins in middle to late adulthood and is relatively common in the older population.

Rovner BW, Shmuely-Dulitzki Y. Screening for depression in low-vision elderly. *Int J Geriatr Psychiatry.* 1997;12(9):955–959.

Organic disorders/dementia

Dementia is a collection of multiple, chronic, and acquired neurocognitive deficits (eg, memory, calculation, orientation, language, construction, purposeful activity, executive planning, or complex behavior control). Acute confusion (ie, delirium), focal deficits (eg, aphasia), and congenital defects (eg, mental retardation) should be excluded. The most common causes of dementia are Alzheimer disease, vascular (multi-infarct) disease, depression (pseudodementia), and frontal lobe disease. (Alzheimer disease is discussed at length in Chapter 12, Behavioral and Neurologic Disorders.) Although less than 15% of dementias are due to reversible causes, these should be ruled out (eg, vitamin B_{12} or folate deficiency, alcohol abuse, normal-pressure hydrocephalus, drug toxicity, thyroid disease, syphilis, seizure, central nervous system infection, tumor).

Some older depressed patients may have pseudodementia. These patients manifest prominent symptoms resembling dementia, with several important differences. Impairment of memory and orientation in pseudodementia has a sudden onset and rapid progression. There is often a prior history of depression, and depressive symptoms are present. Most important, the intellectual deficits are relieved by successful treatment of the depression.

Treatment

Functional disorders in older patients are as treatable as they are in younger patients. Psychotherapy and pharmacologic therapy are effective and should be offered to all patients. Acute mental disorders due to a general medical condition (organic brain syndromes) may also be treatable and thus should be thoroughly worked up.

◉ **Ophthalmic considerations**   Diminishing visual capabilities of any cause can contribute to behavioral disorders in older patients. Depression, paranoia, and organic brain syndromes may be exacerbated. Optimizing visual function through optical correction, medical therapy for vision-impairing disorders, surgical correction of cataract, and low vision rehabilitation can reduce symptoms of behavioral disorders and greatly improve the quality of life.

Osteoporosis

Osteoporosis is defined by the World Health Organization as a disease "characterized by low bone mass and micro-architectural deterioration of bone tissue, leading to bone fragility and a consequent increase in risk of fracture." Osteoporosis is a significant, world-wide public health problem that is becoming increasingly common. It is estimated that 1 of every 2 women and 1 of every 4 men over age 50 will have an osteoporosis-related fracture; 1.5 million fractures related to osteoporosis occur annually in the United States, with the estimated cost of caring for these patients approaching $18 billion. This number is expected to triple by the year 2040. In older patients, a broken hip can increase mortality fourfold. Those with hip fractures are at a 20% risk of entering a nursing home within a year of their fracture. Many patients with hip fractures experience a decline in function, along with increased feelings of isolation, depression, and fear of falling; it is estimated that almost 50% of women with hip fractures do not fully regain previous function.

National Institutes of Health, Osteoporosis and Related Bone Diseases National Resource Center. Available at www.niams.nih.gov/Health_Info/Bone/.

National Registry of Drug-Induced Ocular Side Effects. Available at www.eyedrugregistry.com.

Physician's Guide to Prevention and Treatment of Osteoporosis. Washington, DC: National Osteoporosis Foundation; 2008.

UpToDate. www.uptodate.com.

World Health Organization. Global Strategy on Diet, Physical Activity and Health. Diet, nutrition, and the prevention of chronic diseases. Report of the joint WHO/FAO expert consultation. WHO Technical Report Series, No. 916 (TRS 916). Available at www.who.int.

Bone Physiology

Bone is composed mostly of collagen and calcium phosphate, a combination that makes bone both strong and flexible. The protein collagen provides a soft framework, and the mineral calcium phosphate makes the framework harder and stronger.

Bone is metabolically active and continually remodels throughout life along lines of mechanical stress. During late adolescence, bone mineral content increases rapidly. Bone mass peaks in the third decade of life. With age, the balance between bone resorption and bone formation is altered, and bone mass decreases. By age 60, skeletal mass may be as little as 50% that at age 30. Bone loss for women occurs the fastest after menopause and continues in the postmenopausal years.

Risk Factors

Some risk factors associated with osteoporosis can be modified and others cannot. Risk factors associated with an increased risk of osteoporosis that cannot be modified include

- *Gender:* Women have a greater risk of developing osteoporosis because they usually have less bone mass and lose bone faster after menopause.
- *Body size:* Thin-boned women who are small are at increased risk.
- *Ethnicity:* Caucasian and Asian women are at greater risk than African-American and Hispanic or Latino women.
- *Age:* Older people are at greater risk because bones become thinner with age.
- *Family history:* A history of increased fractures in parents may suggest an inherited cause of reduced bone mass.

Risk factors associated with an increased risk of osteoporosis that can be modified include

- cigarette smoking
- excessive alcohol intake
- inactive lifestyle
- glucocorticoids
- low intake of vitamin D and calcium
- low estrogen and testosterone levels

Clinical Features

The typical clinical picture in osteoporosis includes back pain; spinal deformity; loss of height; and fractures of the vertebrae, hips, and, less commonly, other bones. Multiple vertebral fractures over a period of years can lead to severe kyphosis, with a loss of height of 4–8 inches, and cervical lordosis ("dowager's hump"). The bone loss may occur at first with no symptoms, which is why many people refer to osteoporosis as a "silent disease."

Detection

Measurement of bone mass or bone mineral density (BMD) helps the physician determine a patient's risk of fracture from osteoporosis. The DXA test, a dual-energy radiographic absorptiometry test, is the most widely recognized BMD measure. Bone-density measurements can confirm a diagnosis of osteoporosis in people with a history of one or more fractures, detect low bone density to identify those at risk of fracture, and determine the rate of bone loss to monitor effectiveness of treatment.

Clinical Evaluation

If densitometric studies confirm the diagnosis of osteoporosis, a medical evaluation should be undertaken to rule out secondary causes. Causes of secondary osteoporosis include hyperthroidism, Cushing disease, multiple myeloma, Paget disease, and hypogonadism in men.

Treatment

General considerations

All patients with osteoporosis should adhere to a diet that supplies adequate amounts of calcium, protein, and vitamins. Weight-bearing exercise (eg, walking, jogging, and weight lifting) is important in maintaining bone mass. Limitation of alcohol intake and cessation of smoking are also beneficial, as is avoiding drugs such as glucocorticoids, which can increase bone loss.

McGarry KA, Kiel DP. Postmenopausal osteoporosis. Strategies for preventing bone loss, avoiding fracture. *Postgrad Med.* 2000;108(3):79–88.

Calcium and vitamin D

Calcium supplements are important in maintaining bone mass and preventing fractures related to osteoporosis. The National Osteoporosis Foundation recommends that adults under age 50 take 1000 mg/day of supplemental calcium and that those over age 50 take 1200 mg daily. Vitamin D promotes absorption of dietary calcium and enhances bone mineralization. Vitamin D precursors are synthesized in the skin after exposure to ultraviolet light. People who live in cold climates, people who are homebound, and people who use sunscreens may need to supplement their vitamin D intake. The incidence of hip fractures appears to be significantly less in populations where dietary calcium and vitamin D intake among women is high. Before age 50, calcium supplements should be taken with 400–800 IU of vitamin D_2 or D_3 daily; after age 50, the dose of vitamin D should be increased to 800–1000 IU per day. Calcium and vitamin D supplements have been shown to reduce the incidence of nonvertebral fractures by as much as 23%. Calcium may be obtained from dietary products (eg, milk, yogurt, ice cream, and cheese) and from dark green leafy vegetables (eg, spinach and broccoli). Many foods also come fortified with calcium, such as cereals and orange juice. Calcium and vitamin D supplementation is recommended in patients on long-term corticosteroid therapy. Calcium therapy may cause constipation, nausea, flatulence, bloating, hypercalcuria, and renal stones. Hypercalcemia does not occur in patients with normal renal function, but massive doses of vitamin D can lead to this dangerous condition.

> Clinician's Guide to Prevention and Treatment of Osteoporosis. National Osteoporosis Foundation. Available at http://www.nof.org/prevention/calcium_and_VitaminD.htm.

Pharmacologic therapy

The US Food and Drug Administration has approved a number of drugs for the prevention or treatment of osteoporosis.

Estrogen   Numerous clinical studies have established that estrogen/hormone replacement therapy (ET/HRT) helps to prevent osteoporosis. Estrogens produce significant calcium retention, decrease the imbalance between bone formation and resorption, and tend to decrease the progression of osteoporosis by slowing bone turnover. The Women's Health Initiative (WHI) found that treatment with estrogen can reduce the risk of fracture, but it increases the risk of breast cancer if taken in combination with progestin. Women who started the ET/HRT treatment within 10 years of menopause did not experience an increased incidence of cardiovascular disease. The WHI studied Prempro (conjugated estrogens/medroxyprogesterone) but not ET/HRT at lower doses. In view of the findings from the WHI, patients should be advised of the risks of HRT before starting this treatment for osteoporosis.

> Cauley JA, Robbins J, Chen Z, et al; Women's Health Initiative Investigators. Effects of estrogen plus progestin on risk of fracture and bone mineral density: the Women's Health Initiative randomized trial. *JAMA*. 2003;290(13):1729–1738.

Bisphosphonates   The bisphosphonates alendronate (Fosamax or Fosamax Plus D), risedronate (Actonel), ibandronate (Boniva), and zoledronic acid (Reclast) bind strongly to hydroxyapatite crystals on new bone matrix and prevent bone resorption by inhibiting osteoclast activity. These agents shift the balance between bone formation and resorption toward formation. Bisphosphonates have been shown to increase bone mass in men, and they have been useful for preventing and treating osteoporosis in men and women taking glucocorticoids. Some have been shown to markedly reduce the incidence of vertebral and nonvertebral fractures. The main side effects of bisphosphonates are gastrointestinal, and there have been reports of anterior uveitis as well. As with other therapies for osteoporosis, treatment with bisphosphonates requires adequate calcium and vitamin D intake.

Raloxifene Raloxifene (Evista) is an agent in a class of compounds called *selective estrogen receptor modulators (SERMs)*, which have estrogen-agonistic effects on bone, lipids, and blood clotting and estrogen-antagonistic effects on the breast and uterus. Raloxifene is indicated for the treatment of osteoporosis in postmenopausal women while reducing the risk of invasive breast cancer. Raloxifene has been shown to increase BMD and reduce the risk of vertebral fractures by 30% in women with prior vertebral fractures and by 55% in patients without a previous vertebral fracture.

Calcitonin Calcitonin (Miacalcin, Fortical) is a hormone that inhibits osteoclasts and may increase osteoblast activity, which helps regulate calcium activity via bone, renal, and GI effects. Derived from salmon, it has been used in the treatment of osteoporosis for many years but could be given only by subcutaneous or intramuscular injection. Now, calcitonin nasal spray (Miacalcin) is also available, is well tolerated, and has shown some effectiveness in increasing bone density and reducing fractures, although some patients have reported rhinitis and, less frequently, epistaxis. Adequate concomitant intake of calcium and vitamin D is necessary.

Teriparatide (Forteo) contains recombinant parathyroid hormone (PTH [1-34]), which stimulates new bone formation in men and women and decreases the risk of vertebral and nonvertebral fractures. It is also indicated for use in men with a high risk of fracture from hypogonadal osteoporosis. Treatment with teriparatide should be limited to 2 years or less, as longer courses are not FDA approved.

Falls

The incidence and severity of falls increase with increasing age. Approximately one third of Americans over age 65 fall each year, and falls were the leading cause of nonfatal and fatal injuries treated in hospital emergency departments in 2006. Fall-related direct expenses for persons older than age 65 totaled over $19 billion in 2000, according to the Centers for Disease Control. By 2020, the estimated annual combined direct and indirect costs of fall injuries will approximate $54.9 billion. Traumatic brain injury in the older adult is most commonly caused by falls; falls were the single largest cause of restricted activity in the older population (18%). The mortality rate of a hip fracture is 20% within a year of the fracture. Of all hip fractures, 76% occur in women.

In addition to serious injury or death, falls have a significant psychosocial impact on patients (eg, fear of falling; postfall anxiety; depression; social isolation; and loss of mobility, self-confidence, independence, and function). The 3 most common risk factors for falls are gait or balance disorder, dizziness, or environment-related factors. Visual disorders account for up to 4% of falls. The ophthalmologist's role in fall prevention includes recognition and treatment of visual disorders (including refractive error), multifactorial and multidisciplinary risk reduction, and preventive targeting of risk factors (eg, postural hypotension; multiple medications; and impairments in transferring from chair to chair as well as impairments in strength, balance, and gait). If the ophthalmologist recognizes that a patient is at risk for falls (due to visual disorders or other risk factors), appropriate referral can lead to help in establishing safety and preventive measures in the home (eg, increasing lighting, removing obstacles from the environment, eliminating slippery surfaces, removing loose rugs and electrical cords, using high-contrast colors, handrails, better-fitting and nonskid footwear, and assistive devices. Older adults can help prevent falls by exercising regularly, having regular eye checkups, and improving lighting in their homes.

Kempen JH, Mitchell P, Lee KE, et al; Eye Diseases Prevalence Research Group. The prevalence of refractive errors among adults in the United States, Western Europe, and Australia. *Arch Ophthalmol.* 2004;122(4):495–505.

National Center for Injury Prevention and Control (CDC). Web-based Injury Statistics Query and Reporting System (WISQARS) [online]. Available at www.cdc.gov/injury/wisqars/index.html.

National Center for Injury Prevention and Control (CDC), Division of Unintentional Injury Prevention. (Preventing falls among older adults). Available at www.cdc.gov/ncipc/duip/duip.htm.

US Comsumer Product Safety Commission. Office of Statistics and Programming, National Center for Injury Prevention and Control (CDC). National Electronic Injury Surveillance System-All Injury Program (NEISS-AIP) [online]. Available at www.cdc.gov/ncipc/WISQARS/nonfatal/datasources.htm#5.3.

Systemic Diseases

Ophthalmologists should be aware of the increased incidence of systemic disease in the older population. For example, the prevalence of anemia due to vitamin B_{12} deficiency increases with age. In patients with low to normal serum vitamin B_{12} levels, increased excretion of serum and urinary methylmalonic acid and homocysteine may help with the diagnosis. In addition, 30% of patients with early vitamin B_{12} deficiency have anemia, but 59% may have reversible memory deficits. For the ophthalmologist, patients with vitamin B_{12} deficiency may present with painless, bilateral, progressive visual loss; a central or cecocentral scotoma on visual field testing; and optic atrophy (temporal pallor). Concomitant alcohol and tobacco use should be discouraged.

The prevalence of hypertension, cardiovascular disease, cerebrovascular disease, and diabetes mellitus increases with age; these conditions may affect the eye (eg, homonymous hemianopsia, hypertensive or diabetic retinopathy, amaurosis fugax). Pulmonary diseases such as tuberculosis are more frequent in older persons (who account for 25% of active cases; 60% of deaths related to pulmonary disease occur in patients older than 65 years).

Tuberculosis may cause anterior or posterior uveitis or present with neuro-ophthalmic manifestations. Antituberculosis therapy (eg, ethambutol and isoniazid) may produce toxic optic neuropathy.

The varicella-zoster virus (VZV) can cause a primary infection resulting in varicella (chicken pox); reactivation of latent endogenous VZV is called "herpes zoster" or "shingles." Herpes zoster affects 10% of patients older than age 80 (who have decreased cell-mediated immunity). Herpes zoster ophthalmicus may produce uveitis or CNS manifestations (including ophthalmoplegia) in addition to vesicular dermatomal skin eruption and postherpetic neuralgia (which occurs in 10%–15% of patients). The early use of antiviral agents (eg, acyclovir, famciclovir, and valacyclovir) may reduce both the duration of pain with herpes zoster and the development of postherpetic neuralgia. A currently available vaccine (Zostavax) for individuals aged 60 years and older decreases the chance of developing zoster and postherpetic neuralgia; the vaccine reduced the incidence of postherpetic neuralgia by 67%. The effect was even greater in patients over age 70. Zostavax is not recommended for pregnant women or immunocompromised patients.

Hyperthyroidism and thyroid eye disease may occur in older persons (up to 25% of patients are older than 65 years). Thyroid disease may be iatrogenically precipitated by iodine-containing contrast (eg, contrast-enhanced computed tomography). Older patients with a particular form of hyperthyroidism—apathetic thyrotoxicosis—may present with depression and apathy.

CHAPTER 11

Cancer

Recent Developments

- Biologic therapies using the immune system now play a major role in the treatment of cancer.
- Advances in stem cell biology continue to alter therapeutic strategies for cancer.
- Genetic profiling of tumors and patients may contribute significantly to treatment and identify patients at risk.
- More precise molecular targets for cancer are increasing the effectiveness and reducing the toxicity of chemotherapy.

Introduction

Cancer is the second-leading cause of death in the United States. Each year, over 1 million new cases are diagnosed and some 550,000 deaths occur. More than 3 million Americans have survived cancer, and in more than 2 million of these, the diagnosis was established longer than 5 years ago. About 23% of all deaths in the United States are due to cancer. One in 4 Americans will develop cancer during their lifetime.

Cancer is actually many different diseases; questions of etiology, cancer prevention, and cancer cure must address the specific types of tumors. Nonmelanotic skin cancers are the most common tumors, but these cancers are rarely a cause of death. After skin cancer, the most common forms of cancer in adult Americans (in decreasing order of incidence) are lung, breast, prostate, and colorectal. About 80% of adult cancers arise from the epithelial tissues.

Cancer is the leading cause of death by disease in children under age 15 in the United States. At the same time, death rates have dropped and survival rates have risen. The 5-year survival rate for all childhood cancers is over 90% for many cancers, compared with about 51% in 1973.

Etiology

Cancer is caused by mutations in genes that control cell division. Some of these genes, called *oncogenes*, stimulate cell division; others, called *tumor-suppressor genes,* slow this process. In the normal state, both types of genes work together, enabling the body to replace dead cells and repair damaged ones. Mutations in these genes cause cells to proliferate out of control. Such mutations can be inherited or acquired through environmental insults. Cancer causes, therefore, are explained on the basis of chemical, viral, or radiation-related conditions that occur in a complex milieu, including host genetic composition and immunobiologic status.

Epidemiologic data suggest that as much as 80% of human cancer may be due to exogenous chemical exposure. If these chemicals could be properly identified, a major proportion of human cancers could be prevented by reducing host exposure or by protecting the host. A number of industrial processes or occupational exposures and numerous chemicals or groups of chemicals have been implicated in various forms of human cancer. Specific causes of major cancers, such as large bowel and breast cancer, have not been identified with certainty. Science is looking at a number of issues that need to be resolved before causation is established; these are discussed in the remainder of this section.

Cancer arises from genetic mutations that cause a cell to grow and divide without regard for cell death. The cell cycle is regulated biochemically, and 2 important groups of enzymes involved in this process are the cyclin-dependent kinases (CDKs) and the cyclin-dependent phosphatases. An example of CDK function involves the p53 tumor suppressor gene, which up-regulates the p21 inhibitor of CDK function.

The general population is exposed to both naturally occurring ionizing radiation and man-made ionizing radiation. Man-made sources deliver an average of 106 millirems (mrem) per year to each person. These sources include medical diagnostic equipment and technologically altered natural sources (such as phosphate fertilizers and building materials containing small amounts of radioactivity). The carcinogenic effects of radiation exposure result from molecular lesions caused by random interactions of radiation with atoms and molecules. Most molecular lesions induced in this way are of little consequence to the affected cell. However, DNA is not repaired with 100% efficiency, and mutations and chromosomal aberrations accrue with increasing radiation doses. Although these changes in genes and chromosomes have been postulated to account for the carcinogenic effect of radiation, the precise molecular mechanisms are unknown. Parameters that influence response of the target tissue include the total radiation dose, the dose rate, the quality of the radiation source, the characteristics of certain internal emitters (such as radioiodine), and individual host factors.

The role of viruses in the etiology of cancer has been studied extensively. The inoculation of animals with specific viruses may produce tumors. Several human cancers show a definite correlation with viral infection and the presence and retention of specific virus nucleic acid sequences and virus proteins in the tumor cells (Burkitt lymphoma, nasopharyngeal carcinoma, carcinoma of the cervix, and hepatocellular carcinoma).

All of the DNA virus groups except the parvovirus family have been associated with cancer. This is notable because all the DNA viruses associated with cancer contain double-stranded DNA, whereas the parvoviruses contain only single-stranded DNA.

There are 9 RNA virus groups, but only 1 is associated with oncogenicity: the retrovirus group. The retroviruses differ from all other RNA viruses in that they require a DNA intermediate to replicate. Retroviruses contain and specify an enzyme called *reverse transcriptase*. In the presence of the 4 nucleoside triphosphates, reverse transcriptase can synthesize DNA complementary to the single-stranded RNA contained in the virion, producing an RNA-DNA hybrid. The RNA in this RNA-DNA hybrid is then degraded, and a double-stranded linear DNA molecule forms. This double-stranded DNA molecule moves into the cell nucleus and is integrated into the cellular DNA as a provirus.

The papillomavirus of the papovavirus group has been associated with squamous cell carcinoma, cervical cancer, and laryngeal papilloma in humans. A vaccine is now available against human papillomavirus (HPV). Immunization against HPV can prevent cervical cancer in women. The hepatitis B virus has been associated with primary hepatocellular carcinoma in humans.

The human herpesviruses that are associated with disease include Epstein-Barr virus, herpes simplex virus type 1, herpes simplex virus type 2, cytomegalovirus, and varicella-zoster virus. The Epstein-Barr virus, which causes infectious mononucleosis, has been associated with Burkitt lymphoma and nasopharyngeal carcinoma. The herpes simplex virus type 1, which causes gingivostomatitis, encephalitis, keratoconjunctivitis, neuralgia, and labialis, has been associated with carcinoma of the lip and oropharynx. The herpes simplex virus type 2, which causes genital herpes, disseminated neonatal herpes, encephalitis, and neuralgia, has been associated with cancer of the uterine cervix, vulva, kidneys, and nasopharynx. The cytomegalovirus, which causes cytomegalovirus disease, transfusion mononucleosis, interstitial pneumonia, and congenital defects, has been associated with prostate cancer, Kaposi sarcoma, and carcinoma of the bladder and uterine cervix. The varicella-zoster virus, which causes chickenpox, shingles, and varicella pneumonia, has not yet been associated with specific human cancers.

Finally, cancers may aggregate in a nonrandom manner in certain families. These cancers may be of the same type or dissimilar. Such cancer-cluster families may have several children with soft tissue sarcoma and relatives with a variety of cancers, especially of the breast in young women. Multiple endocrine neoplasia (types 1 and 2) is yet another example of familial cancers. The recognition of family cancer syndromes permits early detection that may be life-saving.

Radiation Therapy

Ionizing radiation interacts with tissues by an energy transfer and a chemical reaction, with the release of free radicals and the decomposition of water into hydrogen, hydroxyl, and perhydroxyl ionic forms. These ionic forms probably react with DNA and RNA in vital enzymes, producing biologic injury.

The injuries noted to date include mitotic-linked death and chromosomal aberrations such as breakage, sticking, and cross-bridging. Consequent cell death occurs in both normal tissue and malignant lesions. In radiotherapy, biochemical recovery and biologic repair occur in the normal host, maintaining the integrity of vital systems.

The poorly differentiated lymphoid cells, intestinal epithelium, and reproductive cells are more readily damaged and recover more quickly than do the highly differentiated normal cells. Lymphocytes are damaged by 1 gray (Gy) of radiation and CNS tissue by 50 Gy. Surface irradiation of approximately 10 Gy produces skin erythema. The most serious damage is the late development of postradiation malignant changes in as many as 21% of patients, manifesting as squamous cell carcinoma and basal cell carcinoma. Bone absorption can produce osteogenic sarcomas and fibrosarcomas as well.

⊙ Ophthalmic considerations   Ocular manifestations of fetal irradiation in the first trimester include microphthalmos, congenital cataracts, and retinal dysplasia. A 0.5-Gy dose may cause congenital anomalies in a fetus. Fetal exposure to approximately 0.30–0.80 Gy doubles the incidence of congenital defects; 5 Gy (the LD_{50} for a human fetus) generally induces an abortion.

Ocular effects of irradiation depend not only on total dose, fractionation, and treatment portal size but also on associated systemic diseases such as diabetes and hypertension. Concomitant chemotherapy has an additive effect.

The lens is the most radiosensitive structure in the eye, followed by the cornea, the retina, and the optic nerve. The orbit is completely included in the treatment portal in diseases such as large retinoblastomas; it is partially included in tumors of adjacent structures, such as the maxillary antrum, nasopharynx, ethmoidal sinus, and nasal cavity. Usual doses range from 20 to 100 Gy. The total dose is usually fractionated during the treatment. With brachytherapy, a low-energy isotope such as radioactive iodine delivers a high dose of radiation within a few millimeters but does not penetrate deep into the tumor. This allows for radioactive episcleral implants to deliver a dose of 100 Gy to the apex of a tumor but much less to the rest of the eye. The sclera can tolerate doses up to 400–800 Gy.

Doses to the lens as low as 2 Gy in 1 fraction may cause a cataract. However, cataracts caused by low doses may be asymptomatic and may not progress. Cataracts caused by higher doses (7–8 Gy) may continue to progress, causing considerable visual loss. The average latent period for the development of radiation-induced cataracts is 2–3 years.

The clinical picture of radiation retinopathy resembles that of diabetic retinopathy. Radiation retinopathy is very rare below the fractionated dose of 50 Gy over 5–6 weeks. At higher fractionated doses (70–80 Gy), however, most patients develop radiation retinopathy. The usual interval between radiation and the development of radiation-induced retinopathy is 2–3 years. Radiation retinopathy may develop earlier in patients who are diabetic or on chemotherapy. The earliest clinical manifestation of radiation retinopathy is usually cotton-wool spots. After several months, these spots fade away, leaving large areas of capillary nonperfusion Telangiectatic vessels grow from the retina into these areas. Microaneurysms may also develop. These ischemic changes may cause rubeosis iridis, which in turn may lead to neovascular glaucoma. The capillary endothelial cell is the first type of cell to be damaged, followed closely by the pericytes and then the endothelial cells of the larger vessels. The new intraretinal telangiectatic vessels have thick collagenous walls. There may be spotty occlusion of the choriocapillaris.

Doses to the optic nerve in the range of 60–70 Gy cause some injury in a small number of patients. Damage to the distal end of the optic nerve is called *radiation optic neuropathy*. Clinically, these patients have disc pallor with splinter hemorrhages. If the injury occurs to the more proximal part of the optic nerve, it resembles retrobulbar optic neuropathy. Affected patients may complain of unilateral headaches and ocular pain; the disc may not reveal edema or hemorrhage. With doses of 60–70 Gy, a dry-eye syndrome sometimes develops. This syndrome usually develops within a year and occasionally progresses to corneal ulceration and severe pain.

Chemotherapy

The goal of cancer chemotherapy is to damage or destroy cancer cells without killing normal cells. The first candidate drugs to selectively target rapidly dividing cells were sulfur and nitrogen mustards that were noted to suppress bone marrow when used in warfare. These compounds bound covalently to DNA, and thus DNA was the first molecular target of chemotherapy. In the 1950s, attention was directed to the precursors of DNA, and drugs such as methotrexate were found effective. The recognition that some tumors were hormonally dependent led to hormonal therapy or suppression as a treatment for cancer. Since the 1970s, many drugs have been developed that inhibit mitotic spindle formation.

Natural Products

Natural products include a wide variety of agents. The most common are vinca alkaloids, podophyllin derivatives, paclitaxel, antitumor antibiotics, and related drugs (Table 11-1). Vinca alkaloids are derived from the periwinkle plant and include vincristine (Oncovin), vinblastine (Velban), and several investigational agents. These agents block incorporation of orotic acid and thymidine into DNA and cause arrest and inhibition of mitosis.

Podophyllin derivatives and semisynthetic plant derivatives arrest cells in the G2 phase. VP-16 (etoposide) and VM-26 (teniposide) are gaining acceptance in many treatment protocols.

Paclitaxel (Taxol) is a compound originally isolated from the bark of the Pacific yew tree. It has been approved by the FDA to treat breast, ovarian, and lung cancers as well as AIDS-related Kaposi sarcoma. Paclitaxel stops microtubules from breaking down. In normal cell growth, microtubules are formed when a cell starts dividing. Once the cell stops dividing, the microtubules are broken down or destroyed. With paclitaxel, cancer cells become clogged with microtubules and cannot grow and divide.

Antitumor antibiotics are compounds produced by species of *Streptomyces* in culture. These agents interfere with the synthesis of nucleic acid. A partial list includes:

- *anthracyclines* (doxorubicin and derivatives), which interfere with template function of DNA (a unique side effect is cardiac muscle degeneration that leads to cardiomyopathy)
- *bleomycin,* which causes DNA-strand scission
- *actinomycin D* (dactinomycin), which inhibits DNA-directed RNA synthesis
- *mitomycin,* which impairs replication by causing cross-linking between DNA strands

The major dose-limiting toxicity of mitomycin is myelosuppression. Mitomycin has also been implicated as a cause of the hemolytic-uremic syndrome.

Table 11-1 Antineoplastic Drugs

Drugs by Class	Mechanism of Action	Tumors Commonly Responsive	Toxicity and Remarks
Alkylating agents Mechlorethamine (nitrogen mustard) Chlorambucil (Leukeran) Cyclophosphamide (Cytoxan) Melphalan (Alkeran) Ifosfamide (Ifex)	Alkylation of DNA with restriction of strands' uncoiling and replication	Hodgkin, malignant lymphoma, small cell lung Ca, Ca of breast and testis, CLL	Alopecia with high IV dosage; nausea and vomiting; myelosuppression; hemorrhagic cystitis (especially with ifosfamide), which can be ameliorated with mesna; muto- and leukemogenic; aspermia; permanent sterility possible
Antimetabolites Folate antagonist methotrexate (MTX)	Folate antagonist with binding to dehydrofolate reductase and interference with (pyrimidine) thymidylate synthesis	Choriocarcinoma (female), Ca of head and neck, ALL, Ca of ovary, malignant lymphoma, osteogenic sarcoma	Mucosal ulceration; bone-marrow suppression; toxicity increased with renal function impairment or ascitic fluid (with pooling of drug). Leucovorin rescue can reverse toxicity at 24 h (10–20 mg q 6 h × 10 doses).
Purine antagonist 6-mercaptopurine (6-MP)	Blocks de novo purine synthesis	Acute leukemia	Myelosuppression, alopecia
Pyrimidine antagonist 5-fluorouracil (5-FU)	Interferes with thymidylate synthase to reduce thymidine production	GI neoplasms, Ca of breast	Mucositis, alopecia, myelosuppression, diarrhea and vomiting, hyperpigmentation. When given after MTX, synergistic effect is significant.
Cytarabine (Ara-C)	DNA polymerase inhibition	Acute leukemia (especially nonlymphocytic), malignant lymphoma	Myelosuppression, nausea and vomiting, cerebellar and conjunctival toxicities at high dosage, skin rash

Drugs by Class	Mechanism of Action	Tumors Commonly Responsive	Toxicity and Remarks
Plant Alkaloids			
Vincas			
Vinblastine (Velban)	Mitotic arrest by alteration of microtubular proteins	Lymphomas, leukemias, Ca of breast, Ewing sarcoma, Ca of testis	Alopecia, myelosuppression, peripheral neuropathy, ileus
Vincristine (Oncovin)	As above	As above	Peripheral neuropathy, SIADH. Dose commonly "capped" at total of 2 mg in adults.
Paclitaxel (Taxol)	Promotes assembly of microtubules	Ca of breast, lung, ovary, head, neck, and bladder	Myelosuppression, alopecia, myalgia, arthralgia, neuropathy
Podophyllotoxins Etoposide (VePesid, VP-16)	Inhibition of mitosis by unknown mechanisms	Lymphoma, Hodgkin, Ca of testis, Ca of lung (especially small cell), acute leukemia	Nausea, vomiting, myelosuppression, peripheral neuropathy. Etoposide cleared by liver (teniposide by kidney); increased toxicity in renal failure.
Antibiotics			
Doxorubicin (Adriamycin)	Intercalation between DNA strands inhibits uncoiling of DNA	Acute leukemia, Hodgkin, other lymphomas, Ca of breast, Ca of lung	Nausea and vomiting, myelosuppression, alopecia. Cardiac toxicity at cumulative dosage >500 mg/m^2. Higher dosage tolerated when given by continuous IV.
Bleomycin	Incision of DNA strands	Squamous cell Ca, lymphoma, Ca of testis, Ca of lung	Anaphylaxis, chills and fever, skin rash; pulmonary fibrosis at dosage >200 mg/m^2; requires renal excretion
Mitomycin	Inhibits DNA synthesis by acting as a bifunctional alkylator	Gastric adenocarcinoma; colon, breast, and lung Ca; transitional cell Ca of the bladder	Local extravasation causes tissue necrosis; myelosuppression, with leukopenia and thrombocytopenia 4–6 wk after treatment; alopecia; lethargy; fever; hemolytic-uremic syndrome

(Continued)

Table 11-1 Antineoplastic Drugs *(continued)*

Drugs by Class	Mechanism of Action	Tumors Commonly Responsive	Toxicity and Remarks
Nitrosoureas			
Carmustine (BiCNU)	Alkylation of DNA with restriction of strands' uncoiling and replication	Brain tumors, lymphoma	Myelosuppression, pulmonary toxicity (fibrosis), renal toxicity
Lomustine (CeeNU)	Carbamoylation of amino acids in proteins	As above	As above
Inorganic ions			
Cisplatin (Platinol)	Intercalation and intracalation between DNA strands inhibits uncoiling of DNA	Ca of lung (especially small cell), testis, breast, and stomach; lymphoma	Anemia, ototoxicity, peripheral neuropathy, myelosuppression, nausea, vomiting
Biologic response modifiers			
IFN (Intron-A, Roferon-A)	Antiproliferative effect	Hairy cell leukemia, CML, lymphomas, Kaposi sarcoma (AIDS), renal cell Ca, melanoma	Fatigue, fever, myalgias, arthralgias, myelosuppression, nephrotic syndrome (rarely)
Enzymes			
Asparaginase (Elspar)	Depletion of asparagine, on which leukemic cells depend	ALL	Acute anaphylaxis, hyperthermia, pancreatitis, hyperglycemia, hypofibrinogenemia
Hormones			
Tamoxifen (Nolvadex)	Places cells at rest: binding of estrogen receptor	Ca of breast	Hot flushes, hypercalcemia, deep vein thrombosis
Flutamide (Eulexin)	Binding of androgen receptor	Ca of prostate	Decreased libido, hot flushes, gynecomastia

ALL = acute lymphocytic leukemia, Ca = cancer, CLL = chronic lymphocytic leukemia, CML = chronic myeloid leukemia, IFN = interferon, SIADH = syndrome of inappropriate antidiuretic hormone secretion.

Adapted from *The Merck Manuals Online Medical Library.* http://www.merck.com/mmpe/sec11.html.

Angiogenesis Inhibitors

Angiogenesis is important to the growth and spread of cancers, as new blood vessels are critical in the formation of tumors. In animal studies, angiogenesis inhibitors have successfully stopped the formation of new blood vessels, causing the tumor to shrink and die. Various angiogenesis inhibitors have been evaluated in human clinical trials. These studies include patients with cancers of the breast, prostate, brain, pancreas, lung, stomach, ovary, and cervix; some leukemias and lymphomas; and AIDS-related Kaposi sarcoma.

Antibodies against vascular endothelial growth factor have proven effective. Aptamers are a new class of drugs that consist of oligonucleotides that bind to specific proteins to inactivate them, much the way that a monoclonal antibody would, but without the problems inherent in injecting foreign protein into a patient.

Biologic Therapies

Biologic therapies (sometimes called *immunotherapy, biotherapy,* or *biologic response modifier therapy*) use the immune system, either directly or indirectly, to fight cancer or to lessen the side effects that may be caused by some cancer treatments. Further, cancer may develop when the immune system breaks down or is not functioning adequately. Biologic therapies are designed to repair, stimulate, or enhance the immune system's responses.

Cells in the immune system secrete 2 types of proteins: antibodies and cytokines. Cytokines are substances produced by some immune system cells to communicate with other cells. Types of cytokines include lymphokines, interferons, interleukins, and colony-stimulating factors. Some antibodies and cytokines, called *biologic response modifiers,* can be used to treat cancer. Other biologic response modifiers include monoclonal antibodies and vaccines.

Interferons are types of cytokines that occur naturally in the body. There are 3 major types of interferons: interferon-α, interferon-β, and interferon-γ; interferon-α is the type most widely used in cancer treatment. Interferons can improve the way a cancer patient's immune system acts against cancer cells. Furthermore, interferons may act directly on cancer cells by slowing their growth or promoting their development into cells with more normal behavior. Interferons may also stimulate natural killer cells, T cells, and macrophages, boosting the immune system's anticancer function. The FDA has approved the use of interferon-α for the treatment of hairy cell leukemia, melanoma, chronic myeloid leukemia, and AIDS-related Kaposi sarcoma.

Interleukins, like interferons, are cytokines; they occur naturally in the body and can be made in the laboratory. Many interleukins have been identified; interleukin-2 has been the most widely studied in cancer treatment. Interleukin-2 stimulates the growth and activity of many immune cells, such as lymphocytes, that can destroy cancer cells. The FDA has approved interleukin-2 for the treatment of metastatic kidney cancer and metastatic melanoma.

Colony-stimulating factors (sometimes called *hematopoietic growth factors*) usually do not directly affect tumor cells but instead stimulate bone marrow production. Colony-stimulating factors allow doses of anticancer drugs to be increased without increasing the risk of infection or need for transfusion.

That a patient has a cancer suggests that there has been a failure in the immune system. Thus, reconstituting the immune system is an attractive approach for treating metastatic tumors. *Monoclonal antibodies (MOABs)* are produced by a single type of cell and are specific for a particular antigen. Researchers are examining ways to create MOABs that are specific to the antigens found on the surface of cancer cells being treated.

MOABs are made by injecting human cancer cells into mice, which stimulates an antibody response. The cells producing antibodies are then removed and fused with laboratory-grown cells to create hybrid cells called *hybridomas*. Hybridomas can indefinitely produce large quantities of these MOABs.

MOABs have many potential uses in cancer treatment, such as linking them to anticancer drugs, radioisotopes, other biologic response modifiers, or other toxins. When the antibodies attach to cancer cells, they can deliver these poisons directly to the cells. MOABs carrying radioisotopes may also prove useful in diagnosing certain cancers, such as colorectal, ovarian, and prostate cancer.

Cancer vaccines are being developed to help the immune system recognize cancer cells. These vaccines are designed to be injected after the disease is diagnosed rather than before it develops. They may help the body reject tumors and prevent cancer from recurring. Vaccines are being studied in the treatment of melanomas, lymphomas, and cancers of the kidney, breast, ovaries, prostate, colon, and rectum.

In the future, other biologic approaches to cancer therapy may include *genetic profiling* of certain tumors. This may prove more helpful and effective than classifying tumors by their organ of origin. An example of this is the differentiation between those tumors with a normal and those with an abnormal tumor suppressor gene p53. Tumor cells with normal p53 genes are far more sensitive to chemotherapy than those with mutant p53.

◉ **Ophthalmic considerations**   The eye and its adnexa are frequently involved in systemic malignancies as well as in extraocular malignancies that extend into ocular structures (including local malignancies of skin, bone, and sinuses). Breast and lung cancers frequently metastasize to the eye and are the second most common intraocular tumors in adults. Acute myelogenous and lymphocytic leukemias frequently have uveal and posterior choroidal infiltrates as part of their generalized disease. In children, these manifestations are often signs of CNS involvement and suggest a poor prognosis. Although malignant lymphomas do not usually involve the uveal tract, histiocytic lymphoma is one type that often involves the vitreous and presents as uveitis. The retina and choroid may also be involved.

Tumors of the eye and adnexa are discussed in several other BCSC books, including Section 4, *Ocular Pathology and Intraocular Tumors*; Section 6, *Pediatric Ophthalmology and Strabismus*; Section 7, *Orbit, Eyelids, and Lacrimal System*; and Section 8, *External Disease and Cornea*.

CHAPTER **12**

Behavioral and Neurologic Disorders

Recent Developments

- Newer therapeutic agents for psychiatric diseases allow more effective treatment with generally fewer side effects compared with older agents. Ophthalmologists should be aware that newer antipsychotic agents have also been associated with an increased risk for diabetes mellitus.
- A recent meta-analysis of the literature on the pharmacologic treatment of dementia indicates that none of the presently available agents can significantly improve cognition, although there may be a mild effect in some patients.
- The Medicare Improvement Act and the Mental Health Parity Act represent an attempt to ensure that psychiatric conditions are given parity with other medical conditions when it comes to insurance coverage.
- The antiepileptic medications topiramate (Topamax) and vigabatrin (Sabril) are associated with ophthalmic side effects. Topiramate can cause angle-closure glaucoma, and vigabatrin can cause visual field loss.

Introduction

Since the 1980s, the World Health Organization (WHO) has focused its efforts on behavioral and neurologic disorders that occur frequently; cause substantial disability; and create a burden on individuals, families, communities, and societies. The WHO approach has been based on epidemiologic evidence: the assessment of disease burden using disability-adjusted life-years. This approach has emphasized the public health importance of behavioral and neurologic disorders, which in 2000 accounted for 12.3% of the world-wide disease burden. It is estimated that such disorders will account for 15% of disability-adjusted life-years in 2030.

In addition to behavioral disorders, the neurologic disorders that significantly affect this disease burden include epilepsy, dementias (in particular, Alzheimer disease), multiple sclerosis, Parkinson disease and other motor system disorders, stroke, pain syndromes, and brain injury.

Behavioral Disorders

Behavioral disorders encompass a wide variety of conditions in which the common factor is disordered functioning of personality. These disturbances range from mild reactions to the events or circumstances of a person's life to debilitating, life-threatening illnesses. Although the practicing ophthalmologist will not be called on to treat mental illness, such disease may profoundly affect the diagnosis and treatment of ophthalmic diseases. In addition, some of the medications used to treat psychiatric disorders may have significant ophthalmic side effects.

It is estimated that roughly 67% of adults and 80% of children requiring mental health services do not receive help, in large part because of discriminatory insurance practices. Two recent pieces of legislation aim to improve this situation. The 2008 Medicare Improvement Act ends a long-standing requirement that affects Medicare beneficiaries who need outpatient mental health services. Currently, they face a discriminatory 50% co-insurance for outpatient therapy. This serves as an incentive to use inpatient or institutional care instead of outpatient services and also causes people who rely on Medicare to forgo needed mental health treatment. The new law establishes mental health parity within the Medicare program. The other law is the Mental Health Parity Act, which recognizes the importance of mental health treatment relative to overall health coverage. It bans employers and insurers from imposing stricter limits on coverage for mental health and substance-use conditions compared to those set for other health problems.

Mental Disorders Due to a General Medical Condition

Formerly called *organic mental syndromes,* this category, *mental disorders due to a general medical condition,* was renamed in the *Diagnostic and Statistical Manual of Mental Disorders,* better known as *DSM-IV*. The essential feature of mental disorders due to a general medical condition is a psychological or behavioral abnormality associated with transient or permanent dysfunction of the brain. Causes include any disease, drug, or trauma that directly affects the CNS and systemic illnesses that indirectly interfere with brain function; Alzheimer disease is included in this category. Orientation, memory, and other intellectual functions are impaired. Psychiatric symptoms may occur, including hallucinations, delusions, depression, obsessions, and personality changes.

Patients with a mental disorder due to a general medical condition with or without cognitive impairment are often unable to remember instructions and therefore unable to comply with treatment regimens. This general inability to understand instructions, integrate information, and perform tasks is referred to as *executive function deficit.* Depression, which frequently accompanies the syndrome, can complicate the situation. Medications with CNS side effects, such as β-blockers and carbonic anhydrase inhibitors, must be used with care, because patients are often sensitive to these agents. See also the discussion of dementia in Chapter 10, Geriatrics.

Schizophrenia

The term *schizophrenia* actually encompasses a group of disorders with similar features. These are some of the most devastating mental illnesses in terms of personal and societal cost. Schizophrenia usually begins when patients are young and continues to a greater or lesser extent throughout their lives. The hallmarks of schizophrenia include "positive" psychotic symptoms such as hallucinations (usually auditory) and delusions, as well as "negative" symptoms such as emotional and cognitive blunting and poor social and occupational functioning. The incidence is estimated at 0.5%–1.0% of the population.

The classic manifestations are delusions, hallucinations, and disorganized speech and behavior. *Delusions* are disturbances in thought: firmly held beliefs that are untrue. Other thought abnormalities include loosening of associations and tangential thinking. *Hallucinations* are abnormal perceptions, experienced without any actual external stimulus. The patient's affect is often flattened or inappropriate.

Motor disturbances range from uncontrolled, aimless activity to catatonic stupor, in which the patient may be immobile, mute, and unresponsive yet fully conscious. Repetitive, purposeless mannerisms and inability to complete goal-directed tasks are also common. Associated illnesses include *schizophreniform disorder,* in which schizophrenic manifestations occur for less than 6 months, and *brief psychotic disorder,* which lasts less than 1 month. Patients with *schizoaffective disorder* have a significant mood disorder, such as depression, that manifests itself independently of the psychotic disorder.

Mood Disorders

Also known as *affective disorders,* mood disorders range from appropriate reactions to negative life experiences to severe, recurrent, debilitating illnesses. Common to all of these disorders is depressed mood, elevated mood (mania), or alternations of the two.

Major depression is far more common than mania and therefore has a greater impact on all aspects of society. The lifetime risk for major depressive disorder is 10% for men and 20%–25% for women. Major depression may occur at any age, but it is most common in middle-aged and older persons. Affective changes include a feeling of sadness, emptiness, and nervousness. Thought processes are typically slowed and reflect low self-esteem, pessimism, and feelings of guilt. Social withdrawal and psychomotor retardation are seen, although agitation also occurs. Basic physical functions are impaired, as manifested by sleep disturbances, changes in appetite with associated weight loss or gain, diminished libido, and an inability to experience pleasure *(anhedonia).* Common somatic complaints are fatigue, headache, and other nonspecific symptoms. Up to 15% of seriously depressed patients may commit suicide. The term *major depressive disorder* is used to describe the condition of patients who have major depressive episodes without any manic symptoms. Patients with *dysthymic disorder* have chronic, less severe depressive symptoms that do not meet the criteria for major depression.

Mania is a period of abnormally and persistently elevated or irritable mood sufficiently severe to cause impairment in social or occupational functioning. Typical symptoms include euphoria or irritability, grandiosity, decreased need for sleep, increased talkativeness, flight of ideas, and increased goal-directed activity. The classic term *manic depression* has been replaced by *bipolar disorder.* Bipolar I disorder describes any illness in which mania is present, whether or not depression occurs. Bipolar II disorder refers to patients with major depressive episodes and at least 1 mild manic episode (hypomania). *Cyclothymic disorder* describes cyclical episodes of mild depression and mania.

For the nonpsychiatric clinician, depression creates a number of problems. In some patients, mood change may not be apparent, and the illness is manifested in somatic complaints leading to time-consuming, expensive workups. Conversely, in patients known to be depressed, an organic disease may be overlooked as psychosomatic. Appropriate recommendations for psychotherapeutic intervention may be met with resistance, anger, or denial, disrupting the patient–physician relationship. Compliance with diagnostic and treatment regimens for medical disorders and surgical procedures can be problematic. A screening study of older patients attending an ophthalmology clinic showed that 1 in 5 patients suffered from depression. It is estimated that up to 30% of patients with macular degeneration have depression, and it is likely that other causes of vision loss contribute to the presence of significant depression in many patients.

Casten RJ, Rovner BW, Tasman W. Age-related macular degeneration and depression: a review of recent research. *Curr Opin Ophthalmol.* 2004;15(3):181–183.

Lee AG, Beaver HA, Jogerst G, Daly JM. Screening elderly patients in an outpatient ophthalmology clinic for dementia, depression, and functional impairment. *Ophthalmology.* 2003;110(4):651–657.

Somatoform Disorders

The essential feature of somatoform disorders is the presence of symptoms suggesting physical disease in the absence of physical findings or a known physiologic mechanism to account for the symptoms. The symptoms in somatoform disorders are considered to be outside the patient's voluntary control. The practicing physician should be aware of these syndromes because encounters with these patients are common.

Several somatoform disorders are recognized. *Conversion disorders* are characterized by temporary and involuntary loss or alteration of physical functioning due to psychosocial stress. Symptoms are typically neurologic and include functional visual loss ("hysterical blindness"). In *somatoform pain disorder,* prolonged, severe pain is the only symptom. Psychotherapy is the primary therapeutic modality.

Somatization disorder is most common in women and consists of multiple somatic complaints. Patients are often histrionic in describing their symptoms and may have undergone multiple hospitalizations and surgery. The incidence of associated psychiatric illness is high. Treatment is aimed at providing psychological support and minimizing the expenditure of medical resources. Psychotherapy is typically met with resistance and is therefore usually unsuccessful. Psychopharmacologic treatment of underlying psychiatric disorders may help.

Hypochondriasis is a preoccupation with the fear of having or developing a serious disease. Physical examination fails to support the patient's belief, and reassurance by the examining physician fails to allay the fear. Treatment principles are the same as for somatization disorder. In *body dysmorphic disorder,* the patient believes that his or her body is deformed, even though there is no physical defect, or the patient has an exaggerated concern about a mild physical anomaly. Ophthalmologists performing reconstructive and cosmetic surgery should be aware of this disorder because surgical repair of the "defect" is rarely successful in the patient's mind.

Two other conditions that are not actually somatoform disorders bear mentioning here. *Factitious disorders* are characterized by willful production of physical or psychological signs or symptoms in the absence of external incentives. It is thought that these patients feign illness solely because of a psychological need to assume the role of a sick person. Treatment requires discovery of the true nature of the physical illness, a carefully planned confrontation, and psychotherapy. Prognosis for recovery is guarded. Chronic conjunctivitis, keratitis, and even scleritis are the usual ophthalmic presentations of factitious disease. *Malingering* is the intentional production of physical or psychological symptoms for the purpose of identifiable secondary gain. Malingering is not considered a primary psychiatric illness. Ophthalmologists should be familiar with techniques for detecting malingerers who feign loss of vision, because such persons are occasionally encountered in practice. (See BCSC Section 5, *Neuro-Ophthalmology,* for some of these techniques.)

The anxiety disorders represent another group of diseases that can significantly interfere with normal functioning. *Generalized anxiety disorder (GAD)* is the most common anxiety disorder and is characterized by unrealistic or excessive anxiety and worry about 2 or more life circumstances. Generalized anxiety disorder is also correlated with depression. Pharmacologic therapy and psychotherapy may be very successful in treating this disease.

Patients with *panic disorder* report discrete periods of intense terror and impending doom that are almost intolerable. These episodes can occur abruptly, either in certain predictable situations or without any situational trigger. Mild cases may be treated with psychotherapy, but more significant disease is often treated with antidepressant medication, especially the selective serotonin reuptake inhibitors (SSRIs).

Post-traumatic stress disorder (PTSD) occurs after an individual has been exposed to a dramatic event that is associated with intense fear. When exposed to reminders of the event, the patient then persistently reexperiences the event through intrusive recollections, nightmares, flashbacks, or distress. The prevalence of PTSD is 8% in the general population and increases to 60% in combat soldiers and assault victims. Treatment usually includes psychotherapy and use of antidepressants. Other anxiety-related conditions that may require pharmacologic intervention include obsessive-compulsive disorder and social phobia.

The various personality disorders merit recognition because of the potential for associated problems to arise, such as poor compliance and substance abuse. Personality disorders are diagnosed when personality traits become inflexible and maladaptive to the point where they create significant dysfunction. Patients usually have little or no insight into their disorder. The personality disorders include *cluster A personality disorders,* which are related to a tendency to develop schizophrenia and include paranoid, schizotypal, and schizoid disorders. *Cluster B personality disorders* include antisocial, borderline, histrionic, and narcissistic personality disorders. These patients may display dramatic or irrational behavior and may be very disruptive in clinical settings. *Cluster C personality disorders* often stem from maladaptive attempts to control anxiety and include avoidant, dependent, and obsessive-compulsive personality disorders. Psychotherapy tends to be the treatment of choice for all of these entities. There is no specific pharmacotherapy, although medication may be used to treat certain symptoms or coexisting mood disorders.

Substance Abuse Disorders

Drug dependence is the abuse of a drug to the point that one's physical health, psychological functioning, or ability to exist within the demands of society is threatened. Common to all types of drug dependence is *psychic dependence*—that is, a psychic drive or a feeling of satisfaction requiring periodic or continuous drug administration in order to avoid discomfort, produce pleasure, relieve boredom, or facilitate social interaction. *Physical dependence* occurs when repeated administration of a drug causes an altered physiologic state in the CNS so that sudden cessation of the drug causes an *abstinence syndrome* (a physical illness whose symptoms are determined by the specific drug). *Tolerance* occurs when increasing amounts of a drug are necessary to achieve the same desired effect. The drugs causing dependence fall into several groups, including opiates, alcohol, sedatives/hypnotics, hallucinogens, cocaine, marijuana, and others.

Drug abuse and addiction are often viewed as strictly social problems. Some believe that drug abusers and addicts should be able to stop taking drugs if they are willing to change their behavior. Recent scientific research provides overwhelming evidence that in addition to short-term effects, drugs also have long-term effects on brain metabolism and activity. At some point, changes occur in the brain, turning drug abuse into the illness of addiction. Those addicted to drugs have a compulsive drug craving and frequently are unable to quit by themselves. Treatment is necessary to end the compulsive behavior.

◉ **Ophthalmic considerations** Pupil changes can occur with drug abuse. For instance, pupil constriction is common with the use of opiates, and pupil dilation occurs with the use of cocaine, amphetamines, or lysergic acid diethylamide (LSD). Pupil dilation can also be seen with opiate withdrawal.

Sustained horizontal gaze-evoked nystagmus can be a sign of sedative or ethanol use. Toxic optic neuropathy is seen in alcohol-dependent patients as a direct effect of the disease or in association with the malnutrition that often accompanies alcoholism. Wernicke disease occurs most often in alcoholics; it is caused by thiamine deficiency, and findings include ocular palsies, nystagmus, memory disturbance, and peripheral neuropathy. Alcohol also crosses the placental barrier, and children born to alcoholic mothers may be affected by fetal alcohol syndrome. Some of the ocular manifestations of this syndrome are blepharophimosis, telecanthus, ptosis, optic nerve hypoplasia or atrophy, and tortuosity of the retinal arteries and veins. (See also BCSC Section 6, *Pediatric Ophthalmology and Strabismus.*)

Vascular occlusion and endophthalmitis can occur in association with intravenous drug abuse, and intravenous drug users are more likely to have HIV infection and associated eye findings. (See BCSC Section 9, *Intraocular Inflammation and Uveitis.*) Optic neuropathy can occur in association with cocaine-induced nasal pathology; intracranial microinfarcts causing internuclear ophthalmoplegia and visual field defects have been reported with cocaine abuse. Cocaine addiction during pregnancy can cause intrauterine growth retardation, microcephaly, developmental delay, and learning disabilities. Affected infants also have an increased risk of strabismus, and neonatal retinal hemorrhages have been reported. Crack cocaine use in particular should be considered in young patients who present with corneal ulcers or epithelial defects without an obvious cause.

Marijuana has a transient lowering effect on intraocular pressure; thus, many patients assume that marijuana is good for treating or relieving the symptoms of glaucoma and other eye problems. However, marijuana has only a temporary effect on ocular pressure (3–4 hours), and the response diminishes with time. Furthermore, the ocular hypotensive effect cannot be isolated from the psychological effect, making this drug clinically useless in ophthalmology.

Pharmacologic Treatment of Psychiatric Disorders

Antipsychotic Drugs

The antipsychotics may be broadly divided into 2 groups—namely, first-generation, or "typical," drugs, and second-generation, or "atypical," drugs. The older term *major tranquilizer* is no longer used. The distinction between the first-generation and the second-generation antipsychotics is based on differences in receptor activity, side effects, and overall efficacy. The first-generation drugs are primarily dopamine receptor blockers; the second-generation antipsychotics, in contrast, have an inhibitory effect on serotonin receptors as well as dopamine-blocking activity. With regard to side effects, most second-generation drugs are better tolerated than are first-generation drugs. Commonly used first-generation antipsychotics include haloperidol (Haldol), fluphenazine (Prolixin), and chlorpromazine (Thorazine). The number of second-generation drugs is continually growing; these are listed in Table 12-1. Clozapine (Clozaril), risperidone (Risperdal), and olanzapine (Zyprexa) are superior to the first-generation agents; whether the other second-generation drugs share this superiority has not yet been demonstrated in controlled trials. Clozapine has an increased risk of agranulocytosis and is reserved for patients with refractory disease. The atypical antipsychotics are also increasingly administered for off-label uses such as treatment of major depression, anxiety disorders, and Alzheimer disease. The FDA has issued a warning that such off-label use has been associated with increased mortality, due usually to heart-related events or infections.

These medications effectively reduce many of the symptoms of acute and chronic psychoses and have allowed many more patients to function outside the walls of psychiatric institutions. A wide range of side effects may occur with these agents, including extrapyramidal reactions, drowsiness, orthostatic hypotension, anticholinergic effects, and tardive dyskinesia. Less common problems include cholestatic jaundice, blood dyscrasias, photosensitivity, and a rare idiosyncratic reaction known as *neuroleptic malignant syndrome (NMS)*. Neuroleptic malignant syndrome is characterized by "lead pipe" muscle rigidity and hyperthermia and can lead to death if not recognized and treated. The atypical

Table 12-1 Antipsychotic Medications

First generation (or typical antipsychotics or classic neuroleptics)
Chlorpromazine (Thorazine)
Fluphenazine (Prolixin)
Haloperidol (Haldol)
Loxapine (Loxitane)
Mesoridazine (Serentil)
Molindone (Moban)
Perphenazine (Trilafon)
Pimozide (Orap)
Thioridazine (Mellaril)
Thiothixene (Navane)
Second generation (atypical)
Aripiprazole (Abilify)
Clozapine (Clozaril)
Olanzapine (Zyprexa)
Paliperidone (Invega)
Quetiapine (Seroquel)
Risperidone (Risperdal)
Ziprasidone (Geodon)
Anticholinergic agents used to minimize extrapyramidal side effects
Benztropine (Cogentin)
Biperiden (Akineton)
Diphenhydramine (Benadryl)
Trihexyphenidyl (Artane)

antipsychotics are far less likely to cause these side effects, although problems may still occur to some extent at higher doses. Some patients may be maintained on first-generation drugs, however, for reasons of cost, effectiveness, and familiarity.

There are some specific issues of concern to ophthalmologists. The atypical agents—especially olanzapine (Zyprexa) and clozapine (Clozaril)—may be associated with initiating or worsening diabetes, and the possibility of secondary refractive and retinal vascular changes should be considered in this patient population. Because of the results of animal studies, the atypical agent quetiapine (Seroquel) was thought to increase the risk of cataracts. For this reason, psychiatrists are instructed to obtain twice-yearly examinations for this patient population. However, because a true causal relationship is unlikely, annual ophthalmic screening examinations are sufficient. Anticholinergic problems such as dry-eye symptoms, accommodative symptoms, and precipitation of angle-closure glaucoma are possible, especially with use of the first-generation agents and the newer drugs olanzapine and clozapine. These problems may be exacerbated if patients are placed on additional anticholinergic medications to minimize extrapyramidal side effects of the antipsychotics (see Table 12-1). Potential ocular side effects of the first-generation drugs include corneal deposition, lens pigmentation, and vision loss from retinal pigmentary degeneration. These adverse effects are most common with use of thioridazine and are more likely to occur with long-term use at high doses (usually higher than 800 mg/day). Blepharospasm and other ocular motility problems can occur in association with extrapyramidal side effects.

Fraunfelder FW. Twice-yearly exams unnecessary for patients taking quetiapine. *Am J Ophthalmol.* 2004;138(5):870–871.

Antianxiety and Hypnotic Drugs

Benzodiazepines

The benzodiazepines are usually the drugs of choice when an antianxiety, sedative, or hypnotic action is needed. Other indications for selected benzodiazepines include preanesthetic medication, alcohol withdrawal, seizures, spasticity, localized skeletal muscle spasm, and nocturnal myoclonus. The benzodiazepines have distinct advantages over other agents with respect to adverse reactions, drug interactions, and lethality. The pharmacokinetics of these medications greatly affects their efficacy and adverse reactions and thus influences drug selection (Table 12-2). Because of their enhanced safety profile, benzodiazepines have largely supplanted the use of barbiturates when antianxiety or hypnotic drugs are required. Barbiturates have been relegated to treatment of seizure disorders and use in anesthesia.

All benzodiazepines alleviate the uncomplicated anxiety of generalized anxiety disorder and improve symptoms of situational anxiety. Long-acting agents such as diazepam

---

Table 12-2 Antianxiety and Hypnotic Drugs

Benzodiazepines
  Compounds with active metabolites
    Chlordiazepoxide (Librium)
    Clorazepate (Tranxene)
    Diazepam (Valium, Valrelease)
    Flurazepam (Dalmane)
    Halazepam (Paxipam)
  Compounds with weakly active, short-lived, or inactive metabolites
    Alprazolam (Xanax)
    Clonazepam (Klonopin)
    Estazolam (Prosom)
    Lorazepam (Ativan)
    Midazolam (Versed)
    Oxazepam (Serax)
    Quazepam (Doral)
    Temazepam (Restoril)
    Triazolam (Halcion)
Barbiturates
    Amobarbital (Amytal)
    Mephobarbital (Mebaral)
    Pentobarbital (Nembutal)
    Phenobarbital (Solfoton)
    Secobarbital (Seconal)
Nonbenzodiazepine-nonbarbiturates
  Antianxiety agents
    Buspirone (BuSpar)
    Hydroxyzine (Atarax, Vistaril)
    Meprobamate (Equanil, Miltown)
  Hypnotic agents
    Chloral hydrate
    Eszopiclone (Lunesta)
    Ethchlorvynol (Placidyl)
    Paraldehyde
    Zaleplon (Sonata)
    Zolpidem (Ambien)

(Valium) are useful for patients requiring chronic treatment. The treatment of insomnia is another common indication for these drugs. Short-acting agents such as estazolam (Prosom), temazepam (Restoril), and triazolam (Halcion) are preferred for this purpose because there is less residual somnolence. Zaleplon (Sonata) and zolpidem (Ambien) are newer, short-acting, nonbenzodiazepine hypnotic agents that are increasingly used in the treatment of insomnia. Eszopiclone (Lunesta), another drug in this class, has the longest half-life, approximately 5–7 hours. All of these drugs, however, have the potential to cause retrograde amnesia and rebound insomnia.

Sedation is the most common initial untoward effect of the benzodiazepines. Other common dose-related adverse effects with oral use include dizziness and ataxia. Respiratory depression can occur, especially if these agents are combined with alcohol. Products available in parenteral form, such as diazepam (Valium) and midazolam (Versed), must be administered with careful monitoring because of an increased risk for apnea and cardiac arrest.

The abuse potential of benzodiazepines is mild compared with that of drugs such as hydromorphone (Dilaudid) and cocaine. Nevertheless, long-term administration of these agents can cause physical dependence. Once physical dependence is established, withdrawal reactions may occur if the drugs are discontinued abruptly. Psychological dependence is more common than physical dependence and can occur with any dose. This type of drug reliance is difficult to distinguish from a recurrence of the original anxiety disorder. Consequently, good medical practice demands that these agents be prescribed initially only when a disorder known to respond to such therapy can be diagnosed with reasonable assurance and that their use be continued only for the shortest time required.

Ocular side effects can occur, although they tend to be dose-related and transient. Decreased accommodation and diplopia from increased phorias have been reported. Transient allergic conjunctivitis with benzodiazepine use has also been seen.

Antidepressants

Psychotherapy, either alone or in combination with antidepressant medication, is the first line of intervention in mild to moderate depression. In patients with major depression, antidepressants can improve symptoms, increase the chances and rate of recovery, reduce the likelihood of suicide, and help social and occupational rehabilitation.

In general, antidepressants take 3–6 weeks to show significant effect. A summary of studies concluded that antidepressants are associated with a 50%–60% response rate among patients with major depression in the primary care setting. These drugs can result in mood elevation, improved appetite, better sleep, and increased mental and physical activity. Treatment is usually necessary for 3–6 months after recovery is apparent.

Table 12-3 shows the various classes of antidepressants. The SSRIs were developed in response to research that implicated specific monoamines such as serotonin in the etiology of depression. They are the most commonly prescribed agents, although a meta-analysis suggested that they are no more efficacious than older tricyclic or heterocyclic antidepressants. The most compelling reason for using SSRIs is lower severity of side effects due to their more targeted mechanism of action. SSRIs are also less dangerous than other antidepressants if

Table 12-3 Pharmacology of Antidepressants

Tricyclics and tetracyclics
Amitriptyline (Elavil)
Amoxapine (Asendin)
Clomipramine (Anafranil)
Desipramine (Norpramin)
Doxepin (Adapin, Sinequan)
Imipramine (Tofranil)
Maprotiline (Ludiomil)
Nortriptyline (Pamelor)
Protriptyline (Vivactil)
Trimipramine (Surmontil)
Selective serotonin reuptake inhibitors
Citalopram (Celexa)
Escitalopram (Lexapro)
Fluoxetine (Prozac)
Fluvoxamine (Luvox)
Paroxetine (Paxil)
Paroxetine CR (Paxil CR)
Sertraline (Zoloft)
Dopamine-norepinephrine reuptake inhibitors
Bupropion (Wellbutrin)
Bupropion SR (Wellbutrin SR)
Bupropion XL (Wellbutrin XL)
Serotonin-norepinephrine reuptake inhibitors
Duloxetine (Cymbalta)
Venlafaxine (Effexor)
Venlafaxine XR (Effexor XR)
Serotonin modulators
Nefazodone (Serzone)
Trazodone (Desyrel)
Noradrenergic and specific serotonergic antidepressant
Mirtazapine (Remeron)
Monoamine oxidase inhibitors
Phenelzine (Nardil)
Tranylcypromine (Parnate)

Modified from Paulsen RH, Katon W, Ciechanowski P. Treatment of depression. In: *UpToDate,* Rose BD (ed), Waltham, MA. Available at www.uptodate.com. Accessed March 1, 2005.

an overdose occurs. Common adverse effects that can occur with use of the SSRIs include restlessness, insomnia, headache, gastrointestinal symptoms, mild sedation, and sexual dysfunction. SSRIs may cause inhibition of platelet function that can increase the risk of gastrointestinal bleeding and possibly increase the risk for transfusions with major surgery. It is not known if this effect is clinically significant in ophthalmic surgery.

The SSRIs also cause nonspecific visual symptoms such as blurred vision in 2%–10% of patients. In addition, patients may complain of "tracking" difficulties, which is more common in younger than older patients and tends to occur upon withdrawal of the drug. The SSRIs can also cause mydriasis, and rare cases of angle-closure glaucoma have been reported, most commonly with paroxetine (Paxil), which tends to have a stronger anticholinergic effect.

Recently, there has been a concern that the SSRIs may initially increase the risk of suicide in some patients, especially in adolescents and children, although the data are controversial. Careful monitoring of patients is recommended when treatment is initiated. Abrupt cessation of SSRIs may result in a "discontinuation syndrome," characterized by dizziness, nausea, fatigue, muscle aches, chills, anxiety, and irritability. This syndrome may be problematic, but it is much more benign than the severe side effects that can occur if heterocyclic or monoamine oxidase inhibitor drugs (discussed later in this section) are abruptly discontinued.

The other major class of antidepressants is the *heterocyclics,* of which the tricyclic antidepressants were the first described. These drugs tend to have more pronounced side effects than the SSRIs, including anticholinergic symptoms such as dry eye and mouth, accommodative changes, constipation, urinary retention, tachycardia, and confusion or delirium. Sedation, weight gain, and orthostatic hypotension may also occur. Most concerning is the toxicity of these medications in overdose. In contrast to the SSRIs, the cyclic antidepressants can be fatal in doses as little as 5 times the therapeutic dose. Mortality is usually due to arrhythmias, although anticholinergic toxicity and seizures can also occur. Sudden cessation may cause pronounced changes in affect, cognition, and cardiac dysrhythmias.

The *monoamine oxidase (MAO) inhibitors* have long been considered second-line drugs in the treatment of mood disorders; however, they can be useful in the treatment of refractory and atypical depression. The significant risk of hypertensive crisis caused by interactions between MAO inhibitors and various foods and drugs must be considered when they are prescribed. When combined with food and beverages of high tyramine content (including cheese, herring, chicken liver, yeast, yogurt, red wine, beer), these drugs may produce severe hypertension that can lead to subarachnoid or cerebral hemorrhage. Because MAO inhibitors prevent catabolism of catecholamines, patients taking these substances have exaggerated hypertensive responses to drugs containing vasopressors, such as cold remedies, nasal decongestants, and even topical or retrobulbar epinephrine.

Other agents have variable effects on other neurotransmitters and do not fall into specific categories. These include bupropion (Wellbutrin), venlafaxine (Effexor), duloxetine (Cymbalta), trazodone (Desyrel), and nefazodone (Serzone). The side-effect profile for each of these drugs, as well as for the SSRIs and heterocyclics, is slightly different from that of the others, thus allowing the selection of an agent that seems to best fit a given patient's constellation of symptoms.

Newer nonpharmacologic treatments for depression are also being evaluated. Vagus nerve stimulation (VNS) uses an implanted stimulator that sends electric impulses to the left vagus nerve in the neck via a lead wire implanted under the skin. In 2005, the FDA approved the use of VNS for treatment-resistant depression, although there is some controversy about its effectiveness. Transcranial magnetic stimulation is a noninvasive method to excite neurons in the brain: weak electric currents are induced in the tissue by rapidly changing magnetic fields. Repetitive transcranial magnetic stimulation (rTMS) can produce longer-lasting changes in neuronal function. Multiple controlled studies support the use of this method in treatment-resistant depression.

Mood stabilizers

Mood stabilizers are a heterogeneous group of medications that do not clearly share a common mechanism of action. These are the drugs of choice for treatment of mania, bipolar disorder, schizoaffective disorder, and cyclothymia. They may also be used for impulse control disorders, symptoms associated with mental retardation, and aggressive behavior. This class consists essentially of lithium carbonate (Eskalith, Lithonate) and various antiepileptic medications. Valproic acid (Depakote) and carbamazepine (Tegretol) are the most commonly used antiepileptic drugs, but many others have been studied and prescribed. The antiepileptic medications are discussed in Epilepsy, later in this chapter.

Lithium is effective in the treatment of bipolar disorder and in some patients with recurrent unipolar depression. It has a very narrow therapeutic ratio, making close monitoring of plasma levels mandatory. Adverse effects include renal, thyroid, parathyroid, cardiac, and neurologic toxicity. Weight gain and gastrointestinal upset are common. Toxic plasma levels due to renal dysfunction, concurrent use of diuretics, or overdose can lead to persistent nausea and vomiting, coma, circulatory failure, and death. Ocular side effects include blurred vision, ocular irritation due to secretion in tears, nystagmus (usually downbeat), and exophthalmos that is often associated with lithium-induced changes in thyroid function.

◉ **Ophthalmic considerations**   Although behavioral disorders do not directly affect the eye, a number of related issues are important to the ophthalmologist. For example, awareness of the potential ocular side effects of the various psychiatric medications is important. Patient education and reassurance may be required because the underlying psychopathology may make anticholinergic ophthalmic side effects such as dry eye and accommodative changes much more frightening and less tolerable for patients with behavioral disorders than for those without such disorders. Noncompliance is another common problem among patients with psychiatric illness, dementia, and depression. Malingering and functional visual loss require a high index of suspicion and special diagnostic skills on the part of the clinician. Some medications used to treat eye disease, including carbonic anhydrase inhibitors, brimonidine, oral corticosteroids, and possibly β-blockers, may induce or exacerbate depression.

Costagliola C, Parmeggiani F, Sebastiani A. SSRIs and intraocular pressure modifications: evidence, therapeutic implications and possible mechanisms. *CNS Drugs.* 2004;18(8): 475–484.

Fraunfelder FT, Fraunfelder FW, Chambers WA. *Clinical Ocular Toxicology: Drug-Induced Ocular Side Effects.* Philadelphia: Elsevier/Saunders; 2008.

Hahn RK, Albers LJ, Reist C. *Psychiatry.* 2008 ed. Current Clinical Strategies. Blue Jay, CA: Current Clinical Strategies; 2008.

Moore DP, Jefferson JW. *Handbook of Medical Psychiatry.* 2nd ed. Philadelphia: Elsevier/ Mosby; 2004.

Neurologic Disorders

Parkinson Disease

Parkinson disease belongs to a group of conditions known as *bradykinetic movement disorders,* which are usually associated with rigidity, postural instability, and loss of automatic associated movements. Parkinson disease strikes men and women in almost equal numbers, usually affecting people older than age 50. The average age of onset is 60 years. However, the number of reported cases of "early-onset" Parkinson disease has increased; it is estimated that 5%–10% of patients are now younger than age 40, and there is also a juvenile form that presents before age 20.

Etiology

The basal ganglia are a complex of deep nuclei that consist of the corpus striatum, globus pallidus, and substantia nigra. These structures regulate the initiation and control of movement. Parkinson disease occurs when neurons in the substantia nigra die or become impaired. Normally, these neurons produce dopamine, a neurotransmitter responsible for transmitting signals between the substantia nigra and the corpus striatum to produce smooth, purposeful muscle activity. Loss of dopamine causes the nerve cells of the striatum to fire out of control, leaving patients unable to direct or control their movements normally. Patients with Parkinson disease have lost 80% or more of dopamine-producing cells in the substantia nigra. An associated pathologic finding is the presence of eosinophilic cytoplasmic inclusion bodies in the substantia nigra that are known as *Lewy bodies.*

Genetic factors are implicated in the pathogenesis. In 15%–20% of patients, a close relative has experienced parkinsonian symptoms. At least 5 possible causative genes have been identified, and the number of Parkinson-like disorders associated with specific genetic defects is growing. Many of these defects appear to be involved in cellular protein metabolism. Overall, Parkinson disease seems to have a multifactorial etiology that includes genetic predisposition, environmental factors, and age-related changes in neuron metabolism. Reports suggest that the frequency of Parkinson disease is actually decreased in patients with a history of cigarette smoking and caffeine consumption.

Symptoms

Usually the first symptom of Parkinson disease is tremor of a limb, especially at rest. The tremor often begins on 1 side of the body, frequently in the hand. Other common symptoms include bradykinesia, rigidity, a shuffling gait, postural instability, and stooped posture. People with Parkinson disease often show reduced facial expression and speak in a soft voice. The disease can also cause depression, personality changes, sexual difficulties, hallucinations, autonomic dysfunction, and dementia.

Treatment

There is currently no cure for Parkinson disease. The main treatment is levodopa (L-dopa), and treatment is generally initiated when symptoms begin to become significant. Neurons use levodopa to make dopamine and replace the brain's diminishing supply.

Dopamine itself cannot be given because it does not cross the blood–brain barrier. Although levodopa helps at least three fourths of Parkinson cases, not all symptoms respond equally to the drug. Bradykinesia and rigidity respond best; tremor may be only marginally reduced. Problems with balance and other symptoms may not be alleviated at all. Usually, patients are given levodopa combined with carbidopa (Lodosyn), often as a combined pill (Sinemet). When added to levodopa, carbidopa delays the conversion of levodopa into dopamine until it reaches the brain, diminishing some of the side effects that often accompany levodopa therapy.

After years of therapy, patients can become acutely aware of a "wearing-off" effect that occurs about 4 hours after a dose of levodopa, when their symptoms return. Alterations in dosing or absorption do not seem to help, although more frequent dosing may decrease symptoms initially. Catechol-O-methyltransferase inhibitors such as entacapone (Comtan) provide a new method of extending the duration of the levodopa effect and reducing the "off" time by inhibiting the methylation of levodopa and dopamine. Long-term levodopa use can also be associated with drug-related dyskinesias and dystonias, which may require changes in dosing and additional medications. In addition, there is ongoing controversy about whether long-term use of levodopa may actually increase the rate of progression of Parkinson disease, and clinical trials are under way to study the effects of levodopa on this progression. In the meantime, levodopa remains the most effective therapy and should be introduced if quality of life or functional ability is sufficiently compromised.

Bromocriptine (Parlodel), pergolide (Permax), pramipexole (Mirapex), and ropinirole (Requip) are 4 drugs that stimulate dopamine receptors in the brain. These drugs can be given alone or in combination with levodopa. They are generally less effective than levodopa in controlling rigidity and bradykinesia, but they may have a neuroprotective effect that may delay the need for levodopa. Trials are under way to evaluate this possibility. Selegiline (Eldepryl) inhibits the activity of the enzyme MAO B, which metabolizes dopamine in the brain. Selegiline may delay the need for levodopa or, when given in combination with levodopa, may enhance and prolong the response of levodopa, although the beneficial effect of this drug appears to be mild and short-lived.

Anticholinergic drugs such as trihexyphenidyl (Artane) and benztropine (Cogentin) were the main treatment for Parkinson disease before the introduction of levodopa. Although their benefit is limited and their effect is usually short-lived, anticholinergics may help control tremor and rigidity. However, only about half of patients respond to anticholinergics, and typical anticholinergic side effects can be problematic.

Amantadine (Symmetrel), an antiviral drug, is often used in the early stages of the disease, either alone or in combination with anticholinergics or levodopa. After several months, the effectiveness of amantadine wears off in a third to a half of patients taking the drug.

Modern surgical treatments consist primarily of pallidotomy and deep-brain stimulation. The dopamine deficiency in Parkinson disease results in excitation of the globus pallidus, which in turn inhibits thalamic activity. Both surgical techniques serve to suppress this excessive globus pallidus activity. Pallidotomy, however, carries the risk of complications such as stroke and hemorrhage, as well as the risk of irreversible side effects. Deep-brain stimulation is safer than pallidotomy initially but requires intensive adjustments and lifelong maintenance, with the risk of hardware complications and infection. Trials are under way to define the role for these therapies.

Experimental transplantation of embryonic dopamine neurons has been attempted with little or no success. A potential complication is "runaway dyskinesia," possibly due to excessive dopaminergic stimulation. Direct brain infusion of glial cell line–derived neurotrophic factor is another approach that is under investigation and may have some utility.

⊚ **Ophthalmic considerations**   There are numerous ophthalmologic findings in patients with Parkinson disease. These findings can be divided into eyelid disorders and ocular motor abnormalities. Eyelid disorders include seborrheic dermatitis and blepharitis, apraxia of eyelid opening, lid retraction, decreased blinking (with secondary dry eye), and blepharospasm. Ocular motor abnormalities include convergence insufficiency, limitation of upgaze, hypometric saccades, saccadic (cogwheel) pursuit, square-wave jerks, and oculogyric crisis. Reading trouble is a common initial complaint, and the ocular surface abnormalities and motor abnormalities may synergize with other ophthalmic and neurologic problems to increase visual difficulties. (The ophthalmic manifestations of Parkinson disease are also discussed in BCSC Section 5, *Neuro-Ophthalmology.*)

Drug-related side effects may also be superimposed, especially for patients on anticholinergic medications, which may exacerbate dry eyes and cause accommodative changes or precipitate angle-closure glaucoma. Visual hallucinations may occur as a result of both the disease and its treatment; this adverse effect has been reported in particular with use of levodopa and anticholinergic agents. Amantadine has been reported to cause corneal infiltrates and edema, although these complications are rare.

Multiple Sclerosis

See BCSC Section 5, *Neuro-Ophthalmology.*

Epilepsy

Epileptic seizures result from synchronized electrical activity of neuronal networks in the cerebral cortex. Epilepsy is characterized by recurrent epileptic seizures due to a genetically determined or acquired brain disorder. More than 2 million people in the United States— approximately 1 in 100—have experienced an unprovoked seizure or been diagnosed with epilepsy. Patients with relatively controlled epilepsy may still have problems with depression, driving, employment, and insurance. In one survey, 31% of respondents with 1 seizure or fewer per year reported that epilepsy had a great impact on their lives; more than 40% of college-educated people with "well-controlled" seizures were unemployed.

Etiology

Epilepsy is a disorder with many possible causes. Any disturbance of normal neuronal activity, including injury, infection, and abnormal brain development, can lead to seizures. Approximately half of all seizures have no known cause. Seizures may develop because of an abnormality in brain wiring, an imbalance of neurotransmitters, or some combination of these factors.

Epilepsy can result from brain damage that can be caused by numerous disorders. Head injury; prenatal injury; developmental problems; and exposure to lead, carbon monoxide, and other poisons have all been associated with seizures. Brain tumors, alcoholism, and Alzheimer disease frequently lead to epilepsy. Strokes and myocardial infarctions that produce cerebral ischemia may account for as much as 32% of all newly developed epilepsy in older persons. Meningitis, AIDS, viral encephalitis, and other infectious diseases can lead to epilepsy. Epilepsy can also be part of a set of symptoms in a variety of developmental and metabolic disorders, including cerebral palsy, neurofibromatosis, tuberous sclerosis, and autism.

Certain types of epilepsy have been shown to be caused by mutations in specific genes. It is likely that genetics plays a more indirect role for many patients, perhaps by increasing a person's susceptibility to seizures that are triggered by an environmental factor or by having subtle effects on neuronal development or physiology that predispose to seizure activity.

More than 30 types of seizures have been described. Typically, seizures are divided into 2 major categories: partial seizures and generalized seizures. *Partial seizures* occur in just 1 part of the brain and are further divided into *simple* (without impairment of consciousness) and *complex* (with impairment of consciousness). Symptoms of simple partial seizures (also called *auras*) depend on the part of the brain from which the seizures originate and include motor symptoms, sensory symptoms, and even autonomic symptoms. Complex partial seizures (previously called *temporal lobe seizures* or *psychomotor seizures*) are the most common type of seizure in epileptic adults. During the seizure, patients appear to be awake but do not interact with others in their environment and do not respond normally to instructions or questions. They often stare into space and either remain motionless or engage in repetitive behaviors, called *automatisms,* such as facial grimacing or gesturing.

Generalized seizures, of which there are 6 main types, almost always produce impaired consciousness and show abnormal activity in both hemispheres at the onset of the seizure. They may be nonconvulsive (absence, or "petit mal") or convulsive (tonic-clonic, or "grand mal," or variations of tonic-clonic). Absence seizures almost always begin in childhood or adolescence and are frequently familial, suggesting a genetic cause. Some patients may make purposeless movements during their seizures, such as jerking an arm or rapidly blinking their eyes. Others have no noticeable symptoms except for brief periods when they are "out of it." Childhood absence epilepsy usually stops when the child reaches puberty. A generalized tonic-clonic seizure is the most dramatic type of seizure. It begins with an abrupt loss of consciousness, often in association with a scream or shriek. All of the muscles then become stiff and the patient may become cyanotic during the tonic phase. After approximately 1 minute, the muscles begin to jerk and twitch for an additional 1–2 minutes, and then the patient goes into in a deep sleep.

The end of a seizure is referred to as the *postictal period* and signifies the recovery period for the brain. This period may last from several seconds up to a few days, depending on factors such as the severity of the seizure and the patient's age. Postictal paresis (Todd paralysis) is a transient focal motor deficit that lasts for hours or, in rare cases, days after an epileptic convulsion and is thought to be related either to neuronal exhaustion (from electrical overactivity during the seizure) or to active inhibition.

Epileptic seizures are distinguished from *nonepileptic seizures (NES),* which are sudden changes in behavior that resemble epileptic seizures but are not associated with the typical neurophysiologic changes characterizing epileptic seizures. Nonepileptic seizures are often caused by medical problems such as hypoglycemia, electrolyte abnormalities, and cerebral anoxia; treatment of the underlying problem controls the seizure activity.

Diagnosis

The electroencephalogram (EEG) is the most common diagnostic test for epilepsy. In most patients with epilepsy, the EEG appears abnormal, although provocative testing (such as sleep deprivation) may need to be done to demonstrate the abnormality. A normal EEG does not rule out epilepsy, however. Computed tomography (CT) and magnetic resonance imaging (MRI) are useful tools for determining structural abnormalities in the brain that cause epilepsy. More sophisticated modalities are being developed that allow imaging of abnormal physiology in addition to anatomy. *Magnetoencephalography (MEG)* detects magnetic fields associated with the intracellular current flow within neurons and can detect signals from deeper in the brain than an EEG can. *Magnetic source imaging (MSI)* is an advanced technique that combines MEG and MRI to measure the magnetic field generated by a series of neurons. MSI is particularly useful for the investigation of patients who may be candidates for epilepsy surgery. Positron emission tomography (PET) and single-photon emission computed tomography (SPECT) are related functional imaging techniques that are also used to locate seizure foci.

Treatment

Currently available treatments control seizure activity at least some of the time in 80% of patients with epilepsy. The other 20% experience intractable seizures or obtain inadequate relief from available treatment. The primary treatment for epilepsy is antiepileptic drugs; the choice of drug is determined by the type of epilepsy. In recent years, a number of new drugs have become available (Table 12-4). The drug dose is titrated up until the disease is controlled; a second agent may be added if necessary, but monotherapy is preferred, if possible, to minimize side effects.

There are 2 main categories of side effects for the antiepilepsy drugs: systemic and neurotoxic. Systemic side effects generally include problems such as nausea, rash, and anorexia. Neurotoxic effects include somnolence, dizziness, and confusion. The neurotoxic effects seem to be an inevitable consequence of the mechanism of action of these drugs and often become the dose-limiting factor.

When medications inadequately control seizures, surgery is a potential option. The most commonly performed surgery for epilepsy is the removal of a seizure focus. This procedure, called *lobectomy* or *lesionectomy,* is appropriate for partial seizures that originate

Table 12-4 Mechanisms of Action of Antiepileptic Drugs

Drug	Mechanism of Action
Carbamazepine (Tegretol, Tegretol XR, Carbatrol)	Blocks voltage-dependent sodium channels
Ethosuximide (Zarontin)	Modifies low-threshold T-type calcium currents
Felbamate (Felbatol)	Blocks NMDA receptor; potentiates GABA-mediated inhibition
Fosphenytoin (Cerebyx)	Water-soluble prodrug of phenytoin
Gabapentin (Neurontin)	Exact mechanism unknown; GABA analogue
Lamotrigine (Lamictal)	Blocks voltage-dependent sodium channels
Levetiracetam (Keppra)	Exact mechanism unknown
Oxcarbazepine (Trileptal)	Blocks voltage-dependent sodium channels
Phenobarbital, mysoline, benzodiazepines	Accentuate GABA-mediated chloride channel openings
Phenytoin (Dilantin)	Blocks voltage-dependent sodium channels
Tiagabine (Gabitril)	Inhibits GABA uptake in neurons and glia
Topiramate (Topamax)	Blocks voltage-dependent sodium channels; inhibits kainate/AMPA receptor; enhances GABA-mediated inhibition at GABA (A) receptors
Valproate (Depakene capsules and syrup, Depakote sprinkle capsules, Depakote delayed-release tablets, Depakote ER, Depacon)	Blocks voltage-dependent sodium channels; enhances postsynaptic GABA-mediated inhibition
Vigabatrin (Sabril)	Irreversible inhibitor of GABA-transaminase
Zonisamide (Zonegran)	Blocks voltage-dependent sodium and T-type calcium channels

Reprinted with permission from Schachter SC. Pharmacology of antiepileptic drugs. In: *UpToDate,* Rose BD (ed), Waltham, MA. Available at www.uptodate.com. Accessed March 1, 2005.

in a single area of the brain. Temporal lobe resection is the most commonly performed type of lobectomy and is successful in 70%–90% of patients. Other surgical procedures for epilepsy include multiple subpial transection, corpus callosotomy, and hemispherectomy. In patients with seizures poorly controlled by medications or surgery, vagus nerve stimulation may be used. The vagal nerve stimulator is a battery-powered device that is surgically implanted under the skin of the chest and is attached to the vagus nerve in the lower neck. The device delivers short bursts of electrical energy to the brain via the vagus nerve. On average, the device reduces seizures by 20%–40%.

◉ Ophthalmic considerations Transient unilateral mydriasis can occur as an expression of minor or major seizure activity, during or after the event. This phenomenon is most common in children. In some patients, the dilated pupil reacts poorly to light. In children, the eyes may deviate to the side of the dilated pupil. Horizontal or vertical gaze deviations are commonly associated with seizure activity. The gaze tends to be directed away from the side of the cortical lesion during a seizure and then toward the side of the lesion after the seizure. Some patients experience conjugate, convergent, or monocular nystagmus during the clonic stage of a seizure. Clonic lid retraction has also been described in patients with petit mal or myoclonic seizures. It is unusual for patients with true seizures to shut their eyes during the episode, whereas patients who are feigning a seizure will often keep their eyes closed.

Certain antiepileptic drugs have the potential for characteristic ocular side effects. Phenytoin (Dilantin) can cause dose-related nystagmus, and maternal use of this medication can cause the fetal hydantoin syndrome (which includes hypertelorism, epicanthal folds, glaucoma, optic nerve hypoplasia, and retinal colobomas). Carbamazepine has been reported to affect saccadic eye movements and has been associated with isolated cases of downbeat nystagmus and oscillopsia. Blurred vision, diplopia, and nystagmus may also occur with this medication. Topiramate (Topamax) has been associated with acute angle-closure glaucoma, anterior chamber shallowing, acute myopia, and choroidal effusions, usually within the first 2 weeks of therapy. These effects may be an idiopathic response related to the presence of sulfa in topiramate. Treatment of the glaucoma includes cessation of the drug and use of cycloplegics and topical hypotensives.

Vigabatrin (Sabril) has recently been approved in the United States for patients unresponsive to other medications. As many as 30%–50% of patients with long-term exposure to vigabatrin have developed irreversible concentric visual field loss of varying severity that is often asymptomatic. Central vision can also be affected. A complete ophthalmic examination and visual field testing should be performed before starting therapy and repeated every 3 months. The onset and progression of vision loss from vigabatrin is unpredictable, and it may occur or worsen precipitously between tests. Once detected, vision loss is not reversible, and it is expected that even with frequent monitoring, some patients will develop severe vision loss. Because of this risk, the drug is available only through a special restricted distribution program.

Stroke

See Chapter 3, Cerebrovascular Disease.

Pain Syndromes

See BCSC Section 5, *Neuro-Ophthalmology.*

Alzheimer Disease and Dementia

Dementia is a disorder characterized by a general decrease in the level of cognition and memory and usually includes behavioral disturbances and inability to remain independent. Dementia is not a specific disease. Although it is common in persons older than age 80, dementia is not a normal part of the aging process. Dementia also differs from delirium. *Delirium,* or an acute confusional state, is an acute or subacute onset of disorientation with alterations in levels of awareness. The major difference between dementia and delirium is that demented patients are alert and without the disturbance of consciousness characteristic of delirious patients.

Alzheimer disease is the most common cause of dementia in people older than age 65, but there are a number of other causes of dementia. Other major dementia syndromes include Lewy body dementia, vascular dementia (previously known as *multi-infarct dementia*), and Parkinson disease with dementia. Most older patients with chronic dementia have Alzheimer disease (approximately 60%–80%). The vascular dementias account for 10%–20%; dementia associated with Parkinson disease, about 5%. Dementia can be associated with trauma (eg, dementia pugilistica, or boxer's syndrome), with infections such as neurosyphilis, tuberculosis (TB), or fungal meningitis, and with AIDS. Metabolic problems such as diabetes mellitus, electrolyte disturbances, and hypothyroidism can cause dementia. Nutritional causes include vitamin B_{12} deficiency and thiamine deficiency (Wernicke-Korsakoff syndrome). Toxic dementia can occur, for instance, with heavy metal exposure or chronic alcoholism. Other causes include drug use, depression, subdural hematoma, and normal-pressure hydrocephalus. A crucial part of the evaluation of a patient with dementia is looking for any potentially treatable factors that may help reverse the problem.

Vascular dementia is associated with findings on neurologic examination consistent with prior strokes; patients often show evidence of multiple infarcts on cerebral imaging. Patients may have an abrupt onset of symptoms followed by stepwise deterioration, unlike the gradual progression that occurs with neurodegenerative conditions such as Parkinson disease. Vascular dementia may also present subsequent to a stroke (poststroke dementia). The incidence of vascular dementia is relatively high in blacks, hypertensive persons, and persons with diabetes. Other causes of vascular dementia include vasculitis, profound hypotension, and lesions caused by cerebral hemorrhages. The term *mixed dementia* refers to patients who have a combination of vascular dementia and Alzheimer disease.

Lewy body dementia (LBD) is the second most common form of neurodegenerative dementia after Alzheimer disease. Lewy bodies are intracytoplasmic inclusions that are also seen in the substantia nigra in Parkinson disease. Lewy body dementia is characterized neuropathologically by the presence of Lewy bodies in the brainstem and cortex. There may be considerable clinical and neuropathologic overlap between LBD, Parkinson disease, and Alzheimer disease, and the clinical distinction among these entities may be difficult at times. Ophthalmologists should be aware of LBD, however, because patients with this syndrome often present with complex formed visual hallucinations. With treatment, patients who have LBD can have marked improvements in cognition and behavioral symptoms, as well as fewer hallucinations. Referral to a neurologist or geriatric psychiatrist is warranted if the disease is suspected.

Alzheimer disease (AD) is an irreversible, progressive disorder that proceeds in stages, gradually destroying memory, reason, judgment, language, and eventually the ability to carry out even the simplest of tasks. Alzheimer disease is the most common neurodegenerative disorder in the United States, affecting an estimated 4 million people. One recent study found that AD was present in almost half of people age 85 and older.

The emotional and financial burden of this disease on individuals and their families and the impact on society are difficult to measure, but currently AD is estimated to cost the nation \$80–\$90 billion a year. Caring for a person with AD is estimated to cost \$47,000 per year, whether the patient lives at home or in a nursing home. It is clear that as life expectancy increases and the United States experiences the demographic impact of the baby boom generation, AD will have an even greater effect on society in coming years.

The pathologic hallmarks of the disease are extraneuronal amyloid plaques (fragmented brain cells surrounded by amyloid-family proteins) and intraneuronal neurofibrillary tangles (tangles of filaments largely composed of protein associated with the cytoskeleton). These 2 findings are associated with neuronal death and decreased levels of the neurotransmitter acetylcholine, as well as with abnormalities in other neurotransmitter systems. Signs of neuronal death first appear in the entorhinal cortex, with eventual extension into the hippocampus (an area essential for memory storage). As the disease progresses, the basal forebrain and eventually the cerebral cortex become involved.

Etiology

The exact etiology of AD is unknown, but both genetic/nongenetic and environmental factors play a role.

Genetic factors   There are 2 types of AD: *familial AD,* which follows a certain inheritance pattern, and *sporadic AD,* in which no inheritance pattern is obvious. Alzheimer disease is further described as *early onset* (occurring in people younger than age 65) and *late onset* (occurring in those older than age 65). Early-onset AD is rare (10% of cases) and generally affects persons between 30 and 60 years of age. Some forms of early-onset AD are inherited and typically progress faster than the more common late-onset forms.

All known familial AD cases have been of early onset, and to date these hereditary forms of AD have mutations that accelerate the production of amyloid-β42 ($A\beta_{42}$). This acceleration occurs either by abnormal production of amyloid precursor protein (APP) or by excessive processing via mutations in the secretase enzymes. For instance, the *APP* gene is on chromosome 21, and patients with Down syndrome have trisomy of chromosome 21 and an excess of APP. As they grow older, such patients usually develop plaques and tangles like those found in AD. There is no evidence that any of these specific familial mutations play a role in the most common sporadic, or nonfamilial, form of late-onset AD.

Nevertheless, there does appear to be a genetic component in the more common form of late-onset AD. Patients who have a first-degree relative with dementia have a 10%–30% increased risk of developing the disorder. A possible marker for the development of AD is the ε4 genotype of the protein apolipoprotein E (APOE). The APOE protein has many functions, including participation in the transport of cholesterol throughout the body. There are 3 alleles of the gene: ε2, ε3, and ε4. People who inherit 2 ε4 genes are 8 times more likely to develop AD than those who inherit 2 of ε3, the most common version. The least common allele, ε2, seems to actually lower the risk for AD.

Nongenetic factors   Numerous factors have been implicated in the cascade of events that produce AD. Oxidative stress from free radicals may damage cells. Unique characteristics of the brain, including its high rate of metabolism and the long life span of its nondividing cells, may make it particularly vulnerable to oxidative stress. Inflammation is another important mechanism that is under intense investigation as a possible cause of AD.

Inflammation in the brain increases with age but is more pronounced in patients with AD. Yet another area of interest involves cerebrovascular disease, including small infarcts in specific regions of the brain that accelerate the findings of AD.

Diagnosis

There is no definitive antemortem diagnostic test for AD other than a brain biopsy. Physicians rely on a variety of methods, including history, physical examination, laboratory tests, brain scans, and assessments of memory, language skills, and other brain functions. Cerebrospinal fluid levels of tau and amyloid protein are under investigation as possible diagnostic markers. A few years ago, some investigators suggested that patients with AD had a more pronounced pupil dilation response to dilute tropicamide, presumably reflecting a generalized cholinergic deficit. Subsequent studies indicated that this was not useful as a diagnostic test, and it is no longer used.

Several imaging techniques are useful, and all may have specific uses in helping to diagnose AD or at least in eliminating other causes of dementia. PET detects changes in glucose metabolism in the parts of the brain most affected by AD. Single-photon emission computed tomography (SPECT) can be combined with genetic and psychological testing to predict which patients with memory loss will eventually develop AD. MRI can be particularly useful in measuring atrophy in the hippocampus, a sign of early AD in patients who demonstrate problems with memory. The precise clinical usefulness of these studies is not yet well defined; as better preventive therapies are developed, early recognition of disease will be more valuable.

Treatment

Given the tremendous toll the disease takes on the patient, caregivers, and society, there is great interest in identifying factors that may prevent onset of the disease. Some epidemiologic studies suggested that NSAIDs may be useful in the prevention of AD. However, more recent studies seem to indicate no significant benefit with these drugs, and they appear to put patients at increased risk for other problems, such as cardiovascular events. Until there is stronger clinical trial evidence of benefit, these drugs have no role in dementia prevention or treatment. The lipid-lowering HMG-CoA reductase inhibitors (statins) may also decrease the risk of developing AD, but definitive studies are pending. Other proposed interventions include exercise, cognitive activity, high n-3 fatty acid intake, consumption of vitamin E–rich foods, use of ginkgo biloba, use of certain antibiotics, and moderate alcohol intake, but none of these has proven conclusively beneficial in a prospective trial.

Once the disease is diagnosed, psychosocial issues need to be addressed. Patients and family members need to deal with matters such as driving and cooking safety, emotional lability, wandering, and falls. A number of resources can assist with these issues, such as the Alzheimer's Association (www.alz.org).

New guidelines for the pharmacologic treatment of dementia have been released based on a systematic review of the evidence for the efficacy of the cholinesterase inhibitors, such as donepezil (Aricept), and the neuropeptide-modifying agent memantine (Namenda). Treatment of dementia with these agents can result in benefits that are statistically significant but that afford clinically marginal improvement in measures of cognition and global assessment of dementia. There is no convincing evidence that one drug is better than another, and treatment choice should be based on a drug's adverse-effect profile, ease of use, and cost. According to the guidelines, the current evidence does not support prescribing these medications to every patient with dementia. The review authors also note that slowing decline in a patient with dementia may not always be a desirable goal, particularly if the patient's quality of life is poor. They recommend that when considering treatment of dementia, clinicians also take adverse effects of these agents into account and balance potential harm against modest—and, in some cases, no—benefit.

Because Alzheimer disease is associated with decreased brain acetylcholine, anticholinergic medications can make it worse. This can occur with commonly used medications such as oxybutynin (Ditropan), tricyclic antidepressants, and even over-the-counter cold medications.

Immunization with amyloid-β (Aβ) peptide has been attempted because it has been shown to reduce the amyloid plaque burden. However, phase 1 testing was suspended because brain inflammation in some of the human subjects led to irreversible CNS damage. Interestingly, a follow-up report of patients without complications found that cognitive decline was significantly less in patients who had an increase in serum Aβ-plaque–related antibodies. Other immunologic-based approaches may be safer and more successful. Efforts are also under way to develop drugs that modify secretase activity and thereby minimize plaque formation.

Qaseem A, Snow V, Cross JT Jr, et al. Current pharmacologic treatment of dementia: a clinical practice guideline from the American College of Physicians and the American Academy of Family Physicians. *Ann Intern Med.* 2008;148(5):370–378.

◉ **Ophthalmic considerations**   Patients with AD may present to the ophthalmologist with vague visual complaints such as poor vision and reading difficulties. In general, AD does not seem to have any direct pathologic effect on the optic nerve and retina, and these visual problems are caused by disruption of central pathways. Specific findings include spatial contrast sensitivity disturbance, fixation instability, saccadic latency prolongation with hypometric saccades, and saccadic intrusions during smooth-pursuit eye movements. Patients with AD can also manifest disorders of higher cortical function, such as visual agnosia and surface dyslexia. Defective motion perception (cerebral akinetopsia) has been described, as has Balint syndrome (simultanagnosia, an inability to recognize 2 or more things at the same time; acquired ocular apraxia; and optic ataxia).

Goetz CG, ed. *Textbook of Clinical Neurology*. 3rd ed. Philadelphia: Elsevier/Saunders; 2007.
Pelak VS, Hall DA. Neuro-ophthalmic manifestations of neurodegenerative disease. *Ophthalmol Clin North Am.* 2004;17(3):311–320.
UpToDate. www.uptodate.com.

The authors would like to thank Michael A. Keys, MD, and James Heckaman, MD, for their contributions to this chapter.

CHAPTER **13**

Preventive Medicine

Recent Developments

- More than 95% of all cervical cancers are positive for human papillomavirus (HPV).
- Virtual colonoscopy with high-resolution computed tomography (CT) is currently being studied as a screening tool for colon cancer.
- Tdap (tetanus toxoid, diphtheria, and acellular pertussis vaccine) is recommended for all unvaccinated health care professionals as a means of avoiding nosocomial outbreaks.
- Newer childhood immunization recommendations include vaccines for hepatitis B, *Haemophilus influenzae* type B, *Pneumococcus, Varicella,* influenza, and hepatitis A.
- New vaccines are now available for meningococcus, Lyme disease, typhoid fever, anthrax, yellow fever, and Japanese encephalitis. Other new vaccines are being evaluated for HIV, cholera, respiratory syncytial virus, rabies, herpes simplex type 2, *Pseudomonas,* plague, rotavirus, malaria, tuberculosis, smallpox, and anthrax.

Screening Procedures

The goal of preventive medicine is not only to reduce premature morbidity and mortality but also to preserve function and quality of life.

Screening techniques can be used both for research and for practical disease prevention or treatment. Screening for nonresearch purposes is useful if the disease in question is

- detectable with some measurable degree of reliability
- treatable or preventable
- significant because of its impact (prevalence or severity)
- progressive
- generally asymptomatic (or has symptoms a patient might deny or might not recognize)

Screening techniques should not be applied to a certain population until the following concerns have been addressed:

- sensitivity and specificity of the test
- convenience and comfort of the test
- cost of finding a problem
- cost of not finding a problem

Cost can and should be measured in both economic and human terms, including the cost of suffering, losing function, or dying.

The term *sensitivity* describes how often a test result is positive among persons with a target disease. *Specificity* measures the test's ability to exclude truly negative results. *Relative risk* is the probability of a disease based on a specific finding divided by the probability of that disease in the absence of that specific finding.

Screening can be done as a 1-time venture or by the sequential application of screening tests. Initially, a more sensitive test is administered; when appropriate, it is followed by a more specific test (which is often more costly or difficult to use). In judging the predictive value of the screens for an individual patient, the physician should account for the patient's clinical history and current medications.

Cardiovascular Diseases

Hypertension

The consequences of uncontrolled hypertension include significantly increased risk of thrombotic and hemorrhagic stroke, atherosclerotic heart disease, atrial fibrillation, congestive heart failure, left ventricular hypertrophy, aortic aneurysm and dissection, peripheral vascular disease, and renal failure. Approximately 30% of end-stage renal disease is related to hypertension. There are more than 65 million cases of hypertension in the United States, about half of which have been diagnosed and a third of which are being treated. Hypertension currently afflicts over 1 billion people worldwide. The prevalence of hypertension in many developed countries is about 20% of the adult population, and it has reached as high as 29% in the United States. It is also becoming a more widely recognized problem in childhood. Hypertension meets all 5 of the criteria mentioned previously for screening: it is detectable, treatable, highly prevalent, progressively damaging, and characteristically asymptomatic until late in its course.

Elevation in either systolic or diastolic blood pressure (BP) is associated with increased cardiovascular risk. *Hypertension* is defined as systolic BP of 140 mm Hg or higher, diastolic BP of 90 mm Hg or higher, or both. *Prehypertension* is defined as systolic BP between 120 and 139 or diastolic BP between 80 and 89 on multiple readings. The classification of hypertension is included in Chapter 2, Hypertension.

The primary screening method is BP measurement, but several prospective studies have shown that ambulatory BP monitoring provides a better prediction of major cardiovascular events. Abnormal measurements, unless urgently high, should be confirmed on two more occasions. Once hypertension is detected, the cause should be sought to allow appropriate treatment. Regular exercise, weight loss, and dietary modifications such as reduction of dietary salt intake and increased dietary potassium and folate intake may enhance BP normalization. Chapter 2 discusses the pharmacologic treatment of hypertension.

Cutler JA, Sorlie PD, Wolz M, Thom T, Fields LE, Roccella EJ. Trends in hypertension prevalence, awareness, treatment, and control rates in United States adults between 1988-1994 and 1999-2004. *Hypertension*. 2008;52(5):818–827.

Krousel-Wood MA, Muntner P, He J, Whelton PK. Primary prevention of essential hypertension. *Med Clin North Am*. 2004;88(1):223–238.

Ram CV. The evolving definition of systemic hypertension. *Am J Cardiol.* 2007;99(8): 1168–1170.

Verdecchia P, Angeli F, Gattobigio R, Porcellati C. Ambulatory blood pressure monitoring and prognosis in the management of essential hypertension. *Expert Rev Cardiovasc Ther.* 2003;1(1):79–89.

Atherosclerotic cardiovascular disease

In the United States, atherosclerosis is responsible for approximately half of all deaths and for one third of deaths between ages 35 and 65. Three fourths of deaths related to atherosclerosis are from *coronary artery disease (CAD)*. Atherosclerosis is the leading cause of permanent disability and accounts for more hospital days than any other illness.

The rationale for early screening emerged when it was shown that reducing risk factors reduces the incidence of coronary disease events. Epidemiologic studies show that each 1% of reduction in total cholesterol produces a 2% reduction in the risk of such events, including fatal and nonfatal myocardial infarctions. Several studies also confirm that reduction in cholesterol results in reduced cardiovascular morbidity and mortality in patients with previous coronary heart disease.

Established clinical risk factors for CAD include family history of early-onset coronary disease, increased age, male sex, hypertension, left ventricular hypertrophy, smoking, diabetes mellitus, physical inactivity, stress, and cocaine abuse. Laboratory risk factors are elevated plasma cholesterol level (also elevated low-density-lipoprotein [LDL] cholesterol and low high-density-lipoprotein [HDL] cholesterol levels), elevated plasma homocysteine level, and increased C-reactive protein. Patients in the top 20th percentile for risk factors experienced approximately 50% of the fatal and nonfatal atherosclerotic events. Counseling on smoking cessation, lifestyle modification, and diet should be an important element of all primary care and preventive care encounters.

Dyslipoproteinemia has become an important concept. We now recognize that excesses or deficiencies of specific lipoproteins and apolipoproteins are more significantly correlated with atherosclerosis than is the more general category of lipids. Indeed, screening for cholesterol and triglycerides alone will miss 50% of cases of hyperlipoproteinemia. Therefore, it is valid and important to measure LDL and HDL cholesterol every 5 years. Total, LDL, and HDL cholesterol screening is recommended for all persons aged 21 and older. If the level is normal (<200 mg/dL), the screen should be repeated every 5 years. If the level is abnormal, the screen should be repeated with a complete cholesterol profile. Hyperlipoproteinemias are discussed in greater detail in Chapter 5 and in Section 8, *External Disease and Cornea*.

Screening for significant coronary artery atherosclerosis is more expensive and time-consuming than screening for associated reversible risk factors. In general, it is reasonable to screen for a history of cardiovascular symptoms and events (chest pain, dyspnea, syncope, arrhythmias, claudication, stroke) and reserve more specific testing (eg, exercise stress testing, dobutamine stress echocardiography, or exercise myocardial scintigraphy) for those in higher risk categories. Single-photon emission computed tomography (SPECT) is a rapid, noninvasive, high-resolution imaging study that detects coronary artery calcium as a means of screening asymptomatic patients for coronary atherosclerosis.

This technique can noninvasively detect and even quantitate the presence of coronary atherosclerosis.

Cosson E, Paycha F, Paries J, et al. Detecting silent coronary stenoses and stratifying cardiac risk in patients with diabetes: ECG stress test or exercise myocardial scintigraphy? *Diabet Med.* 2004;21(4):342–348.

Yokoshima T, Honma H, Kusama Y, Munakata K, Takano T, Nakanishi K. Improved stratification of perioperative cardiac risk in patients undergoing noncardiac surgery using new indices of dobutamine stress echocardiography. *J Cardiol.* 2004;44(3):101–111.

Cancer

In women, the most common cancers are lung, breast, and colorectal. In men, they are lung, prostate, and colorectal. The types of cancer most amenable to screening are cervical cancer, breast cancer, urologic cancer, lung cancer, colorectal cancer, and melanoma. Table 13-1 shows a set of recommendations for early cancer detection.

Table 13-1 American Cancer Society Recommendations for Early Cancer Detection in Asymptomatic Patients

Test or Procedure	Sex	Population Age (Years)	Frequency
Sigmoidoscopy	M, F	>50	After 2 negative exams 1 year apart, perform every 5 years
Colonoscopy	M, F	>50	Every 10 years if not high risk
CT colonography (virtual colonoscopy)	M, F	>50	Every 5 years
Stool guaiac or DNA test	M, F	>50	Annual
Digital rectal examination	M, F	>50	Annual
Papanicolaou test	F	20–65; <20, if sexually active	After 2 negative exams 1 year apart, perform at least every 3 years
Pelvic examination	F	20–40	Every 3 years
		>40	Annual
Endometrial tissue sample	F	Women at high risk* and at menopause	At menopause
Breast self-examination	F	>20	Monthly (now considered optional)
Clinical breast exam	F	20–40	Every 3 years
		>40	Annual
Mammography	F	35–40	Baseline
		>40	Annual
Chest x-ray			Not recommended
Sputum cytology			Not recommended
Health counseling and cancer checkup†	M, F	>20	Every 3 years
	M, F	>40	Annual

*History of infertility, obesity, failure to ovulate, abnormal uterine bleeding, or estrogen therapy.
†To include examination for cancers of the thyroid, testis, prostate, ovary, lymph nodes, oral region, and skin.

Cervical cancer

Cervical cancer is the most common gynecologic cancer in patients between the ages of 15 and 34. Overall, approximately 15,000 cases of invasive cancer of the cervix (about 5000 resulting in death) and 45,000 cases of carcinoma in situ occur each year in the United States. About 80% of the 470,000 cervical cancer cases diagnosed worldwide each year occur in developing countries. Despite advances in the treatment of cervical cancer, approximately half the women with the disease will die. Cervical cancer is the eighth most common cause of cancer mortality in the United States.

The risk factors for cervical cancer are the number of lifetime sexual partners, the presence of high-risk serotypes of HPV, low socioeconomic status, positive smoking history, use of corticosteroid contraceptive hormones, and a history of other sexually transmitted diseases. More than 95% of all cervical cancers are positive for HPV. Early detection and appropriate treatment markedly reduce the morbidity and mortality from invasive cancer of the cervix. In many developed countries, mortality has been reduced by more than 50% by implementation of cytologic screening. Cervical cancer is asymptomatic when it occurs in situ, and the most effective screening technique remains the Papanicolaou test ("Pap smear"). HPV can be detected with PCR assay techniques, and high-risk patients should receive HPV testing at the time of the Pap smear examination. Some researchers now advocate HPV DNA testing over Pap cytology as an initial screening tool. Fourier transform infrared (FTIR) spectroscopy is a new tool for screening cervical cancer, with a sensitivity of 85% and a specificity of 91%. Vaccines to prevent HPV infection and its sequelae are now widely available.

Breast cancer

Though recently surpassed by lung cancer as the most common cause of death in women older than age 40, breast cancer remains the most common malignancy in women. The overall incidence of breast cancer in the United States is 10%–12%; 50% of these patients are curable. The age-adjusted incidence of breast cancer declined by 6.7% in 2003 (12% decline in women over 50 years old). This decrease was mostly due to a 50% reduction in the use of hormone replacement therapy. Nevertheless, in 2004, approximately 215,990 new cases of breast cancer and more than 40,110 related deaths were reported in the United States alone. More than 75% of all breast cancers are cured with current therapy.

The importance of specific screening is increased by the presence of known risk factors, all of which are identifiable by history: (1) first-degree relative with breast cancer, (2) prior breast cancer, (3) nulliparity, (4) first pregnancy after age 30, and (5) early menarche or late menopause. Additional risk factors are elevated serum estrogen levels, elevated testosterone levels, high-fat diet, obesity, and sedentary lifestyle. Fibrocystic disease is not a risk factor unless there is demonstrated hyperplasia or atypia on biopsy.

Hormone replacement therapy (HRT) with estrogen and progesterone was associated with an increased risk of invasive breast cancer and abnormal mammograms in the Women's Health Initiative randomized trial. In the same trial, postmenopausal hormone therapy was also associated with an increased risk for venous thromboembolism, stroke, coronary heart disease, and breast cancer, and these risks have also been reported in other controlled trials. The beneficial effects that were noted in the Women's Health Initiative trial included reductions in the incidence of fractures and colorectal cancer.

Approximately 42% of breast cancers detectable by mammography are not detectable by physical examination alone, and one third of those found by mammographic screening are noninvasive or less than 1 cm in size if invasive. Because mammograms can yield false-negative results, the best detection strategy involves a physical examination plus mammography, with fine-needle aspiration or biopsy if either reveals an abnormality. Mammograms have been shown to be safe as well as effective, with current low-dose radiation not inducing added cancer risk. Clinical breast examination (CBE) and counseling are recommended every 3 years for women with an average risk of breast cancer between the ages of 20 and 39 and annually after age 40 years. Mammographic screening, according to a recent recommendation by the US Preventive Services Task Force, should be performed every 2 years for average-risk women age 40 and older. This ruling is controversial, however, in relation to women 40–49. Newer tools advocated for breast cancer screening include ultrasound, digital mammography, magnetic resonance imaging (MRI), magnetic resonance spectroscopic imaging (MRSI), and positron emission tomography (PET).

Urologic cancer

The prostate, bladder, kidney, and testes yield approximately 16% of new cancer cases per year, with most of the common malignancies in middle-aged and older men. About 230,000 new cases of prostate cancer and nearly 40,000 related deaths occur each year in the United States. Screening remains controversial, but preliminary estimates suggest that it can reduce mortality. Prostate cancer can be detected early by digital examination of the prostate and serum prostate-specific antigen (PSA) measurements. It is now generally accepted that PSA should be measured yearly in men aged 50–74 years with more than 10 years of life expectancy. For patients with a family history of prostate cancer, screening should begin at age 40 or earlier. PSA levels greater than 10 ng/mL strongly suggest metastatic disease; levels less than 4 ng/mL usually suggest benign hypertrophy or a normal prostate, but the false-negative rate varies between 15% and 38%. Also, only about 30% of patients with elevated PSA truly have prostate carcinoma. A trend of increasing PSA levels is an even more sensitive indicator of prostate cancer than an individual elevated PSA level. Men with a PSA velocity greater than 2 ng/mL/year have a significantly higher risk for prostate cancer mortality than those with any other single risk factor. Transrectal ultrasonography assesses prostate volume, which has prognostic value, and helps visualize tumors and facilitate fine-needle biopsy of the prostate.

Although prostate cancer is a potentially lethal illness, many detectable prostate cancers are of little threat to life. Some men with low-grade prostate cancer receive curative treatment, even though their disease may not require treatment. Some studies suggest that more than 75% of men with screen-detected localized disease may not even need treatment. More specific screening methods are needed to allow differentiation between lethal and nonlethal cancers.

Lung cancer

Lung cancer is the leading form of cancer in adults. Among male patients with lung cancer, 93% are smokers. The number and percentage of cases in women have risen with the increased incidence of smoking in women. In one study of lung cancer, 40% of cases were detected by chest radiography and 60% were detected by symptoms. The usefulness of radiographic and sputum cytologic screening is generally considered to be low, but some studies have suggested that annual chest radiography may reduce morbidity and mortality. Chest radiography can be improved with digital radiography, image processing, and computer-aided detection, as these methods have been shown to enhance lung nodule detection. In high-risk patient groups, screening protocols effect a higher yield and may include sputum cytology, low-dose helical chest CT (with possible fine-needle aspiration for suspicious lesions), and bronchoscopy with possible endobronchial biopsy. Fluorescent bronchoscopy is a promising new tool in identifying early malignant changes in the central airways, because it is significantly more sensitive than white-light bronchoscopy. Also, new molecular markers detected in sputum and serum show some promise in the future of lung cancer screening.

Gastrointestinal cancer

The primary risk factors for squamous cell carcinoma of the esophagus are tobacco use and alcohol consumption, accounting for 80%–90% of these neoplasms. The main risk factors for adenocarcinoma of the esophagus are gastroesophageal reflux disease, obesity, and history of Barrett esophagus. Treatment has poor results; thus, prevention or elimination of the risk factors is worthwhile. The incidence of adenocarcinoma of the esophagus is increasing in developed countries, but squamous cell carcinoma remains dominant in underdeveloped areas. Currently, no effective preventative screening programs are available, and most patients present with advanced or metastatic disease. Barrett esophagus is a complication of long-standing gastroesophageal reflux disease (GERD) and is the premalignant condition for the majority of esophageal adenocarcinomas.

Gastric cancer appears to be associated with certain geographic areas (Japan, China, Central and South America, Eastern Europe, and parts of the Middle East), high ingestion of nitrates, loss of gastric acidity, lower socioeconomic status, and blood type A. It remains the second most frequent and lethal malignancy worldwide. Although routine endoscopic screening is not cost-effective, widespread screening for and treatment of *Helicobacter pylori* infection in high-incidence populations could be an effective strategy.

Pancreatic cancer is 2–3 times more common in heavy smokers than in nonsmokers, and it has also been associated with chronic pancreatitis, diabetes mellitus, and obesity. Familial pancreatic cancer represents only about 5% of all cases but carries a higher mortality than sporadic pancreatic cancer. Several genetic mutations have been identified that are responsible for a small percentage of familial cases. Hepatocellular cancer is more common in persons with preexisting liver disease, especially cirrhosis and hepatitis C.

Colorectal cancer

Colorectal cancer is a major killer in Western society, second only to lung cancer in incidence and mortality. The cumulative lifetime probability of developing colon cancer is roughly 6%, with 3% probability of dying from this disease. The chance for survival 5 years after diagnosis remains only 40%, despite the optimistic theory that early detection would lead to curative surgery. Potentially modifiable risk factors such as fiber and fat intake are important in primary prevention.

Most authorities accept the theory that colorectal cancer develops from an initially benign polyp in a mitotic process that occurs over 5–10 years. Studies to date lack the necessary longevity to prove definitively that polyp removal prevents carcinoma. Yet colonoscopic removal or ablation of all polyps has become the standard of care where facilities and trained personnel are available. A national polyp study is under way to define the biology of these tumors, to identify factors that seem to promote invasive carcinoma, and to clarify whether early removal prevents invasive cancer. One study reported characteristics associated with high-grade dysplasia in colorectal adenomas. The major independent risk factors were adenoma size and extent of the villous component in the adenoma.

Increased dietary fiber intake and reduced dietary fat intake have been associated with reduced risk of colorectal cancer. Also, calcium supplementation is associated with a moderate reduction in the risk of recurrent colorectal adenomas.

Detection must be improved with more widespread use of screening studies such as Hemoccult slides, flexible sigmoidoscopy, barium enema, and colonoscopy, with aggressive follow-up of positive cases. It is estimated that widespread adoption of these recommendations could reduce the mortality rate of colorectal cancer by more than 50%. Fecal DNA testing for molecular tumor markers is a new, investigational noninvasive method of colorectal cancer screening with high sensitivity and specificity. Because this testing is easier to use and more sensitive than fecal occult blood testing, patient compliance may be better. Although fecal DNA testing is expensive, initial studies suggest it is cost-effective.

Periodic sigmoidoscopy (every 3 years) and annual digital rectal examination with fecal occult blood testing have been recommended in asymptomatic adults older than 50 years. Recommendations remain controversial because of a lack of randomized trials. Sigmoidoscopy offers good specificity but misses proximal cancers. Nevertheless, several case-control studies have demonstrated a 50%–70% reduction in the risk of colorectal cancer in patients screened with sigmoidoscopy. Similarly, fecal occult blood testing every 2 years has been shown to decrease the mortality rate of colon cancer by up to 40%.

Colonoscopy as a screening test for asymptomatic patients older than age 50 has been gaining popularity. When results are negative, the test is repeated every 10 years in low-risk patients. Colonoscopy is thought to be about twice as sensitive as barium enema for detecting colon cancers, and many of the lesions discovered with colonoscopy would not be detected with sigmoidoscopy. Yearly colonoscopy has been advocated in populations at very high risk, such as patients with familial polyposis and first-degree relatives of patients with colon cancer. The disadvantages of colonoscopy are the increased cost, the number of trained personnel required, and the risks of intravenous sedation and colonic perforation (approximately 0.2%). Virtual colonoscopy with high-resolution CT is currently being evaluated as a screening tool. It may offer the ability to screen out patients without neoplasia, thus allowing colonoscopy to be reserved for patients with significant lesions. Virtual colonoscopy has a high sensitivity for large adenomas and colorectal cancers.

Melanoma

Melanoma is the most deadly form of skin cancer, and its incidence is increasing faster than that of all other cancers. In the United States, about 1 in 75 persons will develop melanoma during his or her lifetime. According to the American Cancer Society, an estimated 62,480 new melanoma cases and 8420 related deaths were reported in the United States in 2008.

Most melanomas probably arise from dysplastic nevi. Risk factors for melanoma include history of melanoma or atypical moles, presence of more than 75–100 moles, positive melanoma family history, history of previous nonmelanoma skin cancer, giant congenital nevus (greater than 20 cm), xeroderma pigmentosum, treatment with UV-A and psoralens, frequent tanning with UV-A light, and a history of 3 or more severe (blistering) sunburns. Other, less significant risk factors are light complexion of the hair and eyes, freckles, inability to tan, indoor occupation with outdoor hobbies, and proximity to the equator.

Ultraviolet damage probably causes most melanomas. Intense intermittent exposures are directly related to melanoma, whereas other skin cancers are more associated with cumulative exposure. Ultraviolet radiation causes DNA damage, which is usually corrected by DNA repair enzymes; however, these DNA repair processes decrease with increasing age.

A pigmented lesion with any of the following characteristics, easily remembered by the *ABCDE* mnemonic, is suggestive of melanoma: *a*symmetrical lesions, *b*order (irregular), *c*olor (variable), *d*iameter (greater than 6 mm), and *e*levation. Other characteristics suggestive of melanoma are pruritus, bleeding, changing morphology, and new lesions or scalp lesions. Everyone should perform self–skin examinations every 1 or 2 months, and suspicious lesions require referral and possible biopsy. Sun avoidance and use of sunblock can reduce the risk of melanoma and other skin cancers. In addition to providing simple visualization, dermoscopy (epiluminescence microscopy) can increase the specificity of clinical examination for the detection of melanomas.

Abbaszadegan MR, Tavasoli A, Velayati A, et al. Stool-based DNA testing, a new noninvasive method for colorectal cancer screening, the first report from Iran. *World J Gastroenterol.* 2007;13(10):1528–1533.

American Cancer Society. What Are the Key Statistics About Melanoma? Last medical review: 06/05/2008. Available at www.cancer.org.

Canto MI. Screening and surveillance approaches in familial pancreatic cancer. *Gastrointest Endosc Clin N Am.* 2008;18(3):535–553.

Centers for Disease Control and Prevention (CDC). Decline in breast cancer incidence— United States, 1999-2003. *MMWR.* 2007;56(22):549–553.

Chlebowski RT, Hendrix SL, Langer RD, et al; WHI Investigators. Influence of estrogen plus progestin on breast cancer and mammography in healthy postmenopausal women: the Women's Health Initiative Randomized Trial. *JAMA.* 2003;289(24):3243–3253.

Cuzick J, Arbyn M, Sankaranarayanan R, et al. Overview of human papillomavirus-based and other novel options for cervical cancer screening in developed and developing countries. *Vaccine.* 2008;26(Suppl 10):K29–K41.

D'Amico AV, Chen MH, Catalona WJ, Sun L, Roehl KA, Moul JW. Prostate cancer-specific mortality after radical prostatectomy or external beam radiation therapy in men with 1 or more high-risk factors. *Cancer.* 2007;110(1):56–61.

Deenadayalu VP, Rex DK. Fecal-based DNA assays: a new, noninvasive approach to colorectal cancer screening. *Cleve Clin J Med.* 2004;71(6):497–503.

El-Tawil SG, Adnan R, Muhamed ZN, Othman NH. Comparative study between Pap smear cytology and FTIR spectroscopy: a new tool for screening for cervical cancer. *Pathology.* 2008;40(6):600–603.

Lin K, Lipsitz R, Miller T, Janakiraman S; U.S. Preventive Services Task Force. Benefits and harms of prostate-specific antigen screening for prostate cancer: an evidence update for the U.S. Preventive Services Task Force. *Ann Intern Med.* 2008;149(3):192–199.

Mak T, Lalloo F, Evans DG, Hill J. Molecular stool screening for colorectal cancer. *Br J Surg.* 2004;91(7):790–800.

Mak T, Senevrayar K, Lalloo F, Evans DG, Hill J. The impact of new screening protocol on individuals at increased risk of colorectal cancer. *Colorectal Dis.* 2007;9(7):635–640.

New York Early Lung Cancer Action Project Investigators. CT screening for lung cancer: diagnoses resulting from the New York Early Lung Cancer Action Project. *Radiology.* 2007;243(1):239–249.

Patel M, Ferry K, Franceschi D, Kaklamanos I, Livingstone A, Ardalan B. Esophageal carcinoma: current controversial topics. *Cancer Invest.* 2004;22(6):897–912.

Pickhardt PJ, Kim DH. CT colonography (virtual colonoscopy): a practical approach for population screening. *Radiol Clin North Am.* 2007;45(2):361–375.

Potential new options for lung cancer screening. *Dis Manag Advis.* 2007;13(6):68–70.

Sharma P. Barrett esophagus: will effective treatment prevent the risk of progression to esophageal adenocarcinoma? *Am J Med.* 2004;117(suppl 5A):79S–85S.

Smith JA, Andreopoulou E. An overview of the status of imaging screening technology for breast cancer. *Ann Oncol.* 2004;15(suppl 1):I18–I26.

Smith RA, Cokkinides V, Brawley OW. Cancer screening in the United States, 2009: a review of current American Cancer Society guidelines and issues in cancer screening. *CA Cancer J Clin.* 2009;59(1):27–41. Full text available at: http://caonline.amcancersoc.org.

Tjalma WA, Arbyn M, Paavonen J, van Waes TR, Bogers JJ. Prophylactic human papillomavirus vaccines: the beginning of the end of cervical cancer. *Int J Gynecol Cancer.* 2004;14(5):751–761.

U.S. Preventive Services Task Force. Screening for prostate cancer: U.S. Preventive Services Task Force recommendation statement. *Ann Intern Med.* 2008;149(3):185–191.

Warren MP. A comparative review of the risks and benefits of hormone replacement therapy regimens. *Am J Obstet Gynecol.* 2004;190(4):1141–1167.

Winawer SJ. Screening of colorectal cancer: progress and problems. *Recent Results Cancer Res.* 2005;166:231–244.

Young GP, Cole S. New stool screening tests for colorectal cancer. *Digestion.* 2007;76(1):26–33.

Infectious Diseases

The major public health screening efforts in the United States have been for tuberculosis and sexually transmitted diseases. Hepatitis screening is used primarily for blood donation, institutionalized populations, and health care workers rather than for the general population. These disorders are discussed in more detail in Chapter 1, Infectious Disease.

Tuberculosis

The prevalence of tuberculosis (TB) has recently increased in the United States, reversing decades of steady decline, and TB skin testing should be performed in high-risk groups. Positive results should prompt chest radiography and consideration of chemoprophylaxis.

Some experts advocate routine skin testing of all people younger than 35 years at the time of routine health examination (for detection as well as for baseline data). The Occupational Safety and Health Administration requires annual TB skin testing of all health care workers.

A PCR assay, the BD ProbeTec ET System (BD, Franklin Lakes, NJ), is capable of rapidly detecting *Mycobacterium tuberculosis* DNA in respiratory specimens and compares favorably with microscopy of smear material using Ziehl-Neelsen stain and with TB cultures. BD ProbeTec ET, in parallel with cultures, can be used to monitor the regression of TB DNA in treated patients. It can also be very useful for rapid detection of *M tuberculosis* complex, especially in smear-negative respiratory specimens.

Several candidate vaccines for TB are currently being developed, including subunit, DNA, microbial vector, and live attenuated vaccines.

Syphilis

Syphilis is almost always transmitted sexually; congenital disease transmitted in utero is now rare. In fact, the incidence of congenital syphilis has dropped 90% since the 1940s because of required premarital screening and pregnancy screening. Better prenatal care and increased syphilis screening during pregnancy improve the chances of detecting infants at risk for congenital syphilis, thus allowing early maternal treatment.

Latent, untreated cases of syphilis in which the primary or secondary mucocutaneous lesion is no longer present can be detected only by screening. It is important to detect early latent disease: in approximately 25% of cases, infectious mucocutaneous lesions reemerge spontaneously in the first 2 years. Late latent disease should be detected and treated because of the long-term destructive effects on the CNS, the aorta, and the skeletal system.

Screening is generally performed with the more sensitive, but less specific, nontreponemal antigen tests (VDRL, RPR). Positive results are then confirmed with treponemal antigen tests (FTA-ABS, MHA-TP, HATTS), which are more expensive.

Centers for Disease Control and Prevention (CDC). Congenital syphilis—United States, 2002. *MMWR Morb Mortal Wkly Rep.* 2004;53(31):716–719.

Hawkridge T, Scriba TJ, Gelderbloem S, et al. Safety and immunogenicity of a new tuberculosis vaccine, MVA85A, in healthy adults in South Africa. *J Infect Dis.* 2008;198(4):544–552.

Hoft DF, Blazevic A, Abate G, et al. A new recombinant bacille Calmette-Guérin vaccine safely induces significantly enhanced tuberculosis-specific immunity in human volunteers. *J Infect Dis.* 2008;198(10):1491–1501.

Källenius G, Pawlowski A, Brandtzaeg P, Svenson S. Should a new tuberculosis vaccine be administered intranasally? *Tuberculosis.* 2007;87(4):257–266.

Immunization

The development of immunization as a means of preventing the spread of infectious disease began in 1796, when Edward Jenner injected cowpox virus, which causes a mild disease, into a child to prevent smallpox, a severe, potentially fatal illness. Immunization today still relies on Jenner's inoculation methods to protect against disease. There are 2 types: active and passive.

In *active immunization,* the recipient develops an acquired immune response to inactivated or killed viruses, viral subtractions, bacterial toxoids or antigens, or synthetic vaccines. Once the immune response to a particular pathogen has developed, it protects the host against infection. The persistence of acquired immunity depends on the perpetuation of cell strains responsive to the target antigenic stimulus, and booster inoculations may be required for certain immunogens.

In general, live inactivated vaccines produce longer-lasting immunity; however, they are contraindicated in immunocompromised persons or pregnant women because the pathogen can potentially replicate in the host. Ideally, active immunization should be completed before exposure; however, life-saving postexposure immunity can be developed through combining active and passive immunization.

The current recommended immunization schedules for the year 2009, developed by the Advisory Committee on Immunization Practices (ACIP), including immunization schedules for persons aged 0–6 years and persons aged 7–18 years, the catch-up schedule for ages 4 months–18 years, and the adult schedule can be found at the Centers for Disease Control website (www.cdc.gov/vaccines/recs/schedules/default.htm). The catch-up protocols are for children who have missed some of the recommended immunization doses.

Passive immunization depends on the transfer of immunoglobulin in serum from a host with active immunity to a susceptible host. Passive immunity does not result in active immunity and sometimes even blocks the development of active immunity. Passive immunity is short-lived and without immune memory; however, it confers immediate protection on the recipient who has been exposed to the pathogen. Pooled human globulin, antitoxins, and human globulin with high antibody titers for specific diseases are the usual products available for passive immunization.

Immunization should be avoided in persons who have allergic reactions to the vaccine or its components. Idiopathic autoantibody or cross-reacting antibody development may occur after vaccination, resulting in systemic disease such as Guillain-Barré syndrome, a rare but devastating complication of vaccination. Immunization should be avoided during a febrile illness. Multidose immunization schedules that are interrupted can be resumed; however, doses given outside the schedule should not be counted toward completion of the vaccination sequence.

Hepatitis B

Approximately 100,000 symptomatic cases of hepatitis B occur annually in the United States. Between 6% and 10% of adult patients with hepatitis B become carriers, and chronic active hepatitis occurs in 25% of these carriers. Of the patients with chronic active disease, 20% will die of cirrhosis and 5% will die of hepatocellular carcinoma.

The available recombinant vaccines based on hepatitis B virus (HBV) surface antigen are Engerix-B, Recombivax HB, and Bio-Hep-B. FENDrix is a new HBV vaccine that is reported to provide higher antibody levels for a longer duration. It is being marketed in Europe for renal dialysis patients because of their high risk of HBV exposure combined with an immunocompromised status. In adults, HBV vaccine is usually administered in 3 sessions, with the second and third occurring 1 and 6 months after the initial injection. On this regimen, 90% of recipients develop protective antibody levels for at least 3 years. The recombinant vaccine can also be given on an accelerated dosing schedule, which requires vaccination at 0, 1, and 2 months followed by a booster dose at 12 months. Antibody levels that are greater than 10 milli-International Units (mIU) per milliliter are considered to be adequate protection. Booster injections are advised for persons whose antibody levels are less than 10 mIU/mL. Repeat vaccination results in the development of protective antibodies in 50% of the nonresponders. Vaccines are also available for hepatitis A and are being developed for hepatitis C and E.

Vaccination before exposure is recommended and cost-effective for all infants and children and in certain high-risk groups: health care workers, hemodialysis patients, residents and staff of institutions for the retarded, household and sexual contacts of chronic carriers of hepatitis B, hemophiliacs, users of illicit injectable drugs, prison inmates, sexually active homosexual men, and HIV-positive patients. Vaccination can be combined with passive immunization for postexposure prophylaxis without affecting the development of active immunity. The incorporation of the vaccine into childhood immunization schedules has resulted in a decrease in the number of new hepatitis B cases reported annually, and there has also been a significant reduction in the number of hepatocellular carcinoma cases reported in children.

Twinrix is a combination hepatitis A and hepatitis B vaccine, combining the antigenic components contained in Havrix (inactivated hepatitis A vaccine) and Engerix-B (recombinant hepatitis B vaccine). When administered in a standard 3-dose schedule at 0, 1, and 6 months, Twinrix provides immunity that is comparable to that of the monovalent vaccines.

Postexposure prophylaxis with hepatitis B immunoglobulin should be considered when there is perinatal exposure of an infant born to a carrier, accidental percutaneous or permucosal exposure to blood positive for HBV surface antigen, or sexual exposure (within 14 days) to a carrier of hepatitis B. Hepatitis B immunoglobulin should be given as soon as possible after exposure in a single intramuscular dose of 0.06 mL/kg body weight; the recombinant HBV vaccine should be concurrently administered in an accelerated dosing schedule.

Lamivudine (Epivir) is a nucleoside analogue inhibitor of reverse transcriptase and was initially developed for the treatment of HIV infection. Interferon-α and lamivudine have been found to be very effective against HBV and are considered the drugs of choice for the treatment of patients with chronic HBV infection. Promising new treatments for hepatitis B include adefovir, entecavir, telbivudine, and peginterferon alpha-2a.

Influenza

Although influenza is usually a self-limited disease with rare sequelae, it can be associated with severe morbidity and mortality in older persons or those with chronic diseases. Influenza vaccines produce long-lasting immunity. However, antigenic shifts, primarily in type A rather than type B influenza virus, necessitate yearly reformulation of the vaccine to contain the antigens of strains considered most likely to cause disease. Protection is correlated with the development of antihemagglutinin and antineuraminidase antibodies, which decrease the patient's susceptibility and the severity of the disease. The influenza vaccine is as effective in HIV-positive patients as it is in HIV-negative patients, regardless of CD4 T-cell counts. Annual vaccination is recommended for adults and children with chronic diseases requiring medical care, immunosuppressed patients (including HIV-infected patients), nursing home residents, children who require long-term aspirin therapy, healthy children younger than 5 years, persons older than age 65, and medical personnel with extensive contact with high-risk patients. The vaccine is well tolerated, and there has been no increased risk of neurologic complications with the vaccines administered after 1991. Influenza vaccine should not be administered to persons with anaphylactic hypersensitivity to eggs or to pregnant women in their first trimester. A trivalent intranasal influenza vaccine (FluMist) is available and provides protection against type A and type B influenza virus. Newer antiviral agents, such as zanamivir (Relenza) and oseltamivir (Tamiflu), were initially very active against influenza types A and B, for prophylaxis as well as treatment. Unfortunately, the major influenza strains encountered during the 2008–2009 season had a very high incidence of resistance to oseltamivir.

Varicella-Zoster

Varivax, an approved varicella-zoster vaccine, is recommended for immunocompetent patients older than 12 months with no history of previous varicella infection. A second dose is given between 4 and 6 years of age. For patients older than 12 years, 2 doses of vaccine are given 4–8 weeks apart. Also, health care workers who have not been exposed to chickenpox should be vaccinated. Varivax is safe and provides immunity for up to 20 years. Data from the Centers for Disease Control confirmed a dramatic decline in the incidence of varicella (87%) from 1995 to 2000.

Zostavax, a live attenuated vaccine given as a single dose, is recommended for persons aged 60 years and older to reduce the risk of development of clinical zoster and postherpetic neuralgia. Zostavax may not be used in place of Varivax in younger persons.

Measles

Vaccination has dramatically reduced the incidence of measles, along with associated encephalitis, mental retardation, and mortality. Introduced in 1963, the initial vaccine was an inactivated virus that did not provide a long duration of protection. In 1967, a live attenuated vaccine that causes long-lasting immunity was introduced. Vaccination with the attenuated strain should be routine not only at age 15 months but also for persons born between 1957 and 1967 who were neither vaccinated nor infected and for persons who received the inactivated viral vaccine. Individuals born before 1957 are considered immune by virtue of natural infection. For persons who cannot have the vaccine (which should be given within 72 hours of exposure), postexposure prophylaxis with immunoglobulin should be considered within 6 days. The vaccine is contraindicated for persons with hypersensitivity to eggs. Measles-mumps-rubella (MMR) vaccination is recommended for all children and is usually given at about age 15 months and again between ages 4 and 6. Past concerns about the adverse effects of thimerosal-containing MMR vaccines are no longer an issue, as the preservative is no longer used in this vaccine. In addition, several studies have refuted previous fears of an association between MMR vaccines and autism.

Mumps

The number of reported cases of mumps in the United States has decreased steadily since the introduction of a live mumps vaccine in 1967. Although mumps is generally self-limited, meningeal signs may appear in up to 15% of cases and orchitis in up to 20% of clinical cases in postpubertal males. Other possible complications include permanent deafness and pancreatitis. Mumps vaccination is indicated in all children and all susceptible adults, particularly postpubertal males.

Rubella

Rubella immunization is intended to prevent fetal infection and consequent congenital rubella syndrome, which can occur in up to 80% of fetuses of mothers infected during the first trimester of pregnancy. The number of reported cases of rubella in the United States has decreased steadily from more than 56,000 in 1969, the year rubella vaccine was licensed, to 10 cases in 2005. A single subcutaneously administered dose of live, attenuated rubella vaccine provides long-term (probably lifetime) immunity in approximately 95% of persons vaccinated.

In 2003, the Pan American Health Organization called for elimination of rubella and congenital rubella syndrome in the Americas by the year 2010. From 1998 to 2006, confirmed rubella cases decreased 98% (from 135,947 to 2,998) in this region. However, in 2007, rubella outbreaks with a total of 13,014 cases were reported in 3 countries (Argentina, Brazil, and Chile), mostly in males not included in previous vaccination campaigns.

Rubella vaccine is recommended for adults, particularly women, unless proof of immunity is available (documented rubella vaccination on or after the first birthday or a positive serologic test result) or the vaccine is specifically contraindicated. Rubella vaccine should be given at least 14 days before administration of immunglobulin or deferred for 3 months after administration. Because of the theoretical risk to the fetus, women of childbearing age should receive the vaccine only if they are not pregnant. A new, nonreplicating rubella virus DNA vaccine is being evaluated and may offer a safer alternative for pregnant patients.

Polio

Before the introduction of the first polio vaccine in 1955, polio caused thousands of cases of paralysis. Despite widespread immunization with oral vaccine in 1962, there has been a steady decline in polio immunization and a growing number of susceptible persons. Although the incidence of polio is low, the possibility of large-scale outbreaks increases as the number of susceptible persons increases. There are 2 forms of the vaccine: an oral form that is a live attenuated virus (oral polio vaccine [OPV], Sabin vaccine) and a subcutaneous injectable form of killed virus (inactivated poliovirus vaccine [IPV], Salk vaccine). Vaccine-associated paralytic poliomyelitis has been associated more with the OPV than with the IPV. Therefore, the American Academy of Pediatrics has recommended that the IPV be administered for all 4 vaccinations in the series, or for the first 2 of the series. Either IPV or OPV can be used for the last 2 vaccinations of the series. OPV is contraindicated in pregnant women, who should receive only the killed virus vaccine.

Tetanus and Diphtheria

The combined tetanus and diphtheria toxoid vaccine (Td) is highly effective; it is used for both primary and booster immunization of adults. The pediatric vaccine, diphtheria-tetanus-pertussis (DTP), has been the standard vaccine for years but has been replaced with the newer pediatric vaccine, DTaP (diphtheria and tetanus toxoid with acellular pertussis). Tdap, which contains a lower concentration of diphtheria toxoid and acellular pertussis than Dtap, is recommended as a 1-time booster for all adults aged 19–64, and particularly for all health care professionals. Young adults should also receive a booster dose of Td every 10 years. If serious doubt exists about the completion of a primary series of immunization, 2 doses of 0.5 mL of the combined toxoids should be given intramuscularly at monthly intervals, followed by a third dose 6–10 months later. Thereafter, a booster dose of 0.5 mL should be given at 10-year intervals.

In wound management of tetanus, previously immunized persons with severe wounds should receive a booster if more than 5 years has elapsed since the last injection. The management of previously unimmunized patients with severe wounds should include tetanus immunoglobulin as well as Td. Although tetanus is uncommon, more than 60% of cases occur in persons older than 60 years. Therefore, older adults should be given a single booster at age 65.

Pneumococcal Pneumonia

Pneumococcal pneumonia is the most serious and prevalent of the community-acquired respiratory infections. Although pneumococcal disease affects children and adults, the incidence of pneumococcal pneumonia increases in persons older than 40 years. Pneumococci that are resistant to penicillin have emerged since 1974. The mortality rate from bacteremic pneumococcal infection exceeds 25% despite treatment with antibiotics.

The current unconjugated pneumococcal vaccine contains polysaccharide antigens from 23 of the types of pneumococci most commonly found in bacteremic pneumococcal disease. The 23-valent vaccine has been designed to induce a protective level of serum antibodies in immunocompetent adults and is highly effective in healthy young adults; however, its effectiveness in older persons and those in poor health has not been precisely determined. Nevertheless, the vaccine is well tolerated and is recommended for older adults, for patients with cardiac or respiratory disease, and for patients who are at high risk for pneumococcal infection, including those with sickle cell disease, splenic dysfunction, renal and hepatic disease, or immunodeficiency. The pneumococcal vaccine is given subcutaneously or intramuscularly as a 0.5-mL dose. In most circumstances, persons who have previously received the 14-valent vaccine should not be revaccinated with the 23-valent vaccine because doing so may lead to increased local and systemic reactions. The duration of protection afforded by primary vaccination with pneumococcal vaccine seems to be 9 years or more. Those who receive pneumococcal vaccine before age 65 should be reimmunized at 65 if more than 6 years has passed since the initial vaccination.

A new conjugated heptavalent pneumococcal vaccine (PCV; Prevnar) has been approved and recommended for all children younger than age 5. It is administered in 4 intramuscular doses at 2, 4, 6, and 12–15 months of age. The vaccine provides coverage for approximately 80% of the invasive pneumococcal diseases in children in the United States. PCV is recommended for all infants and toddlers younger than age 2 and for all children with chronic cardiopulmonary disorders or immune suppression between ages 2 and 5. A recent epidemiologic study revealed that the addition of pneumococcal vaccine to the childhood immunization schedule was associated with a tenfold greater reduction in pneumonia and a 100-fold greater reduction in otitis media when compared with a previously reported reduction in culture-confirmed invasive pneumococcal infections.

Haemophilus influenzae

A vaccine against *H influenzae* type B (Hib) has been endorsed by the American Academy of Pediatrics and the Immunization Practices Advisory Committee. They have recommended that the vaccine be given to all children before age 24 months. The vaccine has significantly reduced the number of infections caused by encapsulated Hib. In the past, approximately 60% of Hib infections were meningitis, amounting to about 10,000 cases each year. The type B capsule enhances the invasive potential of *H influenzae*. These encapsulated strains may result in life-threatening bacteremic infections. A critical factor that determines an individual's susceptibility to systemic Hib infection is the presence or absence of serum antibodies to capsule antigens.

The vaccine significantly reduces the risk of contracting systemic Hib infection and is protective in reducing the incidence of epiglottitis, meningitis, and orbital cellulitis. Hib is one of the safest vaccine products approved for use in children and is estimated to be 90% effective when given before age 24 months. The majority of children who develop these Hib infections are older than 2 years. A newer combination vaccine (Hib-DTaP), which includes Hib conjugate vaccine and DTaP, is available and is effective, safe, and convenient. Other combined vaccines include the tetravalent acellular pertussis combined vaccine (DTacP-IPV; Tetravac), the trivalent Hib-meningococcal-tetanus toxoid vaccine (Hib-MenC-TT), and the pentavalent 2-component acellular pertussis combined vaccine (DTacP-IPV-Hib; Pentavac). The hexavalent vaccine, DTPa-HBV-IPV/Hib, provides immunization for 6 diseases in a series of 3 single injections at 3, 4, and 5 months of age. In trials, the vaccine was shown to be safe, well tolerated, and immunologically equivalent to primary immunization with separately administered vaccines.

Meningococcus

A polysaccharide vaccine (MPSV) and a conjungate vaccine (MCV) for the prevention of meningococcal meningitis are available and are recommended for use in military personnel, college students living in dormitories, travelers to endemic areas, close contacts of infected patients, new outbreaks, and high-risk patients (especially splenectomized and complement-deficient patients). MCV is recommended for high-risk children ages 2–10 years. The vaccine is approximately 85% effective in preventing the spread of group C meningococcal infections but will not prevent infection from strains of meningococcus not represented in the vaccine. The vaccine is used primarily in controlling disease spread and for high-risk patients but is generally not given as a routine immunization.

Travel Immunizations

Precise travel vaccination recommendations depend on the geographic destinations, duration of travel, consumption of local food and untreated water, and likelihood of close contact with local populations. Routine childhood vaccinations should be reviewed in all travelers and updated as needed. Children older than 6 months should be immunized against measles (MMR) prior to travel abroad. Yellow fever vaccination may be required for anyone going to or through a yellow fever endemic area or, to prevent introduction of the disease, for travelers returning from an endemic area. Immunization against HBV should be considered in travelers who expect to have close contact with local populations known to have high rates of hepatitis B transmission. Japanese encephalitis vaccine should be offered to those whose travel plans include prolonged trips to rural areas in Southeast Asia or the Indian subcontinent during the endemic season. Typhoid fever and hepatitis A immunizations are recommended for travelers who may be exposed to potentially contaminated food and water sources. Preexposure rabies vaccination should be considered for travelers whose plans include a prolonged visit in a remote area or for those whose activities might involve working near animals. Travelers planning to visit areas endemic for malaria should consult the CDC website to determine appropriate chemoprophylaxis for the region. The drugs used for malaria prevention include atovaquone/proguanil (Malarone), chloroquine or hydroxychloroquine (Plaquenil), doxycycline, mefloquine (Lariam), and primaquine. All of these medications may cause serious adverse effects. The CDC maintains a website for travelers' health information that includes updated immunization and prevention recommendations for various regions of the world (www.cdc.gov/travel).

New and Future Vaccines

New vaccines are now available for HPV, typhoid fever *(Salmonella typhi)*, anthrax, yellow fever, and Japanese encephalitis. Additional vaccines are currently undergoing clinical trials for HIV, hepatitis C, cholera, dysentery, *Campylobacter,* rotavirus, *Clostridium difficile,* respiratory syncytial virus, Ebola virus, malaria, cytomegalovirus, respiratory syncytial virus, rabies, viral encephalitis, herpes simplex type 2, Epstein-Barr virus, TB, *Pseudomonas aeruginosa, Helicobacter pylori, Staphylococcus, Streptococcus, Propionibacterium acnes,* parainfluenza virus, leishmaniasis, plague, smallpox, and anthrax.

Passive immunization with human hyperimmunoglobulin is currently available to treat or prevent rabies, tetanus, respiratory syncytial virus, cytomegalovirus, hepatitis A, hepatitis B, hepatitis C, herpesvirus, and varicella-zoster infections.

Considering the worldwide impact of many other infectious diseases, there is considerable interest in developing new vaccines for the treatment of TB, AIDS, malaria, gonorrhea, syphilis, toxigenic *Escherichia coli* infection, leprosy, trachoma, and other infectious diseases. It is hoped that ongoing research will lead to safe and effective vaccines for many or all of these illnesses.

American Academy of Pediatrics Committee on Infectious Diseases. Prevention of influenza: recommendations for influenza immunization of children, 2006-2007. *Pediatrics.* 2007; 119(4):846–851.

Centers for Disease Control and Prevention. Progress toward elimination of rubella and congenital rubella syndrome—the Americas, 2003-2008. *MMWR Morb Mortal Wkly Rep.* 2008; 57(43):1176–1179.

Centers for Disease Control and Prevention. Recommended adult immunization schedule—United States, 2009. *MMWR.* 2008;57(53).

Centers for Disease Control and Prevention. Recommended immunization schedules for persons aged 0 through 18 years—United States, 2009. *MMWR.* 2008;57(51&52).

Chumakov K, Ehrenfeld E. New generation of inactivated poliovirus vaccines for universal immunization after eradication of poliomyelitis. *Clin Infect Dis.* 2008;47(12):1587–1592.

de Vries RD, Stittelaar KJ, Osterhaus AD, de Swart RL. Measles vaccination: new strategies and formulations. *Expert Rev Vaccines.* 2008;7(8):1215–1223.

Jackson LA, Janoff EN. Pneumococcal vaccination of elderly adults: new paradigms for protection. *Clin Infect Dis.* 2008;47(10):1328–1338.

Kanoi BN, Egwang TG. New concepts in vaccine development in malaria. *Curr Opin Infect Dis.* 2007;20(3):311–316.

Kotton CN. Vaccination and immunization against travel-related diseases in immunocompromised hosts. *Expert Rev Vaccines.* 2008;7(5):663–672.

Kretsigner K, Broder KR, Cortese MM, et al. Preventing tetanus, diphtheria and pertussis among adults: use of tetanus toxoid, reduced diphtheria toxoid, and acellular pertussis vaccine. Recommendations of the Advisory Committee on Immunization Practices (ACIP) and recommendation of ACIP, supported by the Healthcare Infection Control Practices Advisory Committee (HICPAC), for use of Tdap among health-care personnel. *MMWR Recomm Rep.* 2006;55(RR-17):1–37.

Kundi M. New hepatitis B vaccine formulated with an improved adjuvant system. *Expert Rev Vaccines.* 2007;6(2):133–140.

Lavanchy D. Hepatitis B virus epidemiology, disease burden, treatment, and current and emerging prevention and control measures. *J Viral Hepat.* 2004;11(2):97–107.

Lo Re V III, Gluckman SJ. Travel immunizations. *Am Fam Physician.* 2004;70(1):89–99.

Poehling KA, Lafleur BJ, Szilagyi PG, et al. Population-based impact of pneumococcal conjugate vaccine in young children. *Pediatrics.* 2004;114(3):755–761.

Talbot HK, Keitel W, Cate TR, et al. Immunogenicity, safety and consistency of new trivalent inactivated influenza vaccine. *Vaccine.* 2008;26(32):4057–4061.

Venters C, Graham W, Cassidy W. Recombivax-HB: perspectives past, present and future. *Expert Rev Vaccines.* 2004;3(2):119–129.

Weston WM, Klein NP. Kinrix: a new combination DTaP-IPV vaccine for children aged 4-6 years. *Expert Rev Vaccines.* 2008;7(9):1309–1320.

CHAPTER 14

Medical Emergencies

Recent Developments

- CPR guidelines changed significantly in 2010, with an emphasis on chest compressions first, followed by airway opening and rescue breathing (CAB) and the immediate use of an automated external defibrillator (AED).
- The availability of portable defibrillators in ambulances, public places, and airline jets increases the probability of survival for victims of out-of-hospital ventricular fibrillation.
- Victims of suspected ischemic stroke should be transported to a facility capable of initiating fibrinolytic therapy within 1 hour of arrival unless that facility is more than 30 minutes away by ground ambulance.

Introduction

Although only occasionally called upon to manage a patient in acute distress, the ophthalmologist must be aware of the diagnostic and therapeutic steps necessary for proper care of these emergencies. Infrequent use of these life-support techniques makes periodic review particularly important. Both the American Red Cross and the American Heart Association offer courses in basic life support (BLS), advanced cardiac life support (ACLS), and pediatric advanced life support (PALS).

Cardiopulmonary Arrest

Cardiopulmonary resuscitation (CPR) is intended to rescue patients with acute circulatory failure, respiratory failure, or both. The most important determinant of short-term and long-term neurologically intact survival is the interval from the onset of the arrest to the restoration of effective spontaneous circulatory and respiratory function. Numerous studies have demonstrated that early defibrillation is the most important factor influencing survival and the minimization of sequelae. The sequences included here have been developed to optimize treatment. They are useful guidelines for most patients, but they do not preclude other measures that may be indicated for individual patients. The most crucial aspects of treatment are contained in the mnemonic *CAB*—chest compressions, airway maintenance, and breathing. The most recent published CPR protocols are the 2010 American Heart Association Guidelines for cardiopulmonary resuscitation and emergency cardiovascular care; these basic CPR steps for adults, children, and infants can be found at http://circ.ahajournals.org and www.heart.org. Also, the University of Washington maintains a free website (http://depts.washington.edu/learncpr/) with extensive resources, including text, graphics, and video demonstrations of CPR techniques.

The following steps are performed with an unconscious patient:

1. Determine unresponsiveness. Attempt to arouse the patient by tapping on the victim's shoulder and shouting, "Are you okay?" Do not shake the head or neck unless trauma to this area has been ruled out. Quickly note if breathing is absent or abnormal (gasping).

2. Activate the Emergency Medical Service (EMS) system if there is no response (911 where available). Rescuers should "phone first" for unresponsive adults. Be prepared to give the location and nature of the emergency and condition of the victim. If nearby, an automated external defibrillator (AED) should be retrieved or a second person sent for the AED.

3. Position the victim supine on a firm, flat surface.

4. Determine presence or absence of pulse. Palpate the carotid pulse for no longer than 5–10 seconds. Delays in initiating chest compressions should be minimized.

5. If a carotid pulse is present, rescue breathing should be started at a rate of 10–12 ventilations per minute. Recheck the pulse every 2 minutes. If there is no pulse, begin chest compressions.

6. To ensure good hand placement for chest compressions, place the heel of 1 hand at the midsternal region, with the bottom of the hand 1–2 fingerbreadths above the xiphoid process.

7. "Push hard and push fast." The recommended cardiac compression rate is at least 100 per minute. Cardiac output varies but on average, 30% of normal cardiac output can be expected with CPR. The depth of chest compression is critical; optimal compressions are 1.5 to 2.0 inches for children and at least 2.0 inches for adults. The chest must be allowed to fully recoil after each compression.

8. After delivery of the first 30 chest compressions, open the airway. The head-tilt, chin-lift maneuver is preferred because it is most likely to provide a good airway opening. The rescuer can use the chin lift to tilt the head backward by applying firm pressure to the forehead while placing the fingers of the other hand under the chin, supporting the mandible. The modified jaw thrust without head extension should be used if a neck injury is suspected.

9. If spontaneous respiration is not present, gently pinch the nose closed with the index finger and thumb of the hand that is on the forehead. Make a tight seal over the patient's mouth and ventilate twice with full breaths (1.0 second each). A 2-second pause should be observed between breaths. Visible chest rise should be seen with each breath. Resume chest compressions immediately.

10. For 1- and 2-rescuer CPR: When the victim's airway is unprotected, 30 compressions should be performed before the victim is ventilated twice. About 3–5 seconds should be taken for 2 ventilations, including the pause between ventilations.

11. The rescuer responsible for airway management should assess the adequacy of compressions by periodically palpating for the carotid pulse. Once the patient

is intubated, ventilations are continued at a rate of 8–10 per minute without pausing for compressions. Excessive ventilation should be avoided. The rescuer should stop and check for return of pulse and spontaneous breathing every few minutes. If 2 rescuers are present, chest compression duties should be switched every 2 minutes or 5 compression/ventilation cycles.

12. As soon as the AED is available, the unit should be connected to the patient and instructions followed for assessing the rhythm and potential defibrillation. The second rescuer, who retrieved the AED, may charge and apply the unit to minimize interruptions to chest compressions. Resume chest compressions immediately after the shock.

13. CPR is most effective when started immediately after cardiac arrest. If cardiac arrest has persisted for more than 10 minutes, CPR is unlikely to restore the patient's central nervous system (CNS) to prearrest status. If there is any question about the exact duration of cardiac arrest, the patient should be given the benefit of the doubt and resuscitation should be started.

14. The risk of disease transmission through mouth-to-mouth ventilation is very low, but a variety of face shields and masks are available for the health care professional. Masks are more effective than face shields in delivering adequate ventilation. Alternative airway devices (eg, laryngeal mask airway, esophageal/tracheal Combitube, or King airway device) may also be acceptable for rescuers trained in their use.

15. Patients with suspected stroke should be rapidly transported to a hospital capable of initiating fibrinolytic therapy within 1 hour of arrival unless that facility is more than 30 minutes away by ground ambulance. These patients merit the same priorities for dispatch as patients with acute myocardial infarction or major trauma.

The following adjuncts are helpful in CPR and are suggested components for a medical emergency tray or crash cart:

- oxygen, to enhance tissue oxygenation and to prevent or ameliorate a hypoxic state
- airways, adult and child, oral and nasal, to be used on unconscious or sedated patients
- a barrier device, such as a face shield or mask-to-mouth unit, to prevent disease transmission. Both can be used with supplemental oxygen and are especially useful if the rescuer is inexperienced in using a standard bag-valve device (eg, Ambu bag [Ambu, Ballerup, Denmark]), which should also be included as standard equipment to help secure the airway. Alternative airway devices may also be acceptable when appropriate (see step 14 in the preceding list).
- intravenous drugs (Table 14-1)
- intravenous solutions: 5% dextrose and water, D5 Ringer's lactate, normal saline
- syringes (1, 5, and 10 mL), hypodermic needles (20, 22, and 25 gauge), and venous catheters
- a suction apparatus, tourniquet, taped tongue blade, and tape
- laryngoscope and endotracheal tubes (adult and child)

Table 14-1 Medications Used in Acute Medical Emergencies

Drugs	Indications	Adult Dose	Adverse Effects
Epinephrine (1:1000)	Anaphylaxis	0.3–0.5 mg subcutaneously every 5 minutes	Tachycardia, hypertension
Epinephrine (1:10,000)	Asystole, ventricular fibrillation, EMD	Bolus 0.5–1.0 mg every 5 minutes	Hypertension in excess doses
Lidocaine	PVCs, ventricular tachycardia, ventricular fibrillation	Bolus 1.0 mg/kg with subsequent doses of 0.5 mg/kg to a maximum total dose of 3.0 mg/kg	Focal and grand mal seizures in excess doses
Atropine	Bradycardia, EMD, asystole	Bolus 0.5–1.0 mg every 5 minutes	Induced ventricular fibrillation, ventricular tachycardia, or supraventricular tachycardia
Diphenhydramine HCl (Benadryl)	Anaphylaxis and anaphylactoid reactions	12.5–25 mg (IV)	Drowsiness
Diazepam (Valium)	Seizures	5–10 mg	Sedation
Hydrocortisone sodium succinate (Solu-Cortef)	Anaphylaxis and anaphylactoid reactions	500 mg every 6 hours	Adrenal-pituitary axis suppression
Glucose (D 50)	Profound hypoglycemia	Bolus 10 mL	Hyperglycemia

EMD = electromechanical dissociation, PVCs = premature ventricular contractions.

If there is no 911 community emergency phone system, it is essential to have the phone number of the local paramedic emergency squad posted near all office telephones.

Basic life support also outlines methods for aiding persons who are choking, including the Heimlich maneuver and appropriate manual techniques for removing foreign bodies from the oral pharynx. Epigastric thrusts should be attempted; up to 10–12 thrusts may be necessary. Thereafter, ventilation should be attempted. If these efforts are unsuccessful, the mouth should be cleared with a finger sweep and ventilation attempted again. Transtracheal ventilation by means of cricothyrotomy may be necessary. The increasing availability of portable defibrillators in ambulances, public places, and airline jets improves the probability of survival for victims of out-of-hospital ventricular fibrillation. Recent clinical trials showed that induced hypothermia after cardiac arrest could improve neurologic outcome as well as reduce overall mortality.

In addition to providing guidelines for basic CPR, the American Heart Association has established guidelines and procedures for ACLS. ACLS includes intubations, defibrillation, cardioversion, pacemaker placement, administration of drugs and fluids, and communication with ambulance and hospital systems. Protocols and algorithms have been established in critical cardiac care for ventricular fibrillation, ventricular tachycardia, asystole, electromechanical dissociation, premature ventricular contractions, atrial tachycardia, and bradycardia. The provider of ACLS must precisely understand the actions, indications, doses, and adverse effects of the cardiac drugs used in the specific protocols. Except in dire emergencies, these drugs should be administered to treat cardiac arrhythmias *only* by physicians who use them routinely. Because of the comprehensive and changing nature of ACLS algorithms, these procedures are beyond the scope of this chapter.

Competency in pediatric emergency care may be enhanced with training in PLS (pediatric life support) and PALS (pediatric advanced life support). In addition, ophthalmologists should be familiar with the ophthalmic manifestations of child abuse and shaken baby syndrome. These are discussed in BCSC Section 6, *Pediatric Ophthalmology and Strabismus*.

Berg RA, Hemphill R, Abella BS, et al. Part 5: adult basic life support: 2010 American Heart Association Guidelines for Cardiopulmonary Resuscitation and Emergency Cardiovascular Care. *Circulation.* 2010;122(18 Suppl 3):S685–S705.

Shock

Shock is a state of generalized inadequacy of tissue perfusion that leads to impaired cellular metabolism and—if uncorrected—progresses to multiple organ failure and death.

Classification

Shock is classified according to the 4 primary pathophysiologic mechanisms involved:

1. oligemic or hypovolemic (eg, hemorrhage, diabetic ketoacidosis, burns, or sequestration)
2. cardiogenic (eg, myocardial infarction or arrhythmia)
3. obstructive (eg, pericardial tamponade, pulmonary embolus, or tension pneumothorax)
4. distributive, characterized by maldistribution of the vascular volume secondary to altered vasomotor tone (eg, sepsis, anaphylaxis, spinal cord insult, beriberi, or an arteriovenous fistula)

The type of shock can often be determined by history, physical examination, and appropriate diagnostic tests. Regardless of the event that precipitated the state of shock, microcirculatory failure is the common factor that eventually leads to death in advanced shock. Ventilatory failure appears to be the most significant factor in the morbidity and mortality of shock, with subsequent hypoxemia and metabolic acidosis leading to many complications.

If one rules out vasovagal syncope (by virtue of its short duration and because of knowledge of the situations that produce this condition), the basic life-support measures for the initial emergency care of the unconscious patient are similar. The most important aspects of treatment are the CABs, the same principles used in CPR.

Failure of respiratory gas exchange is the most frequent single cause of death in patients with shock, so respiratory obstruction must be ruled out first. Oxygen is then given by mask; if respiratory movements are shallow, mechanical ventilation is necessary. If laryngeal edema is present, as with anaphylaxis, endotracheal intubation (if possible), tracheotomy, or cricothyrotomy is indicated. Respiratory obstruction can be assumed if there is stridor with respiratory movements or if cyanosis persists even when adequate ventilatory techniques have been applied. A conscious patient in distress who cannot speak but is developing cyanosis may be choking on food or a foreign body; the Heimlich maneuver has been shown to be an effective means of treatment.

Assessment

The vital signs must be monitored. The clinical syndrome is usually characterized by an altered sensorium, relative hypotension, tachycardia, tachypnea, oliguria, metabolic acidosis, weak or absent pulse, pallor, diaphoresis, and cool skin (however, the skin may be warm in septic shock). Decreased pulse pressure is often an early sign of shock, and systolic pressures of less than 90 mm Hg are often associated with vital organ hypoperfusion. Blood pressure, however, is not always a reliable indicator of tissue perfusion.

Treatment

Treatment of shock is often complex; specific guidelines are beyond the scope of this text. General guidelines for the treatment of shock are as follows:

- The patient should be positioned with the legs elevated.
- Supplemental oxygen should be administered to enhance tissue oxygenation. Mechanical ventilation may be necessary to maintain the Po_2 and to prevent respiratory acidosis.
- Volume expansion with an IV infusion is of primary importance in maintaining circulation. Initially, a crystalloid solution (ie, normal saline or Ringer's lactate) should be administered rapidly.
- Sodium bicarbonate, given intravenously over 5–10 minutes, is indicated for correction of severe metabolic acidosis. The dosage should be titrated according to arterial blood gas results.
- Vasopressor drugs (dopamine) may be needed for augmentation of cardiac output and perfusion of vital organs after an adequate circulating volume is established.
- Antibiotic therapy should be initiated promptly if sepsis is suspected.
- Low-dose corticosteroids may hasten the recovery from septic shock in some patients, although there is no improvement in survival in most studies.
- Drotrecogin alfa (Xigris), which is recombinant human activated protein C, is a recently approved drug effective in reducing mortality in severe sepsis with acute organ failure.

Experimental drugs used in treating septic shock include tilarginine, levosimendan, terlipressin, arginine vasopressin, and polyclonal intravenous immunoglobulin (particularly when enriched with IgA and IgM).

Anaphylaxis

One specific cause of shock that requires immediate and specific therapy is anaphylaxis. *Anaphylaxis* is an acute allergic reaction following antigen exposure in a previously sensitized person. It is usually mediated by immunoglobulin E antibodies and involves release of chemical mediators from mast cells and basophils. *Anaphylactoid reactions,* which are more common yet less severe, are the result of direct release of these chemical mediators triggered by nonantigenic agents. Anaphylaxis or anaphylactoid reactions may occur after exposure to pollen, drugs, foreign serum, insect stings, diagnostic agents such as iodinated contrast materials or fluorescein, vaccines, local anesthetics, and food products. The most important parameter for predicting such an attack is a history of a previous allergic reaction to any other drug or possible antigen. Unfortunately, a history of known sensitivity may not always be elicited. A recent study revealed that hospital admissions in the state of New York for anaphylaxis increased fourfold between 1990 and 2006. Other studies confirm an increase in anaphylaxis in recent years.

Anaphylaxis is particularly important to the ophthalmologist, in view of the increasing number of surgical procedures and fluorescein angiograms being performed in the office setting. It is estimated that allergic reactions to fluorescein (including urticaria) occur in up to 1% of all angiograms. In one survey, the overall risk of a severe reaction was 1 in 1900 patients, including a risk of respiratory compromise in 1 in 3800 subjects. Any patient developing diaphoresis, apprehension, pallor, a rapid and weak pulse, or any combination thereof after administration of a drug should be considered to have an allergic reaction until proven otherwise. The diagnosis is certain if there is associated generalized itching, urticaria, angioedema of the skin, dyspnea, wheezing, or arrhythmia. This process may lead rapidly to loss of consciousness, shock, cardiac arrest, coma, or death.

Once an acute allergic reaction is suspected, prompt treatment is indicated:

- Epinephrine (0.3–0.5 mL of 1:1000) injected intramuscularly in a limb opposite to the antigenic agent exposure site is usually effective to maintain circulation and blood pressure.
- Intravenous volume expansion may be needed to restore and maintain tissue perfusion.
- Oxygen should be administered to all patients in respiratory distress.
- Tracheotomy or cricothyrotomy is indicated when laryngeal edema is unresponsive to the previous methods or when oral intubation cannot be performed.
- Hydrocortisone should be administered for serious or prolonged reactions. When given early, corticosteroids help control possible long-term sequelae.
- Antihistamines are also helpful in slowing or halting the ongoing allergic response but are of limited value in acute anaphylaxis.
- All patients with anaphylaxis or anaphylactoid reactions should be observed for at least 6 hours.

In cases of mild allergic reactions, the physician can give 25–50 mg of diphenhydramine (Benadryl) orally or intramuscularly and observe the patient closely to determine whether further treatment is necessary. Pretreating high-risk patients with an antihistamine, corticosteroids, or both prior to a fluorescein angiogram may reduce the risk of an allergic reaction. In all cases of anaphylaxis, supportive treatment should be maintained until the emergency medical team arrives.

For patients with a known history of anaphylaxis, personal emergency kits containing epinephrine are available and can be used until medical help arrives. The kits are designed to allow self-treatment by the patient or administration by a family member or an informed bystander. The Ana-Kit contains a syringe and needle preloaded with 0.6 mL of 1:1000 epinephrine. The physician who prescribes this kit must give detailed instructions concerning the use of the device. The EpiPen and EpiPen Jr (Dey; Napa, California) each contains a spring-loaded automatic injector, which does not permit graduated doses to be given but automatically injects 0.3 mg of epinephrine (0.15 mg in the junior version) when the device is triggered by pressure on the thigh. The epinephrine ampules contained in these self-treatment kits have a limited shelf life and should be replaced when the expiration date is reached or if the solution becomes discolored.

Advanced Cardiac Life Support Provider Manual. Dallas: American Heart Association; 2006.

Annane D, Bellissant E, Cavaillon JM. Septic shock. *Lancet.* 2005;365(9453):63–78.

Cunha BA. Sepsis and septic shock: selection of empiric antimicrobial therapy. *Crit Care Clin.* 2008;24(2):313–334.

Fairbanks RJ, Shah MN, Lerner EB, Ilangovan K, Pennington EC, Schneider SM. Epidemiology and outcomes of out-of-hospital cardiac arrest in Rochester, New York. *Resuscitation.* 2007;72(3):415–424.

Graham CA, Parke TR. Critical care in the emergency department: shock and circulatory support. *Emerg Med J.* 2005;22(1):17–21.

Holmes CL, Walley KR. Arginine vasopressin in the treatment of vasodilatory septic shock. *Best Pract Res Clin Anaesthesiol.* 2008;22(2):275–286.

Laupland KB, Kirkpatrick AW, Delaney A. Polyclonal intravenous immunoglobulin for the treatment of severe sepsis and septic shock in critically ill adults: a systematic review and meta-analysis. *Crit Care Med.* 2007;35(12):2686–2692.

Lin RY, Anderson AS, Shah SN, Nurruzzaman F. Increasing anaphylaxis hospitalizations in the first 2 decades of life: New York State, 1990-2006. *Ann Allergy Asthma Immunol.* 2008;101(4):387–393.

Marik PE, Lipman J. The definition of septic shock: implications for treatment. *Crit Care Resusc.* 2007;9(1):101–103.

Muraro A, Roberts G, Simons FE. New visions for anaphylaxis: an iPAC summary and future trends. *Pediatr Allergy Immunol.* 2008;19(Suppl 19):40–50.

Richardson L, Hunter S. Is steroid therapy ever of benefit to patients in the intensive care unit going into septic shock? *Interact Cardiovasc Thorac Surg.* 2008;7(5):898–905.

Rivers EP, Ahrens T. Improving outcomes for severe sepsis and septic shock: tools for early identification of at-risk patients and treatment protocol implementation. *Crit Care Clin.* 2008; 24(3 Suppl):S1–S47.

Sheikh A, Shehata YA, Brown SG, Simons FE. Adrenaline (epinephrine) for the treatment of anaphylaxis with and without shock. *Cochrane Database Syst Rev.* 2008;(4):CD006312.

Sprung CL, Annane D, Keh D, et al; CORTICUS Study Group. Hydrocortisone therapy for patients with septic shock. *N Engl J Med.* 2008;358(2):111–124.

Steinmetz J, Barnung S, Nielsen SL, Risom M, Rasmussen LS. Improved survival after an out-of-hospital cardiac arrest using new guidelines. *Acta Anaesthesiol Scand.* 2008;52(7):908–913.

University of Washington. A large assortment of free CPR resources with text, graphics, and video is available at http://depts.washington.edu/learncpr/.

Seizures and Status Epilepticus

A *seizure* is a paroxysmal episode of abnormal electrical activity in the brain, resulting in involuntary transient neurologic, motor activity, behavioral, or autonomic dysfunction. Seizures can present with many different clinical manifestations, but most fit into the categories of simple partial, complex partial, or generalized tonic-clonic. See also Chapter 12, Behavioral and Neurologic Disorders, for further discussion.

As in the treatment of all medical emergencies, the first consideration is airway maintenance. This becomes particularly important if the seizure progresses to *status epilepticus,* which is defined as a prolonged seizure or as multiple seizures without intervening periods of normal consciousness. Status epilepticus, like seizures, may have a local onset with secondary generalization or may be generalized from onset. A seizure is considered status epilepticus when it lasts for 30 minutes or longer. Status epilepticus is often found concomitantly with hyperthermia, acidosis, hypoxia, tachycardia, hypercapnia, and mydriasis and, if persistent, may be associated with irreversible brain injury. Status epilepticus that is completely stopped within 2 hours usually has relatively minor morbidity compared with episodes lasting longer than 2 hours.

Major causes of seizures and status epilepticus include

- drug withdrawal, such as from anticonvulsants, benzodiazepines, barbiturates, or alcohol
- metabolic abnormalities, such as hypoglycemia, hyponatremia, hypocalcemia, or hypomagnesemia
- conditions that affect the CNS, such as infection, trauma, stroke, hypoxia, ischemia, or sleep deprivation
- toxic levels of various drugs

In management, it is important not only to stop the seizure activity but also to identify and treat the underlying cause. Following is a general treatment protocol:

1. Note time of seizure onset. Monitor airway, vital signs, and ECG.
2. Establish IV line. Position patient on side to allow gravity drainage of saliva. Insert oral airway if possible. Some experts advocate using a washcloth or taped tongue blade as a bite block.
3. Draw blood immediately; check level of glucose, electrolytes, calcium, and magnesium; and check toxicology screen.
4. Give 50 mL of 50% dextrose IV push (or 1 mL/kg).
5. Administer a benzodiazepine such as diazepam (Valium) or lorazepam (Ativan) slowly by IV line, titrated to an effective dose, usually 5.0 mg/min to a total dose of 0.5 mg/kg. Another option is the newer, short-acting agent, midazolam.
6. Proceed immediately to administer phenytoin (or fosphenytoin) intravenously. Monitor pulse rate, blood pressure, and ECG. Watch especially for hypotension.
7. If seizures continue for 20 minutes, administer a loading dose of phenobarbital.
8. Emergency medical management of seizures is best left to physicians who perform this routinely. Activation of the emergency response (911) team is indicated in all cases of acute seizure onset.

Refractory cases of status epilepticus have responded successfully to repeated electroconvulsive therapy sessions, intravenous sedatives such as ketamine or propofol, surgical ablation and stimulation procedures, and some of the newer agents, topiramate (Topamax) and levetiracetam (Keppra).

Arif H, Hirsch LJ. Treatment of status epilepticus. *Semin Neurol.* 2008;28(3):342–354.

Cline JS, Roos K. Treatment of status epilepticus with electroconvulsive therapy. *J ECT.* 2007; 23(1):30–32.

Knake S, Gruener J, Hattemer K, et al. Intravenous levetiracetam in the treatment of benzodiazepine refractory status epilepticus. *J Neurol Neurosurg Psychiatry.* 2008;79(5):588–589.

Selvitelli M, Drislane FW. Recent developments in the diagnosis and treatment of status epilepticus. *Curr Neurol Neurosci Rep.* 2007;7(6):529–535.

Toxic Reactions to Local Anesthetics and Other Agents

Toxic overdose is another cause of unconsciousness or of acute distress in a conscious patient, and it must be considered whenever a patient is undergoing a procedure that requires local anesthesia. Table 14-2 lists commonly used local anesthetics with their maximum safe dose.

Reactions following administration of local anesthetics are almost always toxic and only rarely allergic. A high blood level of local anesthetic can be produced by the following: too large a dose, unusually rapid absorption (including inadvertent IV administration), and unusually slow detoxification or elimination (especially in liver disease). Hypersensitivity (ie, decreased patient tolerance) and idiosyncratic reactions are rare, but they may occur with local anesthetic agents, as with any drug. Although true allergic or anaphylactic reactions are also rare, they may occur, particularly with agents belonging to the amino ester class.

Toxic reactions cause overstimulation of the CNS, which may lead to excitement, restlessness, apprehension, disorientation, tremors, and convulsions (cerebral cortex effects), as well as nausea and vomiting (medulla effects). Cardiac effects initially include tachycardia and hypertension. Ultimately, however, depression of the CNS and the cardiovascular system occurs, which may result in sleepiness and coma (cerebral cortex effects) as well as in irregular respirations, sighing, dyspnea, and respiratory arrest (medulla effects). Cardiac effects of CNS depression are bradycardia and hypotension.

Injected local anesthetic agents can also produce a direct toxic effect on muscle tissue. In the case of retrobulbar injections, this can result initially in muscle weakness, which

Table 14-2 Maximum Recommended Local Anesthetic Doses

Agent	Commercially Available Concentrations (%) 1% = 10 mg/cc	Plain Solutions, mg	Epinephrine-Containing Solutions, mg
Chloroprocaine	1.0, 2.0, 3.0	800	1000
Lidocaine	0.5, 1.0, 1.5, 2.0, 4.0, 5.0	300	500
Mepivacaine (Carbocaine)	1.0, 1.5, 2.0	300	225
Bupivacaine	0.25, 0.5, 0.75	175	225
Tetracaine	1.0	100	100

in some patients is followed by muscle contracture. Extraocular motility can be affected, resulting in diplopia (usually hypertropia) that may require surgical revision. Hyaluronidase may be partially protective by allowing more rapid diffusion of the anesthetic agent following injection.

Signs of cortical stimulation require immediate treatment, before progressive changes to cortical and medullary function and cardiac depression occur. Increased metabolic activity of the CNS and poor ventilatory exchange lead to cerebral hypoxia. Treatment consists of oxygenation, supportive airway care, and titrated IV administration of midazolam, which is used to suppress cortical stimulation.

In cases of toxic overdose, other emergency procedures must be applied, including suctioning if vomiting occurs and using a taped tongue blade if convulsions develop. If shock develops, the appropriate drugs can be administered by IV infusion.

The addition of *epinephrine* to the local anesthetic can also cause adverse reactions. Epinephrine can produce symptoms similar to early CNS stimulation by local anesthetic, such as anxiety, restlessness, tremor, hypertension, and tachycardia. Unlike local anesthetics, however, epinephrine does not produce convulsions or bradycardia as the toxic reaction proceeds. Oxygen is useful in the treatment of epinephrine overdoses.

The administration of retrobulbar *bupivacaine* has been associated with respiratory arrest. This reaction may be caused by intra-arterial injection of the local anesthetic, with retrograde flow to the cerebral circulation. It could also result from puncture of the dural sheath of the optic nerve during retrobulbar block, with diffusion of the local anesthetic along the subdural space in the midbrain. A large prospective study comparing retrobulbar injection of 0.75% bupivacaine plus 2.0% lidocaine to 0.75% bupivacaine plus 4.0% lidocaine found that patients receiving 4.0% lidocaine mixed with bupivacaine had an almost 9 times greater risk of respiratory arrest than patients receiving 2.0% lidocaine mixed with bupivacaine. (See Chapter 15, Perioperative Management in Ocular Surgery, for further discussion of reactions to local anesthetics.)

The use of *edrophonium chloride* (Tensilon) in the diagnosis of myasthenia gravis can have toxic side effects. The signs and symptoms result from cholinergic stimulation and may include nausea, vomiting, diarrhea, sweating, increased bronchial and salivary secretions, muscle fasciculations and weakness, and bradycardia. Some of these signs may be transient and self-limited because of the very short half-life of IV edrophonium. However, whenever a Tensilon test is to be performed, a syringe containing 0.5 mg of atropine sulfate must be immediately available. (Some physicians routinely pretreat with atropine all patients undergoing Tensilon testing.)

If signs of excess cholinergic stimulation occur, 0.4–0.5 mg of atropine sulfate should be administered intravenously. This dose may be repeated every 3–10 minutes if necessary. The total dose of atropine necessary to counteract the toxic effects is seldom more than 2 mg. If toxic signs progress, the treatment described earlier for toxic overdose may be necessary.

Guyton DL. Strabismus complications from local anesthetics. *Semin Ophthalmol.* 2008;23(5):298–301.

Moorthy SS, Zaffer R, Rodriguez S, Ksiazek S, Yee RD. Apnea and seizures following retrobulbar local anesthetic injection. *J Clin Anesth.* 2003;15(4):267–270.

Ocular Side Effects of Systemic Medications

Because of the development of medical specialties and the proliferation of specific thera-peutic agents, patients frequently have multiple simultaneous drug regimens. Often, no single physician (among the several to whom a patient may relate) is aware of all the drugs the patient is taking. The clinical problem is compounded by several factors. The physi-cian may not be familiar with drugs used outside of his or her specialty. In addition, the patient may have a drug interaction that affects a bodily system not usually monitored by the specialist. Finally, the patient might not associate a symptom with a particular drug that has been used, if that symptom is not related to the system for which the drug was given.

However, the effects of some systemic drugs are widely known. For example, the com-monly prescribed erectile dysfunction agent sildenafil (Viagra) has been noted to block photoreceptor signals, causing electroretinographic changes, visual disturbances, and increased light sensitivity. The spectrum of systemic side effects with commonly used ophthalmic drugs is covered extensively elsewhere in this series (see BCSC Section 9, *Intraocular Inflammation and Uveitis,* and Section 10, *Glaucoma*). The ocular side ef-fects of several commonly prescribed systemic medications are presented in Table 14-3. Drug interactions must always be suspected in patients on multiple topical and systemic medications.

The ophthalmologist can minimize adverse effects from multiple-drug therapy by doing the following:

- Maintain a high level of suspicion for drug interactions.
- Question the patient closely about other drug therapy and general symptoms.
- Encourage all patients to carry a card listing the drugs they use.
- Keep in close communication with the patient's primary care physician.
- Consult with a clinical pharmacologist or internist whenever a question of drug interaction arises.

Unrecognized adverse effects of topical or systemic medications should be reported to the National Registry of Drug-Induced Ocular Side Effects (NRDIOSE) at

Frederick Fraunfelder, MD
Casey Eye Institute
Oregon Health Sciences University
3375 SW Terwilliger Blvd.
Portland, OR 97201-4197
Phone: 503-494-5686
Fax: 503-494-6864

Members of the American Academy of Ophthalmology can access this database free of charge at www.eyedrugregistry.com. The website also has a syllabus from the 2009 AAO Annual Meeting, entitled "Drug-Related Adverse Effects of Clinical Importance to the Ophthalmologist."

Table 14-3 Potential Ocular Effects of Popular Drugs

Drug (Trade Name)	Side Effects*
Antibiotics	
Cefaclor (Ceclor)	Mild inflammation of ocular surface (rare); eyelid problems; nystagmus; visual hallucinations
Cefuroxime axetil (Ceftin)	Mild inflammation of ocular surface (rare)
Ciprofloxacin (Cipro)	Eyelid problems; exacerbation of myasthenia; visual sensations
Moxifloxacin (oral; Avelox)	Iris transillumination; sphincter paralysis
Rifampin (Rifadin and others)	Conjunctival hyperemia; exudative conjunctivitis; increased lacrimation
Tetracycline, doxycycline, minocycline (Dynacin, Minocin)	Papilledema secondary to pseudotumor cerebri; transient myopia; blue-gray, dark blue, or brownish pigmentation of the sclera; hyperpigmentation of eyelids or conjunctiva; diplopia
Antidepressants/anxiolytics	
Alprazolam (Xanax)	Diplopia; decreased or blurred vision; decreased accommodation; abnormal extraocular muscle movements; allergic conjunctivitis
Fluoxetine (Prozac)	Blurred vision; photophobia; mydriasis; dry eye; conjunctivitis; diplopia
Imipramine (Tofranil)	Decreased vision; decreased accommodation; slight mydriasis; photosensitivity
Antiepileptics	
Topiramate (Topamax)	Conjunctivitis; abnormal accommodation; photophobia; strabismus; mydriasis; iritis; acute myopia; secondary angle-closure glaucoma
Analgesics, anti-inflammatory agents	
Aspirin	Transient blurred vision; transient myopia; hypersensitivity reactions
Ibuprofen (Advil)	Blurred vision; decreased vision; diplopia; photosensitivity; dry eyes; decrease in color vision; optic or retrobulbar neuritis
Hydroxychloroquine (Plaquenil)	Maculopathy with decreased vision and color perception
Naproxen (Anaprox, Aleve)	Decreased vision; changes in color vision; optic or retrobulbar neuritis; papilledema secondary to pseudotumor cerebri; photosensitivity; corneal opacities
Disease-modifying agents	
Interferon	Cotton-wool spots
Isotretinoin (Accutane)	Corneal opacities; decreased night vision
Asthma, allergy drugs	
Antihistamines (general)	Decreased vision; may induce or aggravate dry eye; pupillary changes; decreased accommodation; blurred vision; decreased mucoid or lacrimal secretions; diplopia
Corticosteroids (general)	Decreased vision; posterior subcapsular cataracts; increased IOP
Cardiovascular drugs	
Amiodarone (Cordarone, Pacerone)	Photophobia; blurred vision; corneal opacities; subcapsular lens opacities; optic neuropathy
β-Blockers (general)	Decreased vision; visual hallucinations; decreased IOP; decreased lacrimation
α-1a Selective antagonists: tamsulosin (Flomax), alfuzosin (Uroxatral), finasteride (Proscar)	Intraoperative floppy iris syndrome (IFIS), with a sluggish hypotonic iris, miosis, iris prolapse

(Continued)

Table 14-3 *(continued)*

Drug (Trade Name)	Side Effects*
Cardiovascular drugs *(cont)*	
Calcium channel blockers	Decreased or blurred vision; periorbital edema; ocular irritation (general)
Captopril/enalapril (Vaseretic)	Angioedema of the eye and orbit; conjunctivitis; decreased vision
Digitalis glycosides	Decreased vision; color vision defects; glare phenomenon; flickering vision
Diuretics (thiazide-type)	Decreased vision; myopia; color vision abnormalities; retinal edema
Flecainide (Tambocor)	Blurred vision; decreased vision; decreased accommodation; abnormal visual sensations; decreased depth perception; nystagmus
Warfarin (Coumadin)	Retinal hemorrhages in susceptible persons; hyphema; allergic reactions; conjunctivitis; lacrimation; decreased vision
Drugs used in the treatment of impotence	
Cialis (Tadalafil)	Sudden loss of vision; retinal vascular occlusions; decreased
Sildenafil (Viagra)	color perception; conjunctivitis; photophobia
Hormones, hormone-related drugs	
Clomiphene (Clomid and others)	Visual sensations; decreased vision; mydriasis; visual field constriction; photophobia; diplopia
Danazol (Danocrine)	Decreased vision; diplopia; papilledema secondary to pseudotumor cerebri; visual field defects
Estradiol (general)	Decreased vision; retinal vascular disorders; papilledema secondary to pseudotumor cerebri; fluctuations of corneal curvature and corneal steepening; color vision abnormalities
Leuprolide (Lupron)	Blurred vision; papilledema secondary to pseudotumor cerebri; retinal hemorrhage and branch vein occlusion; eye pain; lid edema
Oral contraceptives (general)	Decreased vision; retinal vascular disorders; papilledema secondary to pseudotumor cerebri; color vision abnormalities
Tamoxifen (Nolvadex)	Decreased vision; corneal opacities; retinal edema or hemorrhage; optic disc swelling; retinopathy; decreased color vision; possible optic neuritis or neuropathy

*For ocular side effects of cancer chemotherapy agents, see Chapter 11, Cancer, Table 11-1.

Modified with permission from Doran M. When good drugs go bad. *EyeNet*. 2001;5:43–48. Chart updated 2009.

Cantrell MA, Bream-Rouwenhorst HR, Steffensmeier A, Hemerson P, Rogers M, Stamper B. Intraoperative floppy iris syndrome associated with alpha1-adrenergic receptor antagonists. *Ann Pharmacother.* 2008;42(4):558–563.

Chang DF, Braga-Mele R, Mamalis N, et al. Clinical experience with intraoperative floppy-iris syndrome. Results of the 2008 ASCRS member survey. *J Cataract Refract Surg.* 2008;34(7): 1201–1209.

Doran M. When good drugs go bad. *EyeNet*. 2001;5:43–48.

Fraunfelder FT, Fraunfelder FW. *Drug-Induced Ocular Side Effects.* 5th ed. Boston: Butterworth-Heinemann; 2001.

Issa SA, Dagres E. Intraoperative floppy-iris syndrome and finasteride intake. *J Cataract Refract Surg.* 2007;33(12):2142–2143.

CHAPTER 15

Perioperative Management in Ocular Surgery

Recent Developments

- Use of Universal Protocol is a National Patient Safety Goal designed to eliminate "wrong site surgery."
- Preoperative antibiotics must be considered in every surgical procedure to reduce the risk of postoperative infections.
- Routine preoperative testing is not necessary prior to cataract surgery.
- Dual antiplatelet therapy is indicated in some heart patients during cataract surgery.
- β-Blockers are indicated prior to surgery in some patients.

Introduction

Ocular surgery is generally considered to have low morbidity and mortality, because eye surgery usually is of short duration, with little or no blood loss. The perioperative management of eye patients can be challenging, however. Eye patients are frequently older and have numerous medical conditions. Sometimes the surgery may be directly related to a systemic disease such as diabetes or thyroid disease. Ophthalmic surgery may also be very delicate and may have specific requirements about the level of alertness during the procedure; the level of sedation is particularly important during intraocular surgery. This discussion is divided into the preoperative medical assessment and the intraoperative management of the patient.

Preoperative Assessment

All patients should have a history and physical examination as part of the preoperative assessment (Table 15-1). However, preoperative testing in an asymptomatic patient, including ECG and routine blood tests, is no longer considered necessary. In 2000, a study by Schein and colleagues showed no benefit to routine testing in asymptomatic patients undergoing cataract surgery. In this study, outcomes in both the testing and no-testing groups were the same: 31.3 per 1000 operations. The rates for intraoperative events and

Table 15-1 Joint Commission Standards for History and Physical

History
Presenting diagnosis/condition
History of present illness
Past medical history
Allergies
Current medications
Family history
Social history
Review of systems
Physical examination
Vital signs
General appearance
Eyes, ears, nose, and throat
Head and neck
Cardiovascular
Abdomen
Respiratory
Genitourinary
Musculoskeletal
Skin
Neurologic

postoperative events, considered separately, did not differ significantly. The most frequent medical events in both groups were treatment for hypertension and arrhythmia (mostly bradycardia). The authors concluded that the standard battery of tests should be ordered only when they would have been indicated even if the patient were not planning surgery.

The American Academy of Ophthalmology policy statement on the responsibilities of the ophthalmologist, Appropriate Examination and Treatment Procedures, includes medical diagnosis and preoperative treatment of the patient. Although ophthalmologists may delegate the acquisition of the data required for the preoperative history and physical, the surgical planning and synthesis of information prior to surgery must be done by the operating ophthalmologist.

Avoiding surgical complications begins with the decision to operate. The risks, benefits, and alternatives to surgery are considered and the surgical plan is laid out. Typically, the patient is involved in this process; informed consent is contingent on the patient and legal guardian, when appropriate, receiving a detailed explanation of the surgical plan. In cataract surgery, planning includes an assessment of the patient's functional visual disability, a dilated examination of the fundus, biometry, keratometry, IOL calculations, documentation of informed consent, and identification of the patient with 2 or more identifiers (including name, date of birth, medical record number).

American Society of Anesthesiologists. ASA Physical Status Classification System. Available at www.asahq.org/clinical/physicalstatus.htm.

Ethics Committee. Appropriate Examination and Treatment Procedures. Advisory Opinion of the Code of Ethics. San Francisco: American Academy of Ophthalmology; 2007. Available at www.aao.org/about/ethics/exam_procedures.cfm.

The Joint Commission. Joint Commission E-dition. www.jcrinc.com.

Schein OD, Katz J, Bass EB, et al. The value of routine preoperative medical testing before cataract surgery: study of medical testing for cataract surgery. *N Engl J Med.* 2000;342(3):168–175.

US Department of Health and Human Services, Agency for Healthcare Research and Quality. www.ahrq.gov.

Pediatric Patients

If a child undergoing surgery is healthy and does not chronically take prescribed medications, no laboratory tests are necessary, even for general anesthesia. There is no evidence that abnormalities in a complete blood count affect the choice of anesthetic management for asymptomatic children. However, African-American patients should be screened for sickle cell disease or trait if they have not been tested, because some aspects of anesthetic management will change in patients with hemoglobinopathy. Routine pregnancy testing of female patients of childbearing age, prior to anesthesia, is a complex issue and even more complex in minors, because individual states may have statutes concerning parental notification of test results. The anesthesiologist will likely discuss the need for preoperative pregnancy testing; however, consent for a pregnancy test is required. Preoperative sedation for children can include midazolam or methohexital.

The issue of elective eye surgery in children with an upper respiratory infection requires judgment. A child who is already ill will feel even worse after surgery, and the significance of a postoperative fever may be difficult to interpret. Furthermore, contaminated nasal discharge could possibly enter the ocular area. If the child has a fever above 101°F, has purulent nasal discharge, or appears systemically ill, a bacterial lower respiratory infection should be considered. This circumstance argues for a delay to avoid increased risk of laryngospasm and bronchospasm with general anesthesia. However, in the absence of such findings—such as with a child who appears well except for a runny nose—many anesthesiologists elect to proceed.

Preoperative Medications

In general, medication regimens should not be interrupted during eye surgery. Treatments for asthma, hypertension, angina, and congestive heart failure should be continued throughout the day of surgery. However, as will be discussed later in the chapter, diabetic patients require modification of glucose management. The following are guidelines, although individual practice can vary from locality to locality.

Antihypertensive medications should be continued until the time of surgery to avoid rebound hypertension. Such medications include clonidine (both dermal patch and orally administered), β-blockers, and angiotensin-converting enzyme inhibitors. Oral antihypertensive medications can be taken with a sip of water the day of surgery, whether or not the patient is on NPO status. (See Chapter 2, Hypertension, for a complete discussion of hypertension medications.)

Digoxin can be withheld the day of surgery for many patients, given its long half-life. However, if a patient is receiving digoxin to control the ventricular response to atrial fibrillation, the resting heart rate must be appropriate on the morning of surgery. If the resting heart rate is more than 90 beats per minute, digoxin should be given.

Anticonvulsant medications should be administered (with sips of water) on the patient's usual schedule, because stress and particularly general anesthesia can lower the seizure threshold.

Thyroid medications can be held the day of surgery, given their long half-life.

A patient who has taken systemic corticosteroids for more than 1 month within the 6 months before surgery is customarily "covered" with the equivalent of 300 mg/day of hydrocortisone perioperatively. At the start of the procedure, 100 mg is given intravenously, an additional 100 mg is given at the end of the procedure, and the last 100 mg is administered 6 hours after the end of surgery. Lower doses can be administered for procedures associated with minimal physiologic stress, in the range of 25–30 mg of hydrocortisone intravenously in the first 24 hours after surgery.

It may be desirable to discontinue diuretics on the day of surgery. A patient under local anesthesia may become uncomfortable from a full bladder caused by a preoperative dose of diuretic. A patient undergoing general anesthesia who continues diuretic use on the morning of surgery may become hypotensive because of intravascular volume depletion prior to surgery.

Nicotinic acid should be discontinued before general anesthesia because it can cause an exaggerated hypotensive response from vasodilation. It is generally taught that monoamine oxidase inhibitors should be discontinued 2–3 weeks prior to elective surgery. This is an issue best discussed with the anesthesiologist.

Though echothiophate iodide eyedrops are rarely used today, their use affects the choice of muscle relaxant prior to endotracheal intubations. Ideally, the drops should be stopped 3 weeks before the elective surgery to allow recovery of the cholinesterase enzyme system. However, if echothiophate iodide must be continued, succinylcholine cannot be used during intubations. Alternative medications are available in such cases.

Although it is common to withhold aspirin prior to general surgical procedures, this is not the case in cataract surgery. The risk of significant hemorrhage during cataract surgery is so low that the risk associated with anticoagulant or antiplatelet drugs is minimal. Indeed, stopping antiplatelet therapy may be associated with increased morbidity or mortality. Failure to continue aspirin and other antiplatelet therapy for 6–12 months after a coronary artery stenting has been associated with increased risk of cardiac ischemia.

A number of over-the-counter drugs and nutritional supplements may have antiplatelet activity. Patients taking supplements such as vitamin E and St John's wort and nonsteroidal anti-inflammatory agents such as ibuprofen may fail to report taking these drugs because they are not "prescribed." Many nutritional supplements are not medically indicated and can be stopped prior to surgery.

The management of anticoagulation in the perioperative setting must be individualized because the risk of thrombosis and the strength of the indication for anticoagulation vary greatly, as does the risk of bleeding during various surgical procedures. Therefore, no single regimen satisfies all patient needs. Consultation with the patient's primary physician is advisable if warfarin needs to be stopped. Warfarin can be stopped 5 days before surgery, and if the international normalized ratio (INR) level drops below 2.0, heparin therapy with either IV unfractionated heparin or subcutaneous low-molecular-weight heparin can be given to maintain adequate anticoagulation until just prior to surgery.

Intravenous heparin should be discontinued approximately 12 hours prior to surgery and restarted 24 hours after surgery. If gastrointestinal function is normal, warfarin may be restarted on the day of surgery. If anticoagulation is critical, heparin may be used until therapeutic warfarin levels have been reached.

β-Blockers have been shown to reduce mortality in patients undergoing noncardiac surgery. The surgeries that carry the highest cardiac risk and most benefit from the preoperative use of β-blockers are major operations in older patients. With some ophthalmic surgeries, such as orbital surgery and facial surgery, selected patients may benefit from preoperative use of β-blockers. This group includes patients with previous myocardial infarction, patients with a positive stress test, and patients with 2 or more risk factors for coronary artery disease.

In general, *antimicrobial prophylaxis* of bacterial endocarditis is not necessary in patients with cardiac valvular disease prior to ocular surgery. Guidelines for infective endocarditis prophylaxis can be found in Chapter 1, Infectious Disease, or from the American Heart Association (AHA).

American College of Cardiology. www.acc.org.

American Heart Association. New guidelines regarding antibiotics to prevent infective endocarditis. Available at www.americanheart.org.

Kallio H, Paloheimo M, Maunuksela EL. Haemorrhage and risk factors associated with retrobulbar/peribulbar block: a prospective study in 1383 patients. *Br J Anaesth.* 2000;85(5): 708–711.

Katz J, Feldman MA, Bass EB. Risks and benefits of anticoagulant and antiplatelet medication use before cataract surgery. *Ophthalmology.* 2003;110(9):1784–1788.

Diabetes

Oral hypoglycemic medications are usually withheld the day of surgery. These medications have a relatively long duration of action, which could lead to hypoglycemia late in the day if the patient's oral caloric intake is inadequate.

Management of blood glucose is important in avoiding CNS dysfunction. Whenever possible, insulin-dependent patients should undergo surgery early in the day to minimize disruption of their metabolic status, and glucose levels should be monitored postoperatively. No single regimen works for all patients. Perioperative management of blood glucose during a brief surgical procedure in a diet-controlled diabetic patient generally involves only monitoring of blood glucose immediately perioperatively and every 3 hours until oral intake is resumed.

For patients with relatively well-controlled insulin-requiring diabetes and reasonable glucose control (<250 mg/dL), one option is to hold all short-acting insulin and give half the intermediate- or long-acting insulin the morning of the surgery. It is imperative to provide close preoperative, intraoperative, and postoperative glucose and electrolyte monitoring. For more severe cases of diabetes, titration of a dextrose 5% in water drip with an initial intravenous rate of 75 mL/hour should prevent hypoglycemia or hyperglycemia. Blood glucose should be monitored hourly and the infusion rate adjusted to maintain glucose at 100–200 mg/dL. Alternatively, for patients who are on insulin and undergoing procedures lasting less than 2 hours, the "no insulin, no glucose" regimen works well preoperatively on the morning of surgery. Perioperative monitoring of blood glucose before, during, and after surgery is important. The availability of one-touch monitoring makes such measurements very easy, even in the operating room. During the procedure, intravenous solutions without dextrose (lactated Ringer's or saline) are given. After the surgical procedure, and once oral intake is established, the patient should receive a portion (usually one half or one third) of the usual insulin dose. If a procedure lasts more than 2 hours, insulin may have to be given as an infusion of at least 4 units per hour, with monitoring of the blood glucose level every 30–60 minutes. The anesthesiologist and primary care physician should be involved in managing the blood glucose level in such patients.

Patients using an insulin pump can be easily managed during the perioperative period. The pump is left on the basal rate and, because the patient is not taking meals prior to surgery, the dosing used for meals is not given.

Respiratory Diseases

Chronic obstructive pulmonary disease can pose a distinct problem in ophthalmic surgery. Cessation of smoking is extremely helpful in reducing intra- and postoperative coughing. Preoperative bronchopulmonary care with chest physiotherapy can decrease susceptibility to infection and improve air exchange. General anesthesia may be preferred over local anesthesia because the anesthesiologist may have better control over tracheal bronchial secretions and the cough reflex. (See also Chapter 6, Pulmonary Diseases.)

Preoperative Fasting

Questions often arise as to how long a patient must be kept on NPO status before surgery. A pediatric patient who is kept on NPO status for 10–12 hours preoperatively may become hypotensive as a result of dehydration. It has been shown that use of clear liquids orally up to 2 hours prior to surgery does not lead to any higher incidence of aspiration or other gastrointestinal complications of general anesthesia or local anesthesia.

The purpose of preoperative fasting is to reduce the particulate matter in the stomach and to lower the gastric fluid volume and acidity in case aspiration of stomach contents occurs. Diabetic patients, particularly those with autonomic neuropathy, are at risk for gastroparesis. Pregnant patients have a higher-than-normal risk of aspiration. In addition, patients with known gastroesophageal reflux and those with peptic ulcer disease may also have some increased risk of aspiration.

Oral administration of an H_2 blocker such as ranitidine or famotidine 2–4 hours prior to surgery reduces the percentage of patients with low gastric pH or high gastric volume. Metoclopramide and cisapride (restricted access in the United States) also promote intestinal motility and decrease reflux; these drugs are especially useful in a nonfasting patient who requires urgent surgery. (Table 15-2 lists selected perioperative medications.)

Latex Allergy

The overall prevalence of latex allergy has not been determined, but certain populations appear to be at particular risk for reactions. Health care workers and hospital employees

Table 15-2 Selected Perioperative Medications

Name (Generic and Brand)	Uses
Metoclopramide (Reglan)	Relief of gastric paresis, reduction of gastroesophageal reflux, perioperative antiemetic
Cisapride (Propulsid)	Reduction of gastroesophageal reflux
Midazolam (Versed)	Preoperative sedation
Propofol (Diprivan)	Preoperative sedation/general anesthesia
Diazepam (Valium)	Preoperative sedation
Alfentanil (Alfenta)	Analgesic/anesthetic
Fentanyl citrate (Sublimaze)	Analgesic/anesthetic
Methohexital (Brevital sodium)	Analgesic/anesthetic
Sufentanil (Sufenta)	Analgesic/anesthetic
Ondansetron (Zofran)	Postoperative antiemetic
Ketorolac (Toradol)	Postoperative analgesic

can experience progressive sensitization to latex because of repeated occupational exposure. This sensitivity is accentuated if the health care worker has a history of atopy. Certain medical populations also are at significant risk for latex allergy and anaphylaxis, including patients with myelodysplasia or spina bifida and those who have undergone repeated urinary catheterization or frequent surgical procedures. A cross-reactivity with bananas, avocados, mangoes, and chestnuts has been shown, and allergies to these foods have also been associated with latex allergy. Other implicated foods include apricots, celery, figs, grapes, papayas, passion fruit, peaches, and pineapples. A history of reactivity to balloons also suggests a latex allergy.

Patients suspected of having latex allergy should be clearly identified, and the operating room environment must be evaluated to care for them. Furthermore, an allergic patient should be the first case of the day in that particular operating room.

Universal Protocol

Wrong site surgery includes operating on the wrong site, performing the wrong procedure, or performing a procedure on the wrong person. In ophthalmology, wrong site includes operating on the wrong eye (right/left). Performing the wrong procedure includes implanting a lens with a style and power different from those of the one that was chosen during the preoperative surgical planning. Implanting a monofocal lens during cataract surgery, for example, when the plan was to implant a premium implant is considered the wrong procedure.

The Universal Protocol of the Joint Commission on Accreditation of Healthcare Organizations (www.jointcommission.org/standards_information/up.aspx) is designed to eliminate wrong site surgery; it includes several key elements:

- agreeing on and documenting the procedure to be performed (typically done on the surgical consent form)
- marking the surgical site in the preoperative period (done by a designated member of the team, typically the surgeon)

- pausing prior to beginning of surgery (time-out) to have all members of the surgical team agree that this is the correct patient and correct procedure; that the necessary equipment is present, including implants; that the patient is correctly positioned; that medical information on the patient, including x-rays, is for the correct patient; and that appropriate preoperative antibiotics have been given.

For the time-out to be effective, it is important that members of the surgical team feel empowered to speak up if they do not agree that all elements of the Universal Protocol have been met. Wrong site surgery is considered a sentinel event and in many states must be reported to the state board of medicine.

Intraoperative Complications

The use of balanced general anesthesia—in which small amounts of several different types of medications are titrated to avoid the side effects of a large dose of any one type—has been effective in reducing prolonged anesthesia and prolonged recovery time. Neuromuscular blocking agents of short duration (12 minutes for mivacurium and 30 minutes for atracurium and vecuronium) administered with an infusion pump allow the anesthesiologist to fine-tune the degree of neuromuscular blockade during balanced anesthesia.

The shorter-acting narcotics such as sufentanil have potencies up to 1000 times that of morphine. These agents help provide short-term stability of hemodynamics during intensive stimulation without the cost of prolonged excessive sedation postoperatively. Using such agents immediately before intubation as part of an anesthetic induction has become nearly universal.

Management of postoperative nausea and vomiting after general anesthesia has become easier with more powerful antinausea medications such as ondansetron and metoclopramide. These drugs do not cause sedation, as droperidol does, which means the patient in a same-day surgery setting recovers more quickly.

Postoperative pain can be prophylactically treated during the procedure with IV ketorolac in a 30- to 60-mg dose or with small titrated doses of IV fentanyl in the range of 50–100 µg. Because of the reported gastrointestinal complications of higher doses of ketorolac, patients over the age of 60 should receive a total of no more than 30 mg of IV ketorolac. Longer-acting narcotics, such as morphine or meperidine (Demerol), can delay a patient's discharge because of excessive sedation. Also, there is evidence that IV ketorolac, because of its pain-reducing qualities, can reduce the amount of postoperative nausea and vomiting in patients undergoing strabismus surgery and other procedures requiring general anesthesia. There is no evidence that this particular nonsteroidal anti-inflammatory drug increases postoperative bleeding during ophthalmic surgery.

Sedation is an important part of comfortable regional or general anesthesia in a patient undergoing elective surgery. Anxiolytics such as midazolam can be given intramuscularly (1–4 mg) 30–60 minutes before the procedure or intravenously (0.5–2.0 mg) 2–3 minutes before the stimulus of the anesthetic block. Midazolam is a more appropriate sedative than diazepam for outpatient surgery because its elimination half-life is 2–4 hours; diazepam's half-life is 20–40 hours. Midazolam can also be reversed with flumazenil. Careful IV titration of sedatives and narcotics is important in the older population to avoid oversedation or respiratory depression.

Alfentanil can be given intravenously in titrated doses with appropriate anesthesia monitoring. Its peak effect occurs in 1–2 minutes and lasts 10–20 minutes. Fentanyl citrate, which has a peak effect in 3–5 minutes and lasts about 30 minutes, is also given in titrated doses during regional or topical anesthesia. The effects of narcotics can be reversed with the antagonist naloxone, given intravenously. The duration of naloxone reversal is 1 hour or less.

Thiopental sodium, given in increments every 30 seconds, can be used to ensure amnesia and hypnosis for regional anesthesia or local infiltration of anesthetic agents. However, too rapid or too large a dose can depress hemodynamics and respiration. Methohexital can be similarly used in increments given intravenously every 20–30 seconds.

Propofol is a drug with unique properties of rapid hypnosis and a tendency to produce bradycardia, but it has rapid clearance with very little hangover. It must be given through a large-bore vein or administered after a lidocaine flush of the IV line to avoid significant burning on administration. Propofol is a lipid-based medication that supports rapid bacterial growth at room temperature. Indeed, extrinsically contaminated propofol has been associated with postoperative infections, including endogenous endophthalmitis. It is therefore imperative that hospital personnel involved in the preparation, handling, and administration of this drug adhere to strict aseptic technique during its use.

Local Anesthetic Agents

Screening for possible allergies to local anesthetic agents should be part of the preoperative evaluation. Local anesthetic injection into the retrobulbar space can lead to apnea, respiratory arrest, and cranial nerve palsies on the side being injected, or even on the opposite side. Anatomical studies of the position of the retrobulbar needle in relation to the optic nerve when the adducted or supraducted position of the eye is used during injection show that it is possible to inject anesthetic into the subdural space with a standard Atkinson-type needle. Cases of cranial nerve palsies associated with respiratory difficulties represent actual brainstem anesthesia from injection of the anesthetic agent into the subdural space, with subsequent diffusion into the circulating cerebrospinal fluid.

Several suggestions have been made to avoid such complications, including changing the traditional positioning of the eye during the retrobulbar anesthetic injection so the nerve is rotated away from the track of the needle—for example, by having the patient look straight ahead. Using less sharp, nondisposable retrobulbar needles less than 1¼ inches long also reduces the chance of perforating the optic nerve sheath. Although one series implicated the concentration of anesthetic as the cause of respiratory arrest, it is more likely that a larger volume and, therefore, a larger total dose of anesthetic was delivered to the brainstem through an inadvertent subdural injection. If apnea, respiratory arrest, or cranial neuropathies occur after a retrobulbar injection, the patient's airway must be supported with mask ventilation. Intubation and mechanical ventilation may be necessary. Apnea seldom lasts more than 30–50 minutes, but it is important that experienced medical personnel stabilize the patient's condition during this time. The peribulbar technique was devised, in part, to avoid such complications.

Respiratory distress and dysphagia can result from the Nadbath block, an injection into the stylomastoid foramen that is used to provide facial akinesia. These complications occur when the anesthetic agent is injected deeply into the area of the facial nerve as it exits the stylomastoid foramen, and the anesthetic bathes cranial nerves IX, X, and XI as they exit the jugular foramen. This leads to paralysis of these nerves, and the patient becomes dysphagic, begins to cough or has a hoarse voice, and may develop stridor or severe respiratory insufficiency. The complications tend to occur in thin persons, in whom it is easier to bury the needle deeply. Managing the respiratory distress requires suctioning the pharynx, positioning the patient on his or her side, and supplementing the patient's inspired gases with oxygen or even intubation. This complication can be avoided by use of a short hypodermic needle, advancing it only partway into the area to be injected, and injecting a small volume (<3 mL).

Anesthetic toxicity can occur when high concentrations of anesthetic agent are given. For example, if 4% lidocaine is used for a peribulbar injection, the total volume that can be safely given to a 154-lb (70-kg) patient is limited to 8 mL. A smaller patient would be able to tolerate no more than 5 mL of 4% lidocaine without risking complications of systemic toxicity, including confusion, cardiac arrhythmias, and respiratory depression.

Seizures have occurred from the intra-arterial injection of local anesthetic agent into the ophthalmic artery. Such seizures are instantaneous with injection; supportive measures should include airway maintenance and blood pressure support. The seizures are of short duration.

Rathi V, Basti S, Gupta S. Globe rupture during digital massage after peribulbar anesthesia. *J Cataract Refract Surg.* 1997;23(2):297–299.

Malignant Hyperthermia

A preoperative personal and family history can help determine patients at risk for *malignant hyperthermia (MH)*. Patients determined to be at high risk for MH may require a muscle biopsy for muscle contracture testing or genetic study focused on the *RYR1* gene. Nevertheless, such preoperative screening is not infallible, and the surgeon and anesthesiologist should be prepared to respond to this complication. MH is a disorder of calcium binding by the sarcoplasmic reticulum of skeletal muscles. In the presence of an anesthetic triggering agent, unbound intracellular calcium increases, which stimulates muscle contracture. This increased metabolism outstrips oxygen delivery, and anaerobic metabolism develops, with the production of lactate and subsequent massive acidosis. Hyperthermia thus results from the hypermetabolic state.

The earliest signs of MH include tachycardia that is greater than expected for the patient's anesthetic and surgical status and elevated end-tidal carbon dioxide level when the patient is monitored by capnography. Labile blood pressure, tachypnea, sweating, muscle rigidity, blotchy discoloration of skin, cyanosis, and dark urine all signal progression of the disorder. Temperature elevation, which can reach extremely high levels, is a relatively late sign. Ultimately, respiratory and metabolic acidosis, hyperkalemia, hypercalcemia, myoglobinuria, and renal failure can occur, as can disseminated intravascular coagulation and death.

Although volatile anesthetics such as halothane, enflurane, isoflurane, and intravenous succinylcholine are all known to trigger MH, haloperidol, trimeprazine, and promethazine can also cause this condition.

If a surgeon wishes to avoid the use of succinylcholine, a laryngeal mask airway can be considered for strabismus surgery in adults if muscle relaxation is not otherwise required. The use of the laryngeal mask airway reduces the soreness and irritation of the throat that occurs after oral endotracheal intubation.

Malignant hyperthermia is treated as a medical emergency (Table 15-3 has the treatment protocol). The Malignant Hyperthermia Association of the United States (MHAUS) staffs a 24-hour hotline to advise medical personnel on the diagnosis and treatment of MH at (800) 644-9737.

Kay MC, Kay J. Complications of anesthesia for ocular surgery. In: Charlton JF, Weinstein GW, eds. *Ophthalmic Surgery Complications: Prevention and Management.* Philadelphia: Lippincott; 1995.

Miller RD, Eriksson LI, Fleisher LA, Wiener-Kronish JP, Young WL, eds. *Miller's Anesthesia.* 7th ed. Philadelphia: Elsevier/Churchill Livingstone; 2010.

Van Norman G. Preoperative management of common minor medical issues in the outpatient setting. *Anesthesiol Clin North Am.* 1996;14(4):655–678.

Table 15-3 Malignant Hyperthermia Protocol

1. Stop the triggering agents immediately, and conclude surgery as soon as possible.
2. Hyperventilate with 100% oxygen at high flow rates.
3. Administer:
   a. Dantrolene: 2–3 mg/kg initial bolus with increments up to 10 mg/kg total. Continue to administer dantrolene until symptoms are controlled. Occasionally, a dose greater than 10 mg/kg may be needed.
   b. Sodium bicarbonate: 1-2 mEq/kg increments guided by arterial pH and pCO_2. Bicarbonate will combat hyperkalemia by driving potassium into cells.
4. Actively cool patient:
   a. If needed, IV iced saline (not Ringer's lactate) 15 mL/kg q 10 minutes × 3. Monitor closely.
   b. Lavage stomach, bladder, rectum, and peritoneal and thoracic cavities with iced saline.
   c. Surface cool with ice and hypothermia blanket.
5. Maintain urine output. If needed, administer mannitol 0.25 g/kg IV, furosemide 1 mg/kg IV (up to 4 doses each). Urine output greater than 2 mL/kg/hr may help prevent subsequent renal failure.
6. Calcium channel blockers *should not* be given when dantrolene is administered, as hyperkalemia and myocardial depression may occur.
7. Insulin for hyperkalemia: Add 10 units of regular insulin to 50 mL of 50% glucose and titrate to control hyperkalemia. Monitor blood glucose and potassium levels.
8. Postoperatively: Continue dantrolene 1 mg/kg IV q 6 hours × 72 hours to prevent recurrence. Lethal recurrences of MH may occur. Observe in an intensive care unit.
9. For expert medical advice and further medical evaluation, call the MHAUS MH hotline consultant at (800) 644-9737. For nonemergency professional or patient information, call (800) 986-4287 or go to www.mhaus.org.

CHAPTER **16**

Using Statistics in Practice and Work

The role of clinical research is vital in establishing a standard of care for patients. Such research is best performed using an interdisciplinary approach that combines the efforts of the clinician, statistician, and epidemiologist from the conception of the study through data analyses and interpretation. The choice of study design depends on the research questions to be answered, the population available, and the resources and effort to be expended. If a study finds a statistical association, that association may be considered valid after alternative explanations—such as chance, bias, and confounding—have been ruled out. Furthermore, the association may be more credible if it is a consistent finding in other studies. This chapter is intended to encourage the clinician to critically review the results of clinical research and to apply the results to the clinical practice of ophthalmology.

Obtaining Useful Information From Published Studies

In trying to obtain useful information from studies for resolving either diagnostic or management issues, first assess the question to be answered. Numerous tools are available for obtaining specific factual information from the literature for questions such as the following: What is the prevalence of glaucoma in African Americans? Are African Americans and Mexican Americans at greater risk of having open-angle glaucoma than are Caucasians? Obtaining information on questions like the following, regarding the outcome of specific surgical procedures, can also be relatively straightforward: What is the expected survival of a corneal graft in a person with Fuchs dystrophy? However, responses to other questions, such as, How soon can a person go swimming in the ocean after cataract extraction? are unlikely to be found in any database, because they depend primarily on the experience of experts in the field. Therefore, before attempting to access medical literature, try to determine if the required type of information is likely to be there.

Once that determination has been made, various sources are available from which to choose. These include general textbooks of ophthalmology (eg, *Duane's Ophthalmology*), journals with more detailed information on specific subjects (eg, *Survey of Ophthalmology* [www.ophsource.org/periodicals/sop]), and educational material from the American Academy of Ophthalmology (http://one.aao.org/) (eg, Preferred Practice Patterns [PPP] and Focal Points).

In addition, high-quality meta-analyses of specific management issues (eg, surgery for nonarteritic ischemic optic neuropathy, intervention for involutional lower lid ectropion) can be obtained from the Cochrane Library (www2.cochrane.org/reviews). For more specific, primary sources of information, search Medline/PubMed (www.ncbi.nlm.nih.gov/pubmed). References cited in review articles or other papers of interest and back issues of various journals, such as the following, may be helpful:

- *American Journal of Ophthalmology* (http://ajo.com)
- *Archives of Ophthalmology* (http://archopht.ama-assn.org)
- *Ophthalmology (*www.ophsource.org/periodicals/ophtha)

When performing online searches, refine the search question and use specific keywords; detailed information on using appropriate keywords can be found on the PubMed website. Such searches usually reveal various types of primary sources, from laboratory basic science studies (cell culture, molecular biology) to animal studies (testing new drugs or specific surgical techniques); and from clinical case reports or case series to randomized clinical trials. Searches can be narrowed or widened as needed.

Searches sometimes retrieve articles that suggest different answers to the original question. At this stage, researchers must consider critical issues with regard to each specific study, such as whether the information answers the real question of interest. Such consideration can provide the clinician with the confidence needed to translate the findings into clinical practice.

In evaluating a published study, and before committing time to a critical reading, the clinician must determine if the question being posed in the study aims or introduction is the real question of interest. For example, if the clinician is interested in determining whether use of a prostaglandin is beneficial in patients with open-angle glaucoma (OAG), then examining data from the Early Manifest Glaucoma Trial (EMGT) would not be useful (prostaglandins were not used in EMGT), whereas data from specific drug trials would be important. The key issue here is that the intervention in the 2 studies was different, even though the effect of both interventions was to lower intraocular pressure (IOP). However, if the question of interest is whether lowering IOP is beneficial in patients with OAG, then both types of studies might be useful. Thus, careful evaluation of the question is very important.

Next, determine if the conclusions of the study are believable. There are 2 specific questions to consider:

1. Are the results valid, reliable, and reproducible?
2. Are the results generalizable, or are they applicable to particular patients?

These questions entail examining several additional factors: specific issues related to the participants/patients, sample size, intervention, outcomes, and statistical methodology and inferences.

Participants and Setting

Is there a clear description of the selection process of study participants (which patients were included and excluded)? This description lays the groundwork for understanding the setting of the study. Was it a clinic-based study, was it multicentered, or was it a community-based trial? For therapeutic trials, patient inclusion and exclusion criteria identify the characteristics of those who were or were not treated with an intervention. Specific patient groups may have been excluded because they were considered a vulnerable population. For example, because most ocular hypotensive drug trials exclude children and pregnant women, there is minimal data on the safety and efficacy of most ocular hypotensive agents in these 2 groups. Thus, if a decision needs to be made on whether to use a specific ocular hypotensive agent in a pregnant woman or in a child, most of the evidence can be found only in individual case reports or retrospective case series.

The next consideration is determining if the results of a specific study can be directly applied to particular patients. The first step in this process is determining if there was selection bias in assigning an intervention to certain participants. The questions to be considered here are, Was the intervention randomly assigned? Was the treated group comparable to the control group? The purpose of randomly assigning an intervention to a specific participant is that randomization helps minimize bias. If only those participants with particular characteristics are assigned a particular intervention, and the control group is not, then the intervention effect may be underestimated or overestimated, and the true effect will be difficult to determine. Selection bias can be found when well-meaning clinicians assign a more invasive intervention to patients with more advanced disease, which means the more invasive treatment is likely to have poorer outcomes. Random allocation reduces the likelihood of selection bias. However, it does not always ensure that the participants assigned to each of the intervention groups are similar. To determine this question, study the baseline participant characteristics that may impact the outcome. For example, in a study assessing the effect of lasers for treatment of diabetic retinopathy, the diabetic control, the blood pressure, and the types of medications should be similar in the 2 groups because these factors are likely to have an effect on progression and regression of the retinopathy.

Another consideration in evaluating the generalizability and applicability of a study's results is the severity of disease in the participants included in the study. Was only 1 disease severity group studied, or were the participants representative of different stages of disease, such as mild, moderate, and severe disease? Clinical trials usually study a selected disease severity, making the results applicable and generalizable only to patients with similar disease severity. A common error is extrapolating such data to all patients and their varying degrees of severity of disease. For example, if a particular treatment effect size is noted in patients with mild glaucomatous damage who underwent trabeculectomy but not in those with advanced glaucomatous damage, the application of this study's results should be limited to patients with early glaucoma damage, not generalized to those with advanced glaucomatous damage. Thus, the generalizability of a study's results is guided by the characteristics of the participants included in the study, and any application of the results should be limited to patients with similar characteristics.

Sample Size Determination

Was the sample size (the number of participants in the study) determined before the initiation of the trial and, if so, what criteria were used to determine sample size? The goal of clinical trials is to disprove the null hypothesis, which states that the impact of the intervention in terms of primary outcomes is no different from that of outcomes without the intervention. Sample size is calculated to maximize the likelihood of disproving the null hypothesis. The estimate of sample size is usually based on the expected size of the treatment effect on the primary outcome (eg, improvement in visual acuity, reduction of IOP, proportion of participants with resolution of macular edema). In general, if a large treatment effect is expected, then the sample size needed in a particular study is smaller than that which is needed if a small treatment effect is expected. The estimated effect size is usually based on the available literature. The sample size must be determined carefully. It is not appropriate to change the sample size midway through a study when the initial results do not bear out the prior assumptions of effect size.

Issues Related to Intervention

Was the intervention clearly described, and is it reproducible? In most drug studies, the concentration of the drug is provided in the report, but the details of the other components in the medication may not always be clearly stated. Similarly, in surgical studies, a clear description of the procedure is needed to assess whether and how well other surgeons can perform the procedure. In addition, it is useful to know if the intervention is reproducible, a critical aspect often not addressed. In studies assessing the benefits of drugs, standardization of concentration and content of the drugs is rigorous, as manufacturers have to comply with strict federal guidelines for preparing medications. The concentration and content of the medications can be tested during the course of the trial; testing ensures that the medications have been formulated in a consistent manner.

Unlike with drug studies, similar rigor in ensuring consistency is not generally exercised or reported in surgical studies. The surgical procedure should allow different surgeons to perform it in the same manner in each case. In studies comparing different surgical methods or use of medications versus surgery, the surgical method must be performed in a reproducible manner across all participants who received that intervention. Although surgical standardization cannot be perfect, training all participating surgeons before starting the study, monitoring specific aspects of the surgical procedure during the study, and standardizing postoperative care would help ensure such uniformity.

Issues Related to Outcome

Were the outcome measures clearly defined, and were they measured in a reliable/objective manner? Outcome measures are usually specific for the disease under study. However, most ocular studies also include a measure of visual acuity and may include other clinical measurements, such as an assessment of visual fields, color vision, IOP, or change in a structural abnormality such as macular edema or leakage of fluid in the retina. At the outset of a study, the primary and secondary outcomes should be clearly stated. These outcomes are then used to determine whether the study was able to prove or disprove the null hypothesis. In most studies, the outcome measure, as well as the magnitude of the outcome measure, must be given. For example, if the primary outcome measure is improvement in visual acuity, it is essential to state whether the improvement is 2 lines (or 10 letters) or 3 lines (15 letters). Similarly, the magnitude of the outcome measure can be stated clearly for other measures, such as IOP, intraocular inflammation, and pain relief.

Many outcomes in vision research (eg, vision; IOP; macular thickness, measured with optical coherence tomography [OCT]) are subject to measurement error. Assessment of these outcomes needs to be standardized across different observers and at different centers. For example, when assessing change in the lens, specifically describing its appearance and comparing it to a photographic standard used to assess lens opacification would be useful. Also, those who assess outcome measures should be masked to the intervention, because this reduces the likelihood of measurement bias. Measurement bias is present when an observer assesses a particular outcome variable as either higher or lower than its true value based on the type of intervention. Such an underestimation or overestimation is likely to affect the outcome of the trial.

Validity

The validity of a study is anchored on (1) adequate duration of follow-up, and (2) follow-up of all participants. Thus, in evaluating a study, ask, Was there adequate follow-up of the participants after the intervention? Was the outcome in all participants reported at the conclusion of the study? The duration of follow-up of study participants can determine whether or not a specific outcome is realized. For example, in evaluating the use of atropine eyedrops versus patching in treating amblyopia, a follow-up of 3–6 months may be adequate; similar follow-up periods may be adequate and appropriate in evaluating macular edema resolution after laser or drug therapy or visual acuity improvement after cataract extraction. However, because of glaucoma's slow progression rates, trials assessing visual field loss in glaucoma would require many years of follow-up. Thus, the typical rate of disease progression is an important guide in determining the duration of follow-up required.

Follow-up of all participants in terms of the primary outcome is also critical to a study's validity. This may not be practical or feasible in all cases because of dropout from a study (eg, due to death during follow-up). For cases of dropout not due to death during the follow-up period, determining the reasons for loss to follow-up is essential, as they may suggest problems with the treatments given to those participants. For example, participants in a drug trial may drop out if they frequently get untoward ocular side effects such as burning or stinging from the drug.

Clinical Relevance Issues

Issues related to clinical relevance are central to the decision as to whether a study's results can be applied to the management of patients.

- Is the intervention clinically applicable in the current practice environment?
- Are the outcomes clinically important?
- Are all clinically important outcomes evaluated?
- Is the effect of the treatment both statistically and clinically significant?

The first issue to consider is whether the intervention being studied is likely to be used in practice. If the intervention is too expensive, if it can be performed by only a few physicians, or if it is no longer in general use, then there is little benefit in evaluating the study.

Next, attention should be directed at the outcomes being evaluated. Usually, the statistical tests used to determine the difference between 2 groups depend on the nature of the data. If the data are normally distributed (ie, conform more or less to a bell-shaped curve) and are of a continuous nature (eg, macular thickness in a trial determining the value of intravitreal corticosteroids for treatment of diabetic macular edema), then a Student *t* test comparing the treated and control groups can be performed. For normally distributed data that are expressed as categories (present or absent; small, medium, or large), a χ-square test is used. For data that are not normally distributed, nonparametric tests such as the Wilcoxon rank sum test can be used. All of these tests provide a *P* value that states the likelihood with which a difference between the 2 groups may be from chance alone. Thus, a *P* value of <.05 means that the likelihood that the difference between the 2 groups is due to random chance alone is less than 5%. The lower the P value, the lower the likelihood that the difference is by chance and the more likely it is that the difference is a true difference.

Statistical differences are not the only important factor. Clinically meaningful differences must also be present. In vision research, visual acuity is often a primary outcome variable. However, if the magnitude of the difference being evaluated is an improvement of 3–5 letters, or 1 line or less, on the visual acuity chart, then this difference is within the margin of measurement error and likely does not provide clinically meaningful results. A change of more than 10 letters, or 2 lines, on the visual acuity chart is clinically meaningful. Similarly, in an ocular hypotensive drug trial, an IOP difference of 1 mm Hg is within the measurement error and is likely to not be clinically meaningful, whereas a difference of 3 mm Hg or more may be. Thus, even though a statistical test may suggest a statistically significant difference, the magnitude and nature of the difference are critical to determining if the difference between the 2 interventions is truly clinically meaningful. This point needs to be highlighted because it is useful to consider implementing only those interventions that are both statistically and clinically significant. In addition to evaluating these primary outcome variables, the study should also evaluate secondary clinically important variables related to the safety of the intervention. These variables include dropout rates, pain, allergic reactions, systemic reactions, and death.

Clinical Study Designs

Information about a disease process and its appropriate management can be gained from a wide array of study designs. In *observational studies,* also known as *nonexperimental studies,* people are assessed with respect to their personal characteristics, behaviors, and exposures in relation to their having a particular disease or condition or having a particular complication of the disease. The investigator notes only what has happened and does not directly manipulate the behavior (eg, cigarette smoking) or exposures (eg, use of a medication or treatment with laser) of the patient. In *experimental studies,* typically clinical trials, subjects are assigned a particular treatment, where treatment is used broadly to describe a prescribed behavior (eg, eat a diet high in antioxidant foods) or a therapeutic or preventive intervention (eg, oral neuroprotective agent for patients with glaucoma or antioxidant vitamin supplement for patients with early age-related maculopathy [ARM] at risk of vision loss from the development of late ARM).

When well conducted and appropriately interpreted, each study design yields valuable information. Observational studies are best used for describing the presentation and progression of disease, generating hypotheses, and efficiently assessing data that may already exist for consistency with a hypothesis about an intervention. However, the best evidence on the effects of an intervention is obtained through randomized clinical trials and, when multiple clinical trials have been conducted to address the same or a very similar question, meta-analyses (Fig 16-1).

Case Reports

A report on a single patient can provide valuable information by demonstrating that something unusual can happen under particular circumstances. Reporting unusual presentations of a serious disease may help others recognize the condition. For example, Friedman reported on a patient who presented with retinal vasculitis and who was apparently healthy and free of conditions typically associated with retinal vasculitis, such as toxoplasmosis, syphilis, Behçet syndrome, sarcoidosis, lupus, and herpes. A magnetic resonance image (MRI) scan of the brain revealed findings typical of multiple sclerosis (MS). Although patients with an established history of MS are known to develop retinal vasculitis, this was the first patient who reported with retinal vasculitis as the initial presentation of MS. The author has advised evaluating a patient for MS when the etiology of retinal vasculitis remains unclear after testing for the more common causes.

Case reports cannot provide information on treatment efficacy or on causal mechanisms. At most, they can suggest that a previously unsuspected effect or mechanism might exist. Other study designs, as described in the following sections, can be used to address efficacy and mechanisms.

Friedman SM. Retinal vasculitis as the initial presentation of multiple sclerosis. *Retina.* 2005;25: 218–219.

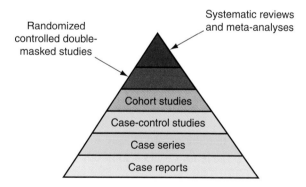

Figure 16-1 The pyramid of evidence from different study designs. *(Adapted from Medical Research Library of Brooklyn. Available at http://library.downstate.edu/ebm/2100.htm.)*

Case Series

Case series are investigations of the presentation, history, and/or follow-up of patients that can provide valuable information on the natural history of a disease or on the prognosis for groups of patients managed in the same way. The methods for subject selection, the assessment of patient characteristics, and the length and completeness of follow-up determine the quality of a case series, and clinicians must consider all of these in deciding if the results of a case series pertain to their particular patients.

Case selection factors

Often, case series are based on patients seen in university-based clinical practices that may serve as tertiary referral centers. These settings may serve patients with particularly severe disease or may have a higher proportion of patients with features that make the disease not amenable to widely available treatments. Characteristics of the presentation and prognosis of patients in a case series may differ dramatically from those of patients seen by a community ophthalmologist. A case series by Margherio and coworkers described the characteristics of consecutive patients with choroidal neovascularization secondary to age-related macular degeneration (AMD) seen in a large practice of retina specialists. The location and composition of neovascular lesions that determined a patient's suitability for either thermal laser treatment or photodynamic therapy with verteporfin may not have been representative of all neovascular lesions that can be seen, because the ophthalmologists whom patients saw for routine care might not have referred all cases, some because they could be treated easily with a thermal laser and some because they were already too large for any treatment. The time period of the collection of the case series may also have a major effect on the prognosis of patients, because of changes in medical management of diseases. A striking example of this is the change in prognosis of HIV patients with cytomegalovirus retinitis after the introduction of highly active antiretroviral therapy (HAART).

> Margherio RR, Margherio AR, DeSantis ME. Laser treatments with verteporfin therapy and its potential impact on retinal practices. *Retina.* 2000;20(4):325–330.

Assessment of patient characteristics

The methods used for measurements, tests, and other evaluations in case series are typically not standardized and may be subject to a high degree of variability. Often, case series are prepared from a review of existing medical records provided by a number of ophthalmologists. Such retrospective collection of data suffers from differing levels of detail across patients and from missing or incomplete information. For example, the technicians, examination rooms, lighting, and/or charts used to measure visual acuity may differ among ophthalmologic offices. In addition to the variability introduced by nonstandardized testing conditions, acuity may be recorded only to the nearest whole line in some charts (20/25) but recorded to the letter (20/25 + 2) in other charts.

Length and completeness of follow-up

Case series that report on the course of patients need to appropriately accommodate the differing lengths of follow-up for patients. Often, cases are collected over a long period, as for example, 1996–2000, so that at the time of chart review in 2005, patients would be expected to have between 5 and 9 years of follow-up. Particularly for characteristics that are likely to change progressively over time (eg, visual fields in patients with glaucoma), reporting on the average change observed among all patients does not provide an adequate description of the course of disease. When the length of follow-up varies, the data should be reported at specific follow-up times, such as at 1, 2, and 3 years after the initiation of treatment. When the outcome measure is an event, such as corneal graft failure, survival analysis can account appropriately for the varying lengths of follow-up. If not all patients are followed for the full length of the possible follow-up period, the reported outlook for the case series may be biased because of losses to follow-up. When a case series is based on review of medical charts, losses to follow-up may be related strongly to how the patient fares over time. For example, in a case series of patients with macular edema from branch retinal vein occlusion, some patients may have chosen not to return because their macular edema resolved and their vision improved; some patients may have suffered further loss of vision and sought care from another ophthalmologist; and some patients may have had no major change in vision and moved to another location. When a large percentage of patients have not returned for complete follow-up, the generalizability of the description of the course of patients becomes limited, because the returning patients may have had an unusually good or unusually bad course.

Case-Control Studies

Case-control studies are observational study designs used to investigate the association between exposures, or potential risk factors (eg, smoking, medical conditions, therapies), and outcomes (eg, loss of visual acuity, development of glaucoma, corneal graft failure, cataract surgery). In case-control studies, one group of participants is selected because these individuals have the disease of interest (cases), and another group of comparable individuals is selected because they are free of disease (controls). The past exposures and characteristics of the cases and controls are compared. If an exposure is more (or less) common in the cases than in the controls, the exposure is considered associated with the disease (Fig 16-2).

Case-control studies are often performed as a first approach to investigating a hypothesis, generated from laboratory findings or from case reports and series, that a factor is associated with a disease. Typically, though not always, the cases and controls are selected from currently available groups, and the history of exposures is obtained through patient interview and/or review of medical records. Thus, compared with cohort studies (discussed later in the chapter), which often require extended periods of subsequent follow-up, case-control studies can be performed relatively quickly and inexpensively. In addition, many potential risk factors can be evaluated simultaneously if the history is gathered while records are reviewed or the patient is questioned.

However, these advantages are often overshadowed by the inaccuracies introduced when exposure data are gathered from records and patients are asked to recall information. In addition to the problems described previously for case series, case-control studies may suffer from bias that distorts the true association between the exposure and the disease.

Case-control study

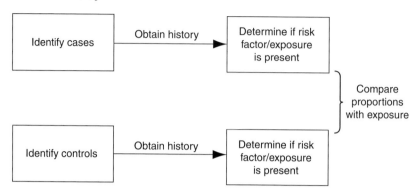

Cohort study

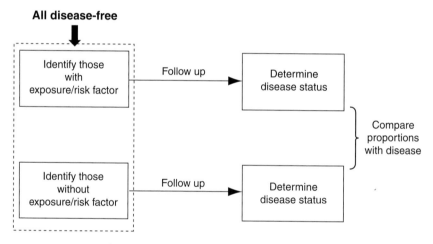

Figure 16-2 Simplified schematics of observational study designs.

For example, patients with retinal vein occlusion (cases) may be much more likely to recall taking medications of any type (eg, aspirin) because of efforts to figure out what caused the occlusion, whereas controls might be less likely to remember taking medications because they have not been motivated to scrutinize their past behavior. Therefore, a higher proportion of cases than controls might report use of aspirin in the past 6 months, even if in truth the proportion of aspirin users was the same in both cases and controls. The apparent increased exposure to aspirin in cases would be attributable solely to recall bias.

Another common challenge in case-control studies is selecting an appropriate control group. For example, if controls for cases with retinal vein occlusion are chosen from a general ophthalmology practice, the proportion of cases with myopia might be much lower than the proportion of controls, because a high proportion of some general ophthalmology practices may be devoted to providing refractive correction for myopic patients. Comparing the proportion of myopic patients in the case and control groups would show an apparent protective effect of myopia. However, the apparent association could be attributable totally to selection bias. A full discussion of the many potential sources of bias is beyond the scope of this chapter; however, such a discussion can be found in most textbooks in epidemiology.

The association between statin use and AMD was investigated by McGwin and colleagues through a database compiled as part of a major study on atherosclerosis. Study participants had fundus photographs taken at one of the required visits; subjects were classified as cases if macular drusen and/or pigmentary changes were present. Electronic records from previous visits were assessed for statin use. Among 871 cases of AMD, 11% had a history of statin use; of 11,717 controls, 12.3% had used statins. After consideration of additional factors known to be associated with AMD, the authors found that the slightly higher proportion of statin users in the control group was statistically significant and concluded that the data supported statin use as a protective factor. In the study, the authors collected data prospectively using standard methods because the patients were involved in an atherosclerosis study. The data were complete and relatively free of bias because of the use of standardized questionnaires that asked about current, rather than past, use of medications. However, in this instance, it is not possible to know whether the drusen and pigmentary changes were present before the drugs were used or if they developed afterward. As patients with early AMD are usually asymptomatic, these subjects may have had the macular changes for a long time before they were photographed.

McGwin G Jr, Xie A, Owsley C. The use of cholesterol-lowering medications and age-related macular degeneration. *Ophthalmology.* 2005;112(3):488–494.

Cross-sectional Studies

Cross-sectional studies also relate exposures and risk factors to the presence or absence of a disease or condition; however, the timing or sequencing of exposure and development of disease is not known. A study in which an ophthalmologist notes the lens status (phakic, pseudophakic, or aphakic) for all scheduled patients arriving for their appointments and in which each of the patients provides a blood sample would be an example of a cross-sectional study. Patients could be classified with respect to whether they have had cataract surgery (case status) and with respect to their cholesterol level and gender (potential risk factors). We might find that the mean cholesterol level in the patients with cataract surgery was much higher than the mean for those without cataract surgery, a finding that would be consistent with the association between high cholesterol level and increased risk of cataract surgery. However, it would not be known whether the cholesterol level was elevated before the onset of lens opacification and the cataract surgery. In addition, as with both case-control and cohort studies (discussed next), there is concern that the apparent association is attributable to confounding factors. For this study, age could be a confounding factor, because cholesterol levels are known to increase with age, as does the likelihood of cataract surgery. Researchers could use stratification and/or regression analyses to adjust for age and then determine if the cholesterol–cataract surgery association persisted.

Cohort Studies

Cohort, or follow-up, studies are another observational study design used to investigate the association between exposures, or potential risk factors, and patient outcomes. In these studies, individuals who are free of the disease of interest are identified and classified by the presence or absence of potential risk factors, and their subsequent development of the disease is assessed (see Fig 16-2).

The Beaver Dam Eye Study has yielded many cohort studies examining several ocular conditions and many different potential risk factors. Approximately 5000 residents of Beaver Dam, Wisconsin, were examined and interviewed and then followed up for 10 years for the incidence of ocular disease. Researchers explored potential risk factors for diseases such as AMD, diabetic retinopathy, glaucoma, and cataract using the residents' exposures at the beginning of the study and the incidence of the diseases 5 and 10 years later. For example, the investigators classified participants without late-stage AMD at the initial examination according to a number of potential risk factors (age, gender, presence of pigmentary changes, drusen characteristics) for progression to that stage. The incidence of late AMD was 15% among eyes with pigmentary changes, 0.4% among eyes without pigmentary changes; the incidence for eyes with soft, indistinct drusen was 20%, compared with 0.8% for eyes without such drusen.

The Beaver Dam Eye Study is an example of a population-based cohort study with prospective data collection. However, groups with and without the potential risk factors may be clinic-based, and the data collection may be retrospective. For example, Strahlman and colleagues were interested in the development of choroidal neovascularization in the second eye of patients who already had neovascularization in the first eye. At the clinical center, retinal photography was available for the fellow eye at the time the patient presented with neovascularization in the first eye. Patients were recalled and examined for the development of neovascularization in the second eye. Patients with large, confluent drusen present at the time of the diagnosis of neovascularization in the first eye were found to have a higher risk of developing neovascularization in the second eye. Because the retinal photographs were retrieved from the patients' medical records, the data collection is considered retrospective; because patients were classified based on their earlier fellow-eye drusen status, and the incidence of neovascularization was compared between the groups with and without confluent drusen, the study is considered a cohort study.

Cohort studies can provide apparently strong links between risk factors and disease. The primary weakness of this study design is that the participants with the risk factor of interest may differ in many ways from those without the risk factor. If those with the risk factor differ from those without it on other factors that affect the incidence of the disease, then the apparent association may have been induced by those other differences. An example of this is the use of interrupted sutures, rather than running sutures, in corneal transplantation. If researchers follow up patients for incidence of graft failure, they find a much higher proportion of graft failure among patients with interrupted sutures.

However, concluding that use of interrupted sutures increases the risk of graft failure would be wrong. Interrupted sutures are often used on patients at high risk of graft failure because of such conditions as stromal vascularization, which increases the risk of immunologic rejection. These eyes are much more likely to have an established, strong risk factor for graft failure; hence, the apparent higher risk of graft failure in the eyes with interrupted sutures. In this example, stromal vascularization is a confounding factor. Statistical analysis techniques, such as stratified analysis and regression analysis, can adjust for the effect of known confounding factors. However, most often, not all of the factors that affect the incidence of disease are known or measured, and confounding factors may be hidden from view. For this reason, although cohort studies may identify strong associations between risk factors and disease incidence, the associations are not considered clear evidence of a causal role.

Klein R, Klein BE, Tomany SC, Meuer SM, Huang GH. Ten-year incidence and progression of age-related maculopathy: the Beaver Dam Eye Study. *Ophthalmology.* 2002;109(10): 1767–1779.

Clinical Trials

Clinical trials are similar to cohort studies (see Fig 16-2) in concept, with 1 major difference: in clinical trials, patients are assigned to treatment groups (exposure groups) randomly (Fig 16-3). Randomized treatment assignment generally yields treatment groups that are similar on all known and unknown risk factors for developing the disease or condition of interest. Randomized treatment assignment is the only way to substantially reduce the effect of confounding variables that bedevil other study designs. Its importance cannot be overstated.

However, randomization alone does not ensure that the information generated from clinical trials on the effects of interventions is valid. All of the features mentioned

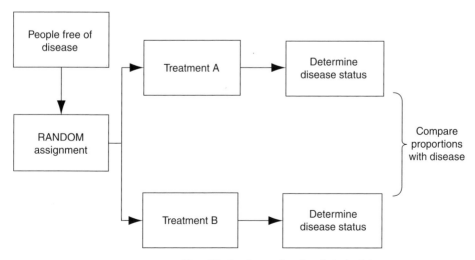

Figure 16-3 Simplified schematic of a clinical trial.

previously as improving the quality of observational studies should be applied to randomized clinical trials:

- well-defined trial objective
- explicit inclusion and exclusion criteria
- adequate sample size
- standardized procedures
- predefined and objective primary and secondary outcome measures
- patients, treaters, and evaluators who are masked to the assigned treatment
- complete follow-up of all patients

The CONSORT (Consolidated Standards of Reporting Trials) guidelines, which have been adopted by most medical journals, provide a comprehensive listing of the features that should be considered when designing trials and that should be included in reports of clinical trials.

Although the results of a properly designed, well-executed, randomized clinical trial should be easy to interpret, 2 complicating issues may arise. The first is excluding patients from data analysis for any of the following reasons: they did not meet all of the eligibility criteria; they had side effects and stopped treatment; or they were noncompliant with the treatment regimen. Exclusion of patients can strongly bias the apparent results of a clinical trial, because the reasons for exclusion are nearly always related in some way to the trial outcome measure. An intention-to-treat analysis includes the data from all patients assigned treatment in a clinical trial and should be the primary analysis.

The second issue is the interpretation of results from subgroups of patients (eg, young versus old; hypertensive vs nonhypertensive). Even if there is no overall benefit of treatment, researchers can almost always identify a subgroup of patients that have a statistically significant benefit of treatment. Minor differences in treatment effect across subgroups are expected because of random variation. Conclusions that a particular subgroup benefits more from treatment than do others are strongest when the subgroup is identified before the trial data are examined; when there is statistical evidence of treatment variability across the subgroups; and when there is a biologically plausible explanation for the finding.

Moher D, Schulz KF, Altman DG. The CONSORT statement: revised recommendations for improving the quality of reports of parallel-group randomised trials. *Lancet.* 2001;357(9263): 1191–1194.

Systematic Reviews and Meta-analyses of Clinical Trials

The strongest evidence for assessing interventions for a particular condition comes from systematic reviews and meta-analyses that combine the evidence from 2 or more clinical trials studying the intervention. In ophthalmology, rarely has more than one high-quality randomized clinical trial of any 1 treatment been carried out, so these types of reviews and meta-analyses are done infrequently. When they are, the Cochrane Eyes and Vision Group often publishes the results. For example, Leyland and Zinicola reviewed the results of 3 multicenter and 5 single-center randomized clinical trials of multifocal versus monofocal intraocular lenses after cataract extraction. Using special statistical methods for combining data from multiple trials, they found no statistically significant difference between the 2 lens types in unaided and aided distance visual acuity; statistically significant better near vision and less need for glasses with multifocal lenses; and significantly more patients experiencing glare, halos, and reduced contrast sensitivity with multifocal lenses.

Leyland M, Zinicola E. Multifocal versus monofocal intraocular lenses after cataract extraction. *Cochrane Database Syst Rev.* 2003;(3):CD003169.

Rothman KJ, Greenland S, Lash TL. *Modern Epidemiology.* 3rd ed. Philadelphia: Lippincott Williams & Wilkens; 2008.

Interpreting Diagnostic or Screening Tests

The best way to learn how to interpret diagnostic or screening tests is to start with the simplest, most straightforward clinical situation: a screening test with a binary (yes/no) outcome that has been well studied by multiple investigators and that has been used in a wide variety of populations; a disease that the patient definitely either has or does not have; and a patient about whom nothing is known at the time of screening. Gradually, insert complicating features, those that often appear in routine ophthalmic practice and in research concerning testing for screening and diagnostic tests. In reporting such research, investigators should have considered these complicating features; in reading these papers, the discriminating reader should ask whether these complicating features were addressed.

The Straightforward Case

Consider a hypothetical screening test for childhood strabismus in 100 children. A thorough examination of this clinic population reveals that 30 children have strabismus and 70 do not. The screening test identifies 60 children with abnormal results and 40 with normal results. Twenty of those failing the screening truly have strabismus; 40 failing the screening do not. Ten strabismic patients pass the screening test. Table 16-1 shows the results.

The data are presented in a 2 × 2 table, from which a great deal can be learned about the screening test. Note that the "truth" is expressed along the horizontal totals row, and the screening test verdict down the vertical column. Accuracy is found by adding "truly normal" and "truly abnormal." The screening test performance is described as follows:

- *Sensitivity:* The test correctly identifies 20 of every 30 children with strabismus (67%).

Table 16-1 Screening Test for Strabismus in Clinic

Screening Test Result	Strabismus	No Strabismus	Totals
Abnormal	Truly abnormal (20)	Falsely abnormal (40)	60
Normal	Falsely normal (10)	Truly normal (30)	40
Totals	30	70	100

- *Specificity:* The test correctly passes 30 of every 70 children who do not have strabismus (42%).
- *Positive predictive value (PPV):* If a child has abnormal test results, there is only a 1 in 3 chance (20/60) that the child actually has strabismus (33%).
- *Negative predictive value (NPV):* If a child passes the screening test, the child has a 3 in 4 chance (30/40) of actually being disease-free (75%).
- *Accuracy:* The screening test is correct in 50 of 100 cases (50%).

Sensitivity and specificity are attractive measures because they are intuitively obvious. *Sensitivity* is the percentage of those who have the disease of interest and fail the test, and *specificity* is the percentage of disease-free persons who pass the test. Confidence limits can be stated for both sensitivity and specificity, based in large part on the sample size used. However, an important caveat is that neither sensitivity nor specificity takes into account the relative frequency of healthy and unhealthy persons in a population. For example, if the hypothetical strabismus test was taken to a shopping center and used to screen children, Table 16-2 might result.

The sensitivity is still 67%, and the specificity is about the same at 41%. However, because of screening failure, 58 disease-free persons and only 2 truly strabismic children would be referred for complete examinations. The PPV and NPV alert us to the problem. For this shopping center population, the PPV (if a person has positive test results, what is the probability that the disease is present?) is 2/(2 + 58), or only 3%. The NPV (if a person has negative test results, what is the probability that the disease is absent?) is 39/(1 + 39), or 98%. However, the point of screening is not to reassure disease-free persons but to detect treatable disease. Clearly, this test, which found 67% of the patients with strabismus and which had a 33% PPV in a clinic population, failed miserably when used in a wider population. PPV and NPV, then, are better parameters to use in assessing a screening test that is to be used in a wider population, because these values take into account the prevalence of disease in the population. Of course, the PPV and NPV are much more relevant when calculated on the basis of disease prevalence in the wider population and not on a disease-rich clinic population.

Complicating Features

Number 1: a screening test with a continuous outcome

Consider the situation in which the screening test has a continuous value, as opposed to a binary outcome. IOP is such a variable. Assume for the moment that people are able to be definitively classified, on the basis of a thorough examination, into those with glaucoma

Table 16-2 **Screening Test for Strabismus in Shopping Center**

Screening Test Result	Strabismus	No Strabismus	Totals
Abnormal	Truly abnormal (2)	Falsely abnormal (58)	60
Normal	Falsely normal (1)	Truly normal (39)	40
Totals	3	97	100

and those without glaucoma. For each value of IOP in mm Hg, individuals above that value of IOP could be classified as having failed the screening, and those below it, as having passed the screening, thus converting the result into a yes/no format at that value of IOP. Percentages for sensitivity and for specificity can be derived for each value of IOP and graphically displayed (Fig 16-4).

Thus, there is a series of paired sensitivity/specificity values, 1 for each level of IOP. This series can be plotted graphically: sensitivity, by convention, is plotted on the y-axis; and (1 – specificity) is on the x-axis. In this form, it is known as a *receiver operating characteristics (ROC) curve*. The ability of IOP to discriminate glaucoma from nonglaucoma is shown in Figure 16-5; data are from the population-based Baltimore Eye Survey. (The data points are actually connected by steps, but the continuous line graph is easier to view.)

It is obvious that IOP is not a very good screening tool for glaucoma, because the graph does not curve strongly toward the upper left of the ROC plot, where good sensitivity is paired with good specificity. The diamond-shaped symbols represent a hypothetical optimal screening test; the triangular symbols represent a test with a 50:50 sensitivity and specificity, nothing better than chance alone. The usual cutoff for "normal" IOP, 21 mm Hg, gives a sensitivity of 91% with a specificity of only 47%. The optimal mix of sensitivity and specificity is at 18 mm Hg, where sensitivity is 65%; specificity, 66%. Despite the inadequate performance of IOP as a screening methodology, it can be seen that for a continuous variable test like IOP, there is a trade-off between sensitivity and specificity. The more specific we want a test result (left side of x-axis), the less sensitive it becomes, and vice versa. An ROC curve can help in the choice of an optimal cutoff point in that the curve selects a sensitivity–specificity pair located toward the upper left of the ROC plot.

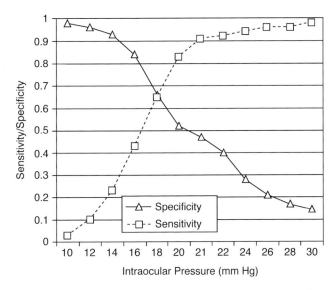

Figure 16-4 Sensitivity/specificity of IOP by IOP level. For each level of IOP along the x-axis, the values for sensitivity and specificity are plotted. *(Data from Tielsch JM, Sommer A, Witt K, Katz J, Royall RM. Blindness and visual impairment in an American urban population: the Baltimore Eye Survey. Arch Ophthalmol. 1990;108(2):286–290.)*

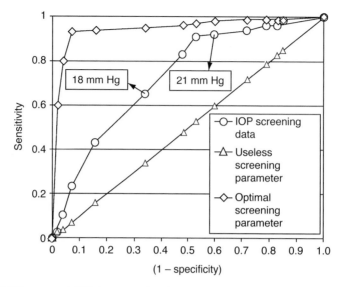

Figure 16-5 ROC curve of IOP in screening for glaucoma. In this ROC curve, the data from Figure 16-4 are replotted, with sensitivity on the y-axis and (1 – specificity) on the x-axis. The middle line shows these pairs. Two of these plotted points are identified with the IOP cutoff represented. *(Data from Tielsch JM, Sommer A, Witt K, Katz J, Royall RM. Blindness and visual impairment in an American urban population: the Baltimore Eye Survey.* Arch Ophthalmol. *1990;108(2):286–290.)*

Other significant factors in choosing a cutoff point are the population to be screened and the fact that sensitivity and specificity may not be equally important. If the consequence of missing a diagnosis is blindness, and the price of a false-positive test is negligible, then a high sensitivity with a poorer specificity would be an appropriate choice. An example of this might be a cutoff value for an erythrocyte sedimentation rate in a person who has recent visual loss and who is suspected of having giant cell arteritis.

Tielsch JM, Sommer A, Witt K, Katz J, Royall RM. Blindness and visual impairment in an American urban population: the Baltimore Eye Survey. *Arch Ophthalmol.* 1990;108(2):286–290.

Number 2: the diagnosis is not yes/no but has arbitrary, consistent criteria

The presence or absence of glaucoma depends on how glaucoma is defined. No test or examination is capable of detecting the first optic nerve axon that is damaged in glaucoma. Therefore, in research, a consistent and verifiable, though arbitrary, criterion for a glaucoma diagnosis must be used. If this criterion is applied, there is a risk of misclassifying an early glaucoma patient as disease-free; a test that correctly identifies such a patient as having glaucoma is misclassified as a false-positive. Therefore, evaluating new diagnostic modalities that may detect glaucoma earlier than do current tests is challenging. The problem is that no gold standard exists against which to compare a new diagnostic test. Even without the benefit of longitudinal follow-up to see who later develops glaucoma, however, a new test can still be evaluated if it is compared with others. ROC curves are useful for comparing the relative efficacy of different screening methods or different diagnostic tests. A good example from the recent literature is shown in Figure 16-6. In this

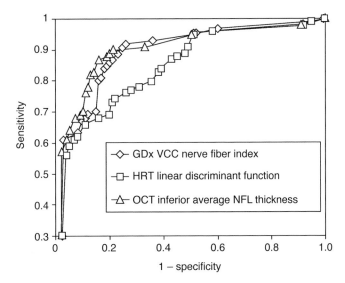

Figure 16-6 ROC curve of 3 glaucoma imaging devices. The single parameter chosen for display for each instrument was the one that performed the best in the authors' study. No statistically significant difference in the area under the ROC curves for these 3 parameters was present. *(The HRT linear discriminant function is from a paper by Bathija et al, referenced by Medeiros et al; the GDx and OCT parameters are standard test outputs provided by the manufacturers. Graph redrawn with data from Medeiros FA, Zangwill LM, Bowd C, Weinreb RN. Comparison of the GDx VCC scanning laser polarimeter, HRT II confocal scanning laser ophthalmoscope, and Stratus OCT optical coherence tomograph for the detection of glaucoma. Arch Ophthalmol. 2004;122(6):827–837.)*

study, 3 devices that image the optic disc and nerve fiber layer were compared on their ability to discriminate between healthy eyes and eyes with glaucomatous visual field loss.

Using ROC curves to compare tests is especially useful when the tests express results in different units or on completely different scales. The area under the ROC curve (AUC) is a summary measure of the relative efficacy of competing tests. The AUC must be better than 0.5, which a useless test can achieve (see Fig 16-5).

Number 3: pretest probability of disease

Now consider the case in which something relevant is known about the patient before the screening or diagnostic test is performed. In the case of glaucoma, perhaps it is known that the patient has a first-degree relative with glaucoma and has a thinner-than-average central corneal thickness (both risk factors for glaucoma). This information lets us know that the patient has a pretest probability of glaucoma 3 times that of a person picked at random from the general population. How much does a diagnostic test improve the ability to diagnose glaucoma in this patient? How much does the relative risk of glaucoma increase as a result of a positive test?

For this problem, apply *Bayes theorem,* which allows the combination of a pretest probability of disease and the test results, producing a posttest probability. Among the statistical applications of this theorem is the very useful *likelihood ratio* and its derived positive and negative predictive values. Although the likelihood ratio sounds complicated, it is simple to understand, because it is calculated using sensitivity and specificity. First, the likelihood ratio of a positive test is the sensitivity divided by (1 − specificity), numbers that can be found in the 2 × 2 table or the ROC curve. For a test with 80% sensitivity and 90% specificity (0.8/1 − 0.9), the positive likelihood ratio is 8. Second, the likelihood ratio of a negative test is (1 − sensitivity) divided by specificity. For the same 80%/90% test, the negative likelihood ratio is (1 − 0.8)/0.9, or 0.22. Positive likelihood ratios start at 1 and continue to infinity—the bigger, the better. Negative likelihood ratios vary from 0 to 1; the smaller, the better. If the interest is in diagnosing disease, the test with the larger positive likelihood ratio is the better test; conversely, if the goal is ruling out disease, the test with the smaller negative likelihood ratio is better.

If the positive likelihood ratio is multiplied by the pretest odds of disease, the result is the *posttest odds of disease.* Thus, for the example patient with the positive family history, thin cornea, and pretest odds of 3: if there is a positive test with a positive likelihood ratio of 8, then the posttest odds of glaucoma are 24 times that of a person drawn at random from the population.

Consider the case of a 65-year-old woman with no risk factors for glaucoma and a pretest probability of disease of 1% (Table 16-3). A positive test result for glaucoma would raise her probability of disease to 7.5%. However, an 85-year-old man with a strong positive family history, thin central corneal thickness, and an IOP of 30 might have a pretest probability of disease of 50%. If his test result were negative, he would still have a posttest probability of 18.2%, greater than that of the 65-year-old woman. This example illustrates how important the pretest probability of disease becomes in deciding whether to employ a diagnostic test.

Often in clinical practice there is an intermediate diagnostic category, such as "glaucoma suspect," between the diseased and the normal condition. Successful statistical treatment of such a category is another advantage that likelihood ratios have and that sensitivity/specificity and ROC curves do not. Sensitivity/specificity and ROC curves require that borderline subjects be placed in 1 of 2 categories: "those with disease" (eg, glaucoma) or "those without disease" (eg, no glaucoma). However, a separate likelihood ratio for the borderline category can be constructed, thereby reflecting the risk of patients exhibiting that characteristic (eg, a "glaucoma suspect").

Number 4: combining tests

Sometimes clinicians may make a diagnosis by using 2 tests, the second employed if the first is positive. Likelihood ratios for each test may be known, because of clinical research

Table 16-3 Example of a Test With 80% Sensitivity/90% Specificity and Changes in PPV and NPV Depending on Pretest Probability

Pretest Probability	Predictive Value of a Positive Test	Predictive Value of a Negative Test
1%	7.5%	99.8%
10%	47.1%	97.6%
50%	88.9%	81.8%
90%	98.6%	33.3%

done independently for each test. It is tempting to use the product of the 2 likelihood ratios and the pretest probability to calculate a posttest probability, but this is unwise because the test results are usually not completely independent of each other.

Consider the following case: the Stratus OCT is used as a diagnostic test, and if the result is positive, the GDx is employed. Reference to Medeiros and colleagues provides likelihood ratios for each test. But both tests measure nerve fiber layer thickness, albeit using different technologies, and are highly correlated. Because the 2 tests are not independent, the actual performance of the 2-test strategy is likely to be disappointing in comparison with the posttest probability calculated from the product of the pretest probability and the 2 likelihood ratios.

Another test combination strategy is performing 2 tests and considering the result positive if either test result is positive. This strategy works best when tests have good specificity (because combining tests this way makes overall specificity deteriorate) and when the 2 tests address different aspects of a disease (such as a functional test and a structural test for glaucoma). A clinical example would be combining an optic nerve imaging test with a visual field test to determine whether glaucoma is present.

Medeiros FA, Zangwill LM, Bowd C, Weinreb RN. Comparison of the GDx VCC scanning laser polarimeter, HRT II confocal scanning laser ophthalmoscope, and Stratus OCT optical coherence tomograph for the detection of glaucoma. *Arch Ophthalmol.* 2004;122(6):827–837.

Number 5: clinical acceptance

So far, it has been assumed that the clinical test under consideration is not burdensome, either physically or financially, on the patient and the test's performance characteristics have been evaluated in a vacuum. However, all tests carry some burden, including the potential for side effects or the need to repeat them and/or order additional tests. A test that produces a small increment in the likelihood ratio of detecting disease, but that is expensive or painful, is not likely to achieve clinical acceptance.

Number 6: generalizability

Most investigations of new screening or diagnostic tests are performed on patients presenting to a clinic. Only after these tests have passed the test of usefulness in that setting are they investigated in a population-based sample (largely because of the high cost of performing population-based research). Because the data for new tests are based on clinic patients, not populations, the generalizability of the results for a screening application is questionable. Even when new tests are being evaluated for diagnostic usefulness, the mix of patients tested may not reflect the usual mix of patients in an office practice. For example, only those patients who clearly have glaucoma and those who are young and disease-free may be studied. This leads to excellent sensitivity and specificity, which would not be replicated in a sample of patients who have borderline glaucoma and are older.

Summary

A variety of measures are available for evaluating the efficacy of screening and diagnostic tests. Sensitivity and specificity are the simplest and easiest to understand, but they suffer from the disadvantage of not considering the prevalence of disease in the target population. PPV and NPV are more useful in that regard. ROC curves can make more comprehensible the relationship of sensitivity and specificity in tests with a continuously variable result; they can also be used for comparing diagnostic tests with one another. Likelihood ratios, and their effect on pretest probability of disease, provide help in critically evaluating screening and diagnostic tests in the context of the clinical setting to which they are to be applied.

Riegelman RK. *Studying a Study and Testing a Test: How to Read the Medical Evidence.* 5th ed. Philadelphia: Lippincott Williams & Wilkins; 2005.

Discussing Benefits, Risks, Probabilities, and Expected Outcomes With Patients

Interpreting results of scientific studies for patients is one of the most important duties of a physician. The origin of the word *physician* in Greek is "to educate." Physicians need to educate patients regarding their disease, including the potential treatments, preventions, and outcomes. Although increasingly complex scientific analyses have made the interpretation of findings challenging at times, physicians must be able to interpret them for patients.

Most clinical studies present research findings as a percentage or as an absolute change in a disease status (eg, presence of AMD) or in a continuous outcome (eg, IOP). Concrete findings such as these can be easily discussed with patients. However, discussing odds ratios and concepts such as absolute and relative risk is more difficult. *Risk* is defined as an expected loss within a distribution of possible outcomes, as when homeowners buy insurance to guard against the risk of a flood. In the context of clinical research, however, risk can often be characterized as the conditional probability of an event, usually an adverse event. The condition might be as basic as survival to a particular point or exposure to some phenomenon—for example, persons "at risk" for disease or "in the risk set."

Two measures may be used to compare risk between groups of individuals. *Risk difference* is the absolute difference in the risk measured between groups. *Relative risk* is the ratio of 2 risk measures. The risk difference depends on the unit of measure, whereas relative risk is dimensionless because it involves division of 2 risk measurements. In the Ocular Hypertension Treatment Study (OHTS), the absolute risk difference of developing glaucoma for subjects who were not treated compared with those who were treated was 5% (9.5% – 4.5%) across 5 years. The relative risk of not being treated compared with treatment was 211% (9.5/4.5). Both of these measures are consistent with the data, but interpreting them can lead to vastly different conclusions. Numerically, a 5% increased risk of glaucoma if ocular hypertension is not treated might seem small to a patient, and a 211% increased risk of glaucoma with untreated ocular hypertension might seem large. A key piece of information that may help in the interpretation is the *baseline probability of the outcome.* In everyday life, people may be willing to board an airplane, doubling their relative risk of accidental death, because the baseline probability of an adverse outcome is so low. In this context, if there is a choice between 2 airlines and the risk difference is

5% per million miles flown, the risk difference would not seem small. Thus, the baseline probabilities or expected outcomes can help people make decisions. This is especially true when the risk ratio is less than 100% and may be wrongly interpreted as a risk difference. For example, a difference in adverse outcome rates of between 10% and 13% could be described as involving a relative risk of approximately 30%, but to those unfamiliar with the baseline probabilities, this 30% figure may sound as though the comparison were between 10% and 40%, when it is not.

In observational studies, investigators may present their results as *odds ratios.* In an odds ratio, the odds of a subject with a disease (case) having an exposure (eg, smoking) are compared with the odds of a subject without the disease (control) having the exposure. When the disease is rare, the odds ratio approximates the relative risk of that exposure, because the denominators for both the odds being compared are close to 1 for rare events. For example, in the meta-analyses on the potential risk factors for late AMD, which occurs relatively infrequently, the odds ratio for smoking is 2.35. This can be interpreted as smokers having a 235% risk of developing late AMD, compared with nonsmokers.

A *risk factor* is a factor to which patients are exposed, either voluntarily or not, and with which an increased or decreased likelihood of a disease is associated. Thus, risk factors influence the occurrence of a disease. Exposures to specific factors may or may not be clinically significant. For example, use of seat belts may not be a clinically significant exposure for AMD, whereas smoking is. One of the subsets of risk factors is *causal risk factors,* which are root causes of the disease. Because it is difficult to distinguish causal risk factors from noncausal risk factors in observational studies, researchers often use inductively oriented causal criteria to determine which risk factors are causal and which are not. The Surgeon General's 1964 report on smoking and health broke new ground by describing criteria for evaluating causal relationships in observational data.

When research findings from clinical trials or observational studies are being interpreted, the generalizability of the findings to individual patients must be considered. Questions to raise are, Do the study inclusion criteria include factors that would be applicable to the patient? Can the findings be extrapolated to the patient? The distinction between an *individual effect* and an *average effect* is important. For example, in the OHTS, the investigators reported that a 1 mm Hg increase in IOP was associated with an approximately 10% increase in the risk of developing glaucoma. Does this necessarily mean that lowering the IOP 1 mm Hg in all ocular hypertensive patients would decrease the overall risk of glaucoma in each patient by 10%, or does it mean that some patients would have more than a 10% risk reduction, and others less? The answer is that this statement refers to an average effect in the overall population of ocular hypertensive patients and not to an individual patient. The concept is population-based and analogous to the health advantages of lower cholesterol levels. Medicine has a history of finding an average effect from a treatment in a study and then administering that treatment to everyone who has the disease or condition being studied, in the hope that this helps. Thus, in general, lowering IOP is useful as an overall goal for ocular hypertensive patients, but its benefits may differ from one patient to another.

The literature on causal inference makes clear that it is impossible to draw inferences about individual effects unless an assumption is made that individual effects are the same in a subgroup of patients as in the population studied. A goal of research should be to continue refining estimates of individual effects so that they are tailored as closely as possible to individual characteristics. A goal of patient care should be that treatment decisions are made so that both patient and physician have a clear understanding of the risks involved.

Kass MA, Heuer DK, Higginbotham EJ, et al. The Ocular Hypertension Treatment Study: a randomized trial determines that topical ocular hypotensive medication delays or prevents the onset of primary open-angle glaucoma. *Arch Ophthalmol.* 2002;120(6):701–713.

Rubin DB. Bayesian inference for causal effects: the role of randomization. *Ann. Statist.* 1978; 6:34–58.

Smoking and Health: Report of the Advisory Committee to the Surgeon General of the Public Health Service. Washington, DC: US Dept of Health, Education, and Welfare, Public Health Service; 1964. Public Health Service Publication 1103.

Tomany SC, Wang JJ, Van Leeuwen R, et al. Risk factors for incident age-related macular degeneration: pooled findings from 3 continents. *Ophthalmology.* 2004;111(7):1280–1287.

Applying Statistics to Measure and Improve Clinical Practice

As awareness of the variation in the practice and quality of eye care increases, insurers, professional organizations, physician practices, hospitals, and patients will need to understand and use systems that both measure and seek to improve care. Donabedian organized quality into 3 distinct elements—structure, process, and outcomes—that provide an organizational framework within which eye care can be monitored. *Structure* refers to how the care system is designed, such as whom the patient sees initially, what pathways exist for obtaining various diagnostic tests, and what the financial arrangements are for care reimbursement. *Process* is the content of care: what the provider does or does not do. The principle that drives process quality is "doing the right thing at the right time," to which structure adds "by the right person at the right place." *Outcomes* are the results of care, or the completion of the principle "so that the right results occur."

Several important statistical principles and techniques are applied in creating and using a system that enhances care. At the outset, when the system is being planned or designed, issues of validity, reliability, and population bias are essential considerations. If the system is not designed to measure every occurrence, sampling concerns and nonresponse and missing data issues will need to be addressed when the system is implemented. Analysis of results, particularly comparisons across different providers, can raise important questions about statistical and clinical significance, confounders and adjustments, use of appropriate comparisons, and the extent to which the observed variability of the results is explained through the analyses being used. The final component needed to improve the system is methods of data presentation that facilitate a continual feedback process whereby performances can be tracked and then improved over time. Issues related to comparisons over time thus become important to understand.

Committee on Quality of Health Care in America, Institute of Medicine. *Crossing the Quality Chasm: A New Health System for the 21st Century.* Washington, DC: National Academies Press; 2001.

Donabedian A. Evaluating the quality of medical care. *Milbank Mem Fund Q.* 1966;44(3): Suppl:166–206.

Issues in Designing a Measurement System

The first requirement of a useful system is that proposed indicators actually reflect the quality or characteristic to be assessed. This is referred to as *validity*. One question commonly faced by ophthalmologists is whether a patient's eye was dilated during an eye examination, as several national assessments of quality of care measure whether a retinal examination is performed on a patient with diabetes at least every year or two. What might indicate that a dilated examination was done? The single best way, also referred to as the gold standard, is to have every ophthalmic examination videotaped, so that a reviewer, through observing the use of an indirect ophthalmoscope or a mirrored contact lens after dilating drops had been placed, could note that a dilated examination was indeed done. An alternative gold standard, according to practice guidelines, is to see that photographs of the retina, including the periphery, were obtained. The following also could lead to the conclusion that a dilated examination was performed: (1) documentation indicating that dilating drops were placed in the eye; (2) chart notations indicating that a peripheral dilated examination was performed, such as "P" or "periphery," noted as being "normal" or "abnormal"; (3) a diagram or drawing of the retina, on which the periphery or peripheral findings are indicated. All of these would be considered "valid" measures in that their presence in the chart would most likely indicate that a dilated examination had been done; their absence, that it had not. The use of proxies for a gold standard is referred to as *construct validity*.

Once there is a valid measure, *reliability* needs to be determined—that is, whether the measure gives the same answer when it is repeated under a different set of assessment conditions but without a change in the underlying document or service being assessed. How exactly might conditions change? First, a clinician reviewing a medical chart may be distracted or tired. When the test or review is repeated by the same clinician at a different time, does the analysis show the same results? Measures that are designed to minimize errors when repeated are noted to have good test–retest reliability, or reproducibility. Are the same results obtained when the measure is made with the same instrument the second time and the third? Second, if the person doing the measurement gets the same results on the same subject, with multiple attempts, then there is good intrarater reliability. Third, measures should be designed (as should the training system and support system that capture and analyze the data) so that many different people can use the measure and obtain the same results. Measures that have this characteristic are said to have good interrater reliability.

Two common statistical techniques are used to determine whether there is "good" agreement. One method is to simply tally the number of identical answers between 2 different tests and then divide that number by the total number of items being assessed, thereby yielding a "percent agreement." A second method is to use the κ (kappa) statistic, a measure of agreement between 2 or more persons or entities which takes into account that sometimes observers agree through chance alone. Kappas greater than 0.70 are thought to denote good agreement; those from 0.50 to 0.70, only moderate agreement; those from 0.31 to 0.49, poor agreement; and those 0.30 or less, no agreement.

Once a valid and reliable measure has been established, the population in which the measure is to be used must be considered. First, inclusion criteria and exclusion criteria (who is in and who is out of the population to be measured) need to be carefully defined.

For example, a study of the quality of care provided by ophthalmologists might exclude retina specialists (exclusion criterion) and include only comprehensive ophthalmologists who see patients at least 50% of the time (inclusion criterion).

Second, it needs to be ascertained whether the population is one in which there is sufficient frequency of occurrences for meaningful differences to be found. Or are the events so rare ("floor effect") or so common ("ceiling effect") that little value is to be gained in using such a measurement system? Often, issues like this do not become apparent until after at least a pilot analysis is done; but more often, these issues are overlooked when the system is designed. However, even rare events (eg, endophthalmitis or appropriate workups obtained in patients with third nerve palsies) can be meaningful clinically, as can common events (eg, patients surviving surgery or having their vision checked postoperatively). Both, therefore, should be measured on that basis. Such decisions should be made with an understanding of the number of observations (sample size) needed to find statistically and clinically significant differences.

Third, the measures should be easily obtained in the population of interest (including validity and reliability). Systems that do not require much additional work are more practical for the purpose of monitoring practices. Thus, billing files may provide sufficient information on the likelihood of specific process quality steps, such as the performance of regular visual field testing in patients with glaucoma; or of outcomes, such as suprachoroidal hemorrhage after intraocular surgery.

Implementing a Monitoring System

An ideal monitoring system would capture every patient of interest for a given practitioner. Doing so gives the maximum number of cases for statistical analyses and thus provides maximum statistical power while allowing for more reliable estimates of uncommon or rare events. In addition, a 100% analysis minimizes bias due to missing patients. For administrative data, 100% review is made feasible by the presence of data in accessible electronic formats. For example, every patient who had intraocular surgery in a practice (defined by specific CPT codes) can be identified during a specified period, and then subsequent surgeries (again defined by CPT codes) within the next 30 or 90 days can be determined, as can a subsequent diagnosis of a specific complication (by ICD codes) such as retinal detachment or endophthalmitis.

In contrast, questions about process quality—such as whether a target pressure range was set for every patient with glaucoma—are not amenable to a 100% review because that type of data (target pressure ranges) is not captured in current administrative databases (but registration and billing data are). Also, a trained reviewer is required to abstract that type of information from charts. Other process quality measures that are separately billed services, such as gonioscopy, are identifiable by analyses of billing databases.

Thus, to the extent that many structure, process, and outcomes quality indicators are not included in electronic databases, it may be feasible to use them only when the care of a limited number of patients is reviewed. As electronic medical records become more popular, such reviews will become more feasible, because specific process steps would then be electronically accessible.

The review of a smaller population of interest requires sampling of the larger pool of patients. First, the universe of patients of interest is clearly defined, with explicit inclusion and exclusion criteria. Second, a list of eligible patients (as complete as possible) is compiled. Third, ideally, the sample for review is drawn in a random fashion by a disinterested party or method. Allowing providers to select the patient sample creates substantial selection bias, because the providers are likely to pick patients whose charts show the most complete data. Using a convenient sample of the last 20 or so consecutive patients also raises the concern that the sample is not truly representative (eg, during the period of interest, the clinic may have been overbooked, causing providers to defer certain steps of the examination).

Once the sample is drawn, the records are reviewed. What standards should be used for a review? What criteria should be used? Evidence suggests that explicit criteria with yes/no or limited categories (eg, optic nerve documentation could include a statement of the nerve's condition or a measure of the vertical cup-to-disc ratio or a drawing or photograph) are more reliable than implicit criteria (the reviewer's judgment that overall quality was good or not good), particularly for interrater reliability. For ophthalmology, the American Academy of Ophthalmology (AAO) provides the Preferred Practice Patterns and Summary Benchmarks series, both of which can be used to obtain explicit criteria. Similarly, the American Board of Ophthalmology (ABO) has explicit criteria in the Office Record Review module for board maintenance of certification. These are available at one. aao.org/CE/default.aspx and at www.abop.org/maintain/orr/index.asp, respectively.

In many reviews, charts may not be available, or they are incomplete, with missing data or visits. Efforts should be made to obtain unavailable charts. If, after reasonable effort, these charts remain unavailable, the number of unavailable charts is recorded, and replacement charts from the randomization should be reviewed. If the missing-chart rate exceeds a specific rate (eg, the typical rate for missing charts in a particular clinic for patient visits), then issues of bias (perhaps intentional) are more likely to be present. For charts with missing visits, specific review criteria may be answered completely from available visits. For review criteria that require every visit to be checked, the options are to (1) exclude that patient; (2) exclude that patient only for analyses needing that missing visit data; (3) impute the missing values by statistical modeling of available data; or (4) treat the missing visit as either meeting or not meeting the criteria (generally the latter). The key steps are to make a decision on what to do and then apply that decision consistently over time (and report the decision with the data and results). Finally, patients with missing data from a specific visit are typically treated as having not met the review criteria—which is, in essence, determining if something is or is not documented in the chart.

One concern is the number of charts that should be reviewed. The sample size required depends on the underlying rates of performance and the amount of difference sought. In general, rates at either extreme (very rare or very common) require a greater sample size. The smaller a difference (eg, in how one provider performs compared with the group average) the researcher wishes to determine to be statistically significant, the greater the sample size required. An important element of establishing a monitoring system for quality of care is performing power calculations to determine sample sizes, as these calculations provide confidence that a nonsignificant difference is truly that (and not due to having insufficient sample size).

A related concern is the route of administering the measure, as the route or method used can have significant effects on the results. The dilated eye examination quality indicator in patients with diabetes can be used as an example. McGlynn and colleagues (2004) noted that use of a chart review format (as described previously) yielded an annual dilated eye examination rate of only 19% among patients with diabetes. Yet a rate of approximately 50% resulted when billing levels were used, specifically, when an appropriate eye examination was imputed to those who had had any eye visit with an eye care professional at a billing level sufficient to support that a dilation could have been done. Clearly, there are significant validity issues with the measure that uses claims data.

Regardless of the method used, systematic errors may occur. The data may have been recorded incorrectly, on the part of either the observer or the person abstracting the data from the data source. Errors related to administrative databases include coding issues, data entry problems, and incorrect diagnoses. Errors for chart review approaches, in addition to the above-mentioned, include those made by the abstractor and those made later in calculating quality scores. These errors can be minimized by (1) upfront training of all personnel; (2) review of cases with values outside the expected range; and (3) duplicate review of a 5%–10% sample of cases.

McGlynn EA, Asch SM, Adams J, et al. The quality of health care delivered to adults in the United States. *N Engl J Med.* 2003;348(26):2635–2645.

Analyzing the Results

Once the results have been compiled, they must be interpreted and used appropriately. For projects designed to detect important deviations from expected performance, it is important to use statistical tests that determine statistical significance. For many measures, comparisons of mean performance are satisfactory—as in the percentage of AAO benchmark process indicators for cataract that every provider has achieved. However, for others, the best way to compare performance may be to use the number of persons whose care meets a given threshold. For example, investigators may want to know the percentage of patients who have at least a 90% quality score. Once they have obtained that measure, they can then compare it among providers.

Even if differences are found to be statistically significant, they still may not be clinically meaningful. The greater the sample size, the more likely it is that a statistically significant difference can be found. However, are such differences truly meaningful? For example, one provider may document the optic nerve 78% of the time; another provider, 81% of the time. With a large enough sample size, this difference can be statistically significant. However, is it clinically meaningful? Does this difference show that one doctor is technically of higher quality than the other? Indeed, an appreciation of clinically significant differences is very useful for calculating the sample sizes in the first place.

In addition, factors beyond the provider's control may result in a finding that, although clinically significant, also needs to take these other factors into account. For process steps such as taking a history or performing a dilated examination, the only likely confounders are the patient's refusal or inability to allow that step and the patient's inability to afford any additional tests. For outcomes of chronic diseases, however, the weight of confounders and other factors may often overwhelm the provider's ability to influence the results by doing the right thing, especially over a longer period. For example, the rate of blindness from glaucoma over 20 years is subject to the physiologic severity on presentation and the risk for progression of the pool of patients. Even beyond this concern for "case-mix" of severity, however, many other issues are at play, such as the ability of patients to return for regular care and to use their recommended treatments regularly, and the impact of their socioeconomic and cultural states. Thus, measuring whether the provider performs specific examination steps, such as examining the optic nerve (process) is appropriate, whereas looking at rates of blindness over 20 years (outcomes) may not be appropriate.

In other words, even if adjustments are made for case-mix and other confounders, caution still needs to be exercised so that appropriate comparisons are used. The fundamental question is whether it is fair to hold the provider accountable for the indicator in question. Where the criterion is wholly or even largely within the control of the provider, it certainly is. Where the criterion is within the control of an agent or factor independent of the provider, it most likely is not. If providers are held accountable, they are, in essence, being made responsible for the behaviors of their patients and the patients' families. Under such a circumstance, providers would most likely find a strong disincentive to accept poorer, less compliant patients, instead focusing on only those with the attitudes, skills, and resources to follow recommended care. For example, a provider caring for indigent patients in an inner-city neighborhood may be penalized relative to a lower-quality provider in a wealthy suburb, unless such adjustments and appropriate comparisons are made.

In making statistical comparisons and including confounding factors, investigators specify a defined set of factors and conditions that may be helpful in understanding the results of the analyses. A key step, often overlooked, is to see how important these indicators are to the overall quality of care and thence to how the patient fares (the AAO Preferred Practice Patterns grade each process indicator as to the "importance to care"). If a step is not truly crucial to defining a condition, in relating to overall quality, or to assessing how a patient does over time, then its nonperformance may be less of a problem.

One technique commonly used to perform this key analysis is looking at how much of the variance in the dependent variable of interest is accounted for by all of the independent variables in the analysis. This is often stated as the percent of variance that is "explained" by the variables included in the analysis. Where the proportion of variability explained is high, paying greater attention to the specific criteria in the analysis is important; where the proportion of variability explained is low, less weight is given to the criteria. From a statistical perspective, one shorthand method of expressing variance explained is assessing the R^2 (proportion of variance explained) of the variables in the analysis. The fundamental question is, How much do the statistically (and clinically) meaningful variables explain the dependent variable of interest?

Methods of Data Presentation to Facilitate Continuous Improvement of Practices

Once the initial system has been designed, implemented, and analyzed, the results from the analyses must be disseminated and used to improve care processes and structures. Just measuring and feeding back results have been shown to improve subsequent care by between 3% and 6% in the performance indicators. Delivery systems that make continual quality improvements demonstrate significantly greater performance gains. A discussion of the methods of continuous quality improvement (CQI) and total quality management (TQM) is beyond the scope of this chapter; however, several useful tools for data analysis and presentation have broader use.

First, plotting the data on a frequency distribution, or histogram (Fig 16-7), or using a scatter diagram (Fig 16-8) to show the distribution along 2 or more variables is vital to understanding the nature of the data. Are the data "normally distributed" in a bell-shaped curve, or are they skewed? The answer to this question affects the choice of statistical tools and analyses, and it can also provide important insights into potential underlying factors. Or, 2 distinct subgroups may be found in the data and these subgroups need to be defined. For example, care in solo practices is likely to differ significantly from that in large single-specialty groups for a particular disease area.

Second, use of a Pareto chart (Fig 16-9) provides insights into a cumulative distribution of key factors of interest. The chart combines a histogram with a cumulative frequency line, making it possible to assess performance across the range of values for the variable of interest.

Third, the rates of events, especially uncommon ones, can fluctuate over time. Are the fluctuations significant, both statistically and clinically, compared with those of prior periods and other institutions or practices? The use of run diagrams, or control charts (Fig 16-10), in which event rates are plotted over time with both SD (standard deviation) and benchmark lines, enables reviewers to determine (1) if an aberrant data point is really

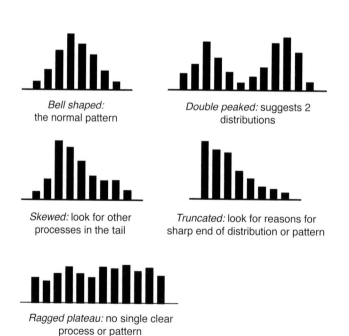

Bell shaped:
the normal pattern

Double peaked: suggests 2
distributions

Skewed: look for other
processes in the tail

Truncated: look for reasons for
sharp end of distribution or pattern

Ragged plateau: no single clear
process or pattern

Figure 16-7 Types of histograms. *(Reproduced from the Quality Assurance Project. Available online at www.qaproject.org.)*

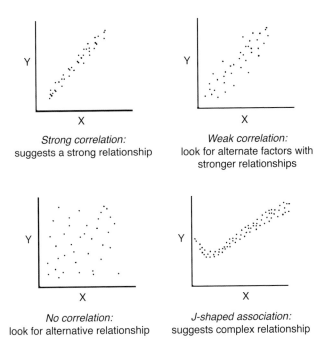

Figure 16-8 Scatter diagram interpretation. *(Reproduced from the Quality Assurance Project. Available at www.qaproject.org.)*

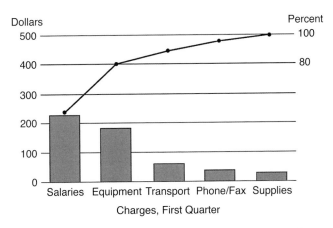

Figure 16-9 Pareto chart. *(Reproduced from the Quality Assurance Project. Available at www.qaproject.org.)*

a meaningful finding or due to random error and (2) how the organization is faring compared with peer organizations.

The purpose of these data analyses is to identify variation in the factor of interest. Factors that are due to the way the system is established and that are inherent in its current state of operations are referred to as *common cause factors*. To improve performance in this area, the system will have to be redesigned and reengineered. For example, there

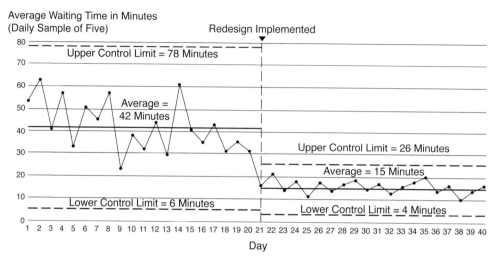

Average Waiting Time in Minutes
(Daily Sample of Five)

Figure 16-10 Control chart of average wait time before and after a redesign. *(Reproduced from the Quality Assurance Project. Available at www.qaproject.org.)*

may be a known rate of "unreliable" visual fields in glaucoma, despite the best training of technicians and screening of patients. In contrast, there are "special causes" of variation that are due to a specific, identifiable factor, often a specific provider or person. Rapid identification of "special cause" variance allows for quick correction of variation that exceeds normal rates. However, it is improving the performance of the overall system and reducing the common cause variation that can improve care and impact the most patients. By "shifting the curve," care for every patient may be improved, as opposed to just identifying the outlier providers and assisting in their rehabilitation.

> Fremont AM, Lee PP, Mangione CM, et al. Patterns of care for open-angle glaucoma in managed care. *Arch Ophthalmol.* 2003;121(6):777–783.

Other Features of Continuous Quality Improvement

Use of continuous quality improvement tools requires significant thought on how to improve care structures and processes. An essential step in improving care processes, before or after initial analyses, is developing a checklist of the steps and parties involved and then creating a flowchart (Fig 16-11) of the care system involved. By looking at the overall process for a specific outcome (eg, making sure a patient with diabetes gets an annual eye examination), researchers can identify opportunities for streamlining the process.

Another tool is the fishbone, or cause-and-effect, diagram (Fig 16-12), which provides detailed information on the different factors, including personnel, that are significant inputs to each step of the care process. Mapping each of these important steps can help clarify where problems may occur and where work may be improved. Changes in those steps can then be measured and the results monitored. Those interested in improving the quality of care are, in this way, provided with continuous feedback.

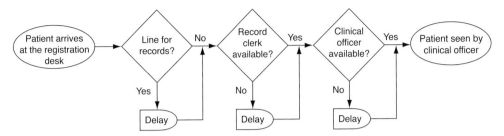

Figure 16-11 Flowchart of patient registration. *(Reproduced from the Quality Assurance Project. Available at www.qaproject.org.)*

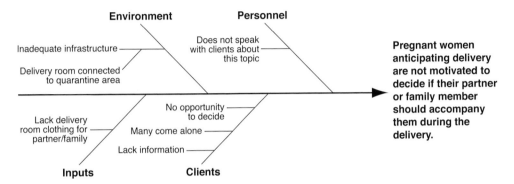

Figure 16-12 Fishbone diagram used at a hospital. *(Reproduced from the Quality Assurance Project. Available at www.qaproject.org.)*

Summary

Efforts to improve the quality of care—and ensuring that fair and meaningful quality measures are part of this endeavor—bring key statistical concepts to the forefront. Because quality is likely to become an important component of reimbursement for federal government programs as well as for private managed-care companies (Physician Quality Reporting Initiative, PQRI), creation and maintenance of an appropriate system are essential. Indeed, to the extent quality measures are also used to select providers for participation in provider panels of insurance companies, having meaningful systems that entail appropriate statistical approaches in their design and implementation is even more important. Thus, statistics is useful not only for understanding the scientific literature and providing care for patients, but also for influencing the practices and livelihoods of providers, including ophthalmologists.

Giaconi JA, Coleman AL. Evidence-based medicine in glaucoma. *Focal Points: Clinical Modules for Ophthalmologists.* San Francisco: American Academy of Ophthalmology; 2008, module 3.

Schuster MA, McGlynn EA, Brook RH. How good is the quality of health care in the United States? *Milbank Q.* 1998;76(4):517–563.

Sloan FA, Brown DS, Carlisle ES, Picone GA, Lee PP. Monitoring visual status: why patients do or do not comply with practice guidelines. *Health Serv Res.* 2004;39(5):1429–1448.

The BCSC faculty wishes to acknowledge the following individuals for their contributions to this chapter: Paul P. Lee, MD, JD; Maureen Maguire, MD; and Richard P. Mills, MD, MPH.

Dr Lee states that he receives financial compensation from Pfizer and from Allergan. Dr Mills states that he has an affiliation with Pfizer and with Allergan.

Basic Texts

General Medicine

Advanced Cardiac Life Support Provider Manual. Dallas: American Heart Association; 2006.

Beers MH, Porter RS, Jones TV, eds. *The Merck Manual of Diagnosis and Therapy.* 18th ed. Hoboken, NJ: John Wiley; 2006.

Cancer: Rates and Risks. 4th ed. Bethesda, MD: National Institutes of Health; 1996.

Cooper DH, Krainik AJ, Lubner SJ, Reno HEL, eds. *The Washington Manual of Medical Therapeutics.* 32nd ed. Philadelphia: Lippincott Williams & Wilkins; 2007.

Cush JJ, Kavanaugh AF, Stein CM. *Rheumatology: Diagnosis and Therapeutics.* 2nd ed. Philadelphia: Lippincott Williams & Wilkins; 2005.

DeVita VT Jr, Lawrence TS, Rosenberg SA, eds. *DeVita, Hellman, and Rosenberg's Cancer: Principles and Practice of Oncology.* 8th ed. Philadelphia: Lippincott Williams & Wilkins; 2008.

Diabetes in America. 2nd ed. Bethesda, MD: National Institutes of Health; 1995.

Duthie EH Jr, Katz PR, Malone ML. *Practice of Geriatrics.* 4th ed. Philadelphia: Elsevier/Saunders; 2007.

Fauci AS, Braunwald E, Kasper DL, et al, eds. *Harrison's Principles of Internal Medicine.* 17th ed. New York: McGraw-Hill; 2008.

Firestein GS, Budd RC, Harris ED Jr, McInnes IB, Ruddy S, Sergent JS, eds. *Kelley's Textbook of Rheumatology.* 8th ed. Philadelphia: Elsevier/Saunders; 2008.

Fraunfelder FT, Fraunfelder FW, Chambers, WA. *Clinical Ocular Toxicology: Drug-Induced Ocular Side Effects.* Philadelphia: Elsevier/Saunders; 2008.

Goetz CG, ed. *Textbook of Clinical Neurology.* 3rd ed. Philadelphia: Elsevier/Saunders; 2008.

Goldman L, Ausiello DA, eds. *Cecil Medicine.* 23rd ed. Philadelphia: Elsevier/Saunders; 2007.

Henderson KE, Baranski TJ, Bickel PE, et al, eds. *The Washington Manual Endocrinology Subspecialty Consult.* 2nd ed. Philadelphia: Lippincott Williams & Wilkins; 2008.

Kronenberg HM, Melmed S, Polonsky KS, Larsen PR, eds. *Williams Textbook of Endocrinology.* 11th ed. Philadelphia: Elsevier/Saunders; 2007.

Libby P, Bonow RO, Mann DL, Zipes DP, eds. *Braunwald's Heart Disease: A Textbook of Cardiovascular Medicine.* 8th ed. Philadelphia: Elsevier/Saunders; 2007.

Mandell GL, Bennett JE, Dolin R, eds. *Mandell, Douglas, and Bennett's Principles and Practice of Infectious Diseases.* 7th ed. Philadelphia: Elsevier/Churchill Livingstone; 2010.

McPhee SJ, Papadakis M, eds. *Current Medical Diagnosis and Treatment.* 49th ed. New York: McGraw-Hill; 2009.

Miller RD, Eriksson LI, Fleisher LA, Wiener-Kronish JP, Young WL, eds. *Miller's Anesthesia.* 7th ed. Philadelphia: Elsevier/Churchill Livingstone; 2010.

Moore DP, Jefferson JW. *Handbook of Medical Psychiatry.* 2nd ed. Philadelphia: Elsevier/ Mosby; 2004.

Rakel RE, Bope ET, eds. *Conn's Current Therapy 2009.* 52nd ed. Philadelphia: Elsevier/ Saunders; 2008.

Ropper AH, Samuels MA, eds. *Adams and Victor's Principles of Neurology.* 9th ed. New York: McGraw-Hill; 2009.

Volberding PA, Sande MA, Lange J, Greene WC, Gallant JE, eds. *Global HIV/AIDS Medicine.* Philadelphia: Elsevier/Saunders; 2008.

Credit Reporting Form

Basic and Clinical Science Course, 2012–2013
Section 1

The American Academy of Ophthalmology is accredited by the Accreditation Council for Continuing Medical Education to provide continuing medical education for physicians.

The American Academy of Ophthalmology designates this enduring material for a maximum of 10 *AMA PRA Category 1 Credits™*. Physicians should claim only the credit commensurate with the extent of their participation in the activity.

If you wish to claim continuing medical education credit for your study of this Section, you may claim your credit online or fill in the required forms and mail or fax them to the Academy.

To use the forms:

1. Complete the study questions and mark your answers on the Section Completion Form.
2. Complete the CME Activity Evaluation.
3. Fill in and sign the statement below.
4. Return this page and the required forms by mail or fax to the CME Registrar (see below).

To claim credit online:

1. Log on to the Academy website (www.aao.org/cme).
2. Select Review/Claim CME.
3. Follow the instructions.

Important: These completed forms or the online claim must be received at the Academy by June 1, 2013.

I hereby certify that I have spent _____ (up to 10) hours of study on the curriculum of this Section and that I have completed the study questions.

Signature: _____
                                                           Date

Name: _____

Address: _____

City and State: _____ Zip: _____

Telephone: (_____) _____ Academy Member ID# _____
                   area code

Please return completed forms to: **Or you may fax them to:** 415-561-8575
American Academy of Ophthalmology
P.O. Box 7424
San Francisco, CA 94120-7424
Attn: CME Registrar, Customer Service

2012–2013
Section Completion Form

Basic and Clinical Science Course

Answer Sheet for Section 1

Question	Answer	Question	Answer
1	a b c d	19	a b c d
2	a b c d	20	a b c d
3	a b c d	21	a b c d
4	a b c d	22	a b c d
5	a b c d	23	a b c d
6	a b c d	24	a b c d
7	a b c d	25	a b c d
8	a b c d	26	a b c d
9	a b c d	27	a b c d
10	a b c d	28	a b c d
11	a b c d	29	a b c d
12	a b c d	30	a b c d
13	a b c d	31	a b c d
14	a b c d	32	a b c d
15	a b c d	33	a b c d
16	a b c d	34	a b c d
17	a b c d	35	a b c d
18	a b c d		

CME Activity Evaluation

To comply with guidelines from the Accreditation Council for Continuing Medical Education and the American Medical Association and to assist us in planning future activities, please provide us accurate and important feedback as requested below.

1. Has this activity enhanced your professional abilities?

   ☐ Yes

   ☐ No

2. Because of my participation in this activity, I will make the following change to my practice:

3. How effective was the activity at meeting the stated objectives?

   ☐ All objectives were met.

   ☐ Most objectives were met.

   ☐ Few objectives were met.

   ☐ No objectives were met.

   ☐ I do not recall the objectives for this activity.

4. To what degree is this activity likely to have a positive impact on health outcomes of your patients?

   ☐ Extremely likely

   ☐ Highly likely

   ☐ Somewhat likely

   ☐ Not at all likely

   ☐ Not applicable

5. Was this activity free of commercial bias?

   ☐ Yes

   ☐ No

   If you selected "No," please comment:

6. How might we improve this activity to make it more relevant to your practice?

Study Questions

Although a concerted effort has been made to avoid ambiguity and redundancy in these questions, the authors recognize that differences of opinion may occur regarding the "best" answer. The discussions are provided to demonstrate the rationale used to derive the answer. They may also be helpful in confirming that your approach to the problem was correct or, if necessary, in fixing the principle in your memory. The Section 1 faculty would like to thank the Self-Assessment Committee for reviewing the study questions and discussions.

1. Which of the following is associated with Lyme disease?
   a. The infection is carried by mosquito larvae.
   b. The infectious pathogen is *Borrelia burgdorferi*.
   c. Nervous system involvement does not occur.
   d. All patients present with a typical rash known as erythema chronicum migrans.

2. In relation to HIV infection, the CCR5 receptor gene is important because
   a. it is required for attachment of HIV to T lymphocytes
   b. a defective CCR5 gene allows HIV infection to flourish
   c. all long-term survivors of HIV infection have the CCR5 gene defect
   d. CCR5 receptor inhibitors have proven ineffective in clinical trials to treat HIV infection

3. Which of the following is a risk factor for breast cancer?
   a. fibrocystic disease
   b. first-degree relative with breast cancer
   c. late menarche
   d. multiple previous pregnancies

4. What is the most effective screening technique for cervical cancer?
   a. Fourier transform infrared
   b. PCR assay
   c. HPV DNA testing
   d. Pap smear

5. Which of the following is a component of the 2009 Recommended Childhood, Adolescent, and Adult Immunization Schedules?
   a. Initial hepatitis B immunization should be given between 3 and 4 years of age.
   b. DTaP (diphtheria and tetanus toxoids and acellular pertussis vaccine) is first administered at age 6 weeks or older.
   c. The first dose of MMR (measles, mumps, rubella) vaccine is given between 4 and 6 months of age.
   d. The varicella vaccine should always be given during pregnancy.

6. What is the most important parameter in predicting anaphylaxis?
   a. past use of many antibiotics
   b. sensitivity to epinephrine
   c. sensitivity to hydrocortisone
   d. history of previous allergic reactions

7. In patients with shock, what is the most frequent single cause of death?
   a. hemorrhage
   b. myocardial infarction
   c. ventilatory failure
   d. sepsis

8. What is the initial consideration in treating status epilepticus?
   a. airway maintenance
   b. blood glucose levels
   c. blood pressure
   d. toxicology status

9. Which of the following is a potential adverse effect of anticytokine drugs such as etanercept (Enbrel) and infliximab (Remicade)?
   a. disc edema
   b. angle-closure glaucoma
   c. optic neuropathy
   d. increased risk of diabetes

10. Which of the following is most effective for treating Wegener granulomatosis?
    a. acetaminophen
    b. nonsteroidal anti-inflammatory agents
    c. cyclophosphamide
    d. methotrexate

11. Which of the following is a major ocular manifestation of systemic lupus erythematosus?
    a. retinal and choroidal microvascular lesions
    b. heliotrope rash of eyelids
    c. recurrent unilateral anterior uveitis
    d. conjunctivitis

12. The preferred test for diagnosing type 2 diabetes is
    a. hemoglobin A_{1c}
    b. fasting plasma glucose
    c. oral glucose tolerance test
    d. urine glucose and ketones

13. Which of the following classes of oral hypoglycemic agents has been associated with worsening macular edema?

   a. sulfonylureas

   b. α-glucosidase inhibitors

   c. biguanides

   d. thiazolidinediones

14. Patients with multiple endocrine neoplasia syndrome type 2B (MEN 2B) are likely to have which of the following ophthalmic findings?

   a. prominent corneal nerves

   b. bitemporal hemianopsia

   c. exophthalmos

   d. hypertensive retinopathy

15. What is currently the main treatment for Parkinson disease?

   a. dopamine

   b. pramipexole

   c. levodopa

   d. benztropine

16. Which of the following ophthalmic findings suggests that a patient is feigning a grand mal seizure:

   a. monocular nystagmus

   b. gaze deviation

   c. eyelid closure

   d. diminished saccades

17. Which of the following types of dementia is more likely to present with formed visual hallucinations:

   a. Alzheimer's disease

   b. Lewy body dementia

   c. vascular dementia

   d. dementia associated with Parkinson's disease

18. Which of the following is the leading cause of mortality among women in the United States?

   a. atherosclerotic heart disease

   b. breast cancer

   c. ovarian cancer

   d. stroke

19. The first line of treatment in reducing serum cholesterol should be

    a. drug therapy

    b. aerobic exercise

    c. weight loss

    d. dietary therapy

20. When LDL goals are not achieved by lifestyle changes alone in a patient with hypercholesterolemia, what is the next step?

    a. begin nicotinic acid

    b. begin bile acid sequestrants

    c. begin statin medications

    d. change the LDL goal

21. Adverse ocular reactions seen with use of digoxin include which of the following?

    a. glare phenomenon and xanthopsia

    b. corneal microdeposits

    c. keratoconjunctivitis sicca

    d. bull's-eye maculopathy

22. Prophylactic implantable cardioverter-defibrillators are indicated treatment for which of the following groups?

    a. patients with chronic atrial fibrillation

    b. survivors of a hemodynamically unstable episode of ventricular tachycardia

    c. patients not expected to survive more than 6 months regardless of treatment

    d. patients without inducible ventricular arrhythmias on electrophysiologic testing

23. The JUPITER study suggests that

    a. statins may be of value in patients with normal serum lipid and an elevated C-reactive protein level

    b. statin use may increase the risk of age-related macular degeneration

    c. statin therapy is not indicated in patients whose LDL-C has failed to respond to therapeutic lifestyle changes

    d. statins may rarely cause liver failure, rhabdomyolysis, or polyneuropathy

24. The metabolic syndrome is diagnosed on the basis of the presence of a constellation of findings, including

    a. normal fasting glucose

    b. elevated HDL (>50 mg/dL)

    c. blood pressure of 110/70 mmHg

    d. increased abdominal obesity

25. You suspect that an older patient who presents with a hyphema has been abused. What is your first step?

    a. Call the patient's primary care physician about the suspected abuse.

    b. Treat the suspected eye injury and address the nature of the injury on a follow-up examination, after obtaining further information from the family.

    c. Advise the caregiver to watch the patient for unstable balance and possible falls.

    d. Complete a written report promptly, document any suspicious injuries, and report your suspicions to the appropriate authorities.

26. Two months ago, a 90-year-old patient was informed by her ophthalmologist that her macular degeneration was progressing. At her follow-up visit, she seemed withdrawn and thin and talked about having lived too long. The most likely diagnosis is

    a. depression

    b. fear of living alone, as her spouse just passed away

    c. progressive dementia

    d. occult malignancy

27. The severity and frequency of falls increase as we age. Which of the following is the most likely?

    a. The older patient who suffers a fall will most likely develop dementia.

    b. Traumatic brain injury in older adults is most commonly caused by falls.

    c. Vision loss does not affect the incidence of falls in the older population.

    d. An older patient who falls should always be taken to an emergency room.

28. Widespread, cost-effective screening is best for diseases that

    a. are not treatable or preventable

    b. are difficult to diagnose

    c. have a high prevalence

    d. are very rare

29. Monitoring for hypertension should begin at what age?

    a. 3 years

    b. 18 years

    c. 35 years

    d. 40 years, barring suggestive symptoms or signs

30. Carotid endarterectomy has been proven to be of benefit in reducing stroke following nondisabling symptomatic events in patients with which of the following:

    a. ipsilateral 0%–29% carotid artery stenosis

    b. ipsilateral 30%–69% carotid artery stenosis

    c. ipsilateral 70%–99% carotid artery stenosis

    d. ipsilateral 100% carotid artery stenosis

31. Magnetic resonance imaging is more sensitive than computed tomography in the diagnosis of which of the following?

    a. intracranial hemorrhage

    b. early cerebral infarction

    c. ischemic stroke

    d. transient ischemic attack

32. The single most effective measure that can be instituted to reduce the risk of chronic obstructive pulmonary disease is

    a. weight loss

    b. exercise

    c. reduction of respiratory infections by hand washing

    d. smoking cessation

33. Which of the following is the best test to monitor heparin therapy?

    a. prothrombin time

    b. partial thromboplastin time

    c. bleeding time

    d. platelet count

34. If the risk of endophthalmitis is 1% per year in one hospital and 0.01% in another over a 1-year period, the risk difference is

    a. 0.01% over 1 year

    b. 100%

    c. 100% over 1 year

    d. 0.99% over 1 year

35. In a screening test applied to 250 patients, the sensitivity was estimated to be 80%. If 100 patients have the disease, then how many patients were false-negatives?

    a. 75

    b. 180

    c. 20

    d. 170

Answers

1. **b.** The infectious pathogen of Lyme disease is *Borrelia burgdorferi*. The carrier is the *Ixodes* genus of tick. Many patients present with erythema chronicum migrans but not all.

2. **a.** CCR5 is a surface receptor required for the attachment of HIV to lymphocytes. Patients with a defective CCR5 gene have natural immunity to HIV infection. Approximately 50% of long-term survivors of HIV infection are heterozygous for the CCR5 defect.

3. **b.** Nulliparity, early menarche, and history of a first-degree relative with breast cancer are all risk factors for breast cancer. Fibrocystic disease is not a risk factor for breast cancer.

4. **d.** The most effective screening technique remains the Papanicolaou test ("Pap smear"). Fourier transform infrared (FTIR) spectroscopy is a new tool for screening cervical cancer and has a sensitivity of 85% and a specificity of 91%. PCR DNA techniques can be used to help detect concomitant HPV infection.

5. **b.** The minimum age for administration of DTaP is 6 weeks. The first hepatitis B immunization should be given at birth, before discharge from the hospital. If the mother is HBsAg positive, the infant should receive hepatitis B immunoglobulin as well. The first dose of MMR (measles, mumps, rubella) vaccine is given between 12 and 15 months of age. Pregnancy is a contraindication for the varicella vaccine.

6. **d.** The most important parameter for predicting anaphylaxis is a history of a previous allergic reaction to another drug or antigen. The others are not risk factors for anaphylaxis.

7. **c.** Ventilatory failure is the most significant factor in the morbidity and mortality of shock, with subsequent hypoxemia and metabolic acidosis leading to many complications.

8. **a.** The airway must be maintained in the treatment of status epilepticus prior to any other treatment or diagnostic measures.

9. **c.** Etanercept and infliximab have been associated with demyelinating disease and optic neuritis. The antiepileptic medication topiramate (Topamax) has been associated with acute angle-closure glaucoma. The newer atypical antipsychotic agents, such as olanzapine (Zyprexa) and clozapine (Clozaril), may be associated with initiating or worsening diabetes. Cyclosporine (Neoral, Sandimmune) has been associated with disc edema.

10. **c.** Aspirin and nonsteroidal anti-inflammatory agents may be helpful in managing many forms of arthritis and other inflammatory disorders. Methotrexate is beneficial as a disease-modifying agent for patients with rheumatoid arthritis and other autoimmune diseases. Wegener granulomatosis is a potentially fatal systemic disease and usually requires aggressive treatment, including cyclophosphamide and prednisone.

11. **a.** Retinal and choroidal microvascular lesions are one of the more common manifestations of ocular involvement with systemic lupus erythematosus (SLE). Discoid lesions of the skin of the eyelids and keratitis sicca from secondary Sjögren syndrome are also common when the eye is involved. Recurrent unilateral anterior uveitis would be unusual with SLE; it is much more common with HLA-B27–associated diseases such as ankylosing spondylitis. A heliotrope rash of the eyelids, although rare, is almost pathognomonic for dermatomyositis. Autoimmune conjunctivitis can be a feature of reactive arthritis.

12. **b.** Fasting plasma glucose (FPG) is the preferred test. The oral glucose tolerance test may be more sensitive than the FPG, but it is not routinely used because it is costlier, inconvenient, and difficult to reproduce. The hemoglobin A_{1c} measurement is not currently recommended for diagnosing diabetes, although this may change when the test becomes more standardized. Although measuring urine glucose is much easier than measuring blood glucose, it is not sensitive, because blood glucose levels need to be quite elevated before glucose appears in urine. Measurement of urinary ketones is useful during periods of illness or stress, because any positive value suggests the presence of ketonemia; however, measurement of urinary ketones is not used for the diagnosis of diabetes.

13. **d.** The thiazolidinediones (rosiglitazone [Avandia] and pioglitazone [Actos]) have been implicated in contributing to macular edema in some patients. They can also cause fluid retention, and in 2010 the FDA significantly restricted the use of rosiglitazone because of increased risk of cardiovascular complications. The most common side effect of the sulfonylureas is hypoglycemia, especially with the longer-acting agents. α-Glucosidase inhibitors can cause flatulence, which can limit compliance. The only available biguanide is metformin (Glucophage), and it has the potential to cause severe lactic acidosis in the setting of renal insufficiency. The drug should therefore be avoided in patients with early renal disease and should not be used concomitantly with intravenous contrast agents that can precipitate renal failure.

14. **a.** Prominent corneal nerves are reported to occur in 100% of affected patients. This finding is significant because almost all affected patients will develop medullary thyroid cancer; however, because this may not appear until the patient's second or third decade, the ophthalmic manifestations may be the initial indication that the syndrome is present. Bitemporal hemianopsia can occur with pituitary tumors, which are part of multiple endocrine neoplasia syndrome type 1 (MEN 1). Exophthalmos can occur in Graves disease but is not part of the spectrum of the MEN syndromes. Hypertensive retinopathy can occur in patients with pheochromocytoma, which can be part of MEN 2A and 2B.

15. **c.** The main treatment is levodopa (L-dopa), which is generally initiated when symptoms become significant. Usually patients are given levodopa combined with carbidopa (Lodosyn), often as a combined pill (Sinemet). Dopamine itself cannot be given because it does not cross the blood–brain barrier. Pramipexole (Mirapex) stimulates dopamine receptors in the brain and can be given alone or in combination with levodopa, but it is less effective than levodopa. Benztropine (Cogentin), an anticholinergic drug, was a common treatment for Parkinson disease before the introduction of levodopa. Anticholinergics may help control tremor and rigidity, although their benefit is limited and their effect is usually short-lived.

16. **c.** It is unusual for patients experiencing a genuine seizure to shut their eyes during the episode, whereas patients who are feigning a seizure often keep their eyes closed. Patients who are having seizures may commonly have either horizontal or vertical gaze deviations. The gaze tends to be directed away from the site of the cortical lesion during a seizure and then toward the site of the lesion after the seizure. Monocular nystagmus can occur during the clonic stage of a seizure. Diminished saccadic movement is a side effect of the antiseizure medication carbamazepine (Tegretol).

17. **b.** Lewy body dementia is the second most common form of neurodegenerative dementia after Alzheimer's disease, and patients with this syndrome often present with complex, formed visual hallucinations. Although there may be considerable clinical and neuropathologic overlap among the various types of dementia, visual hallucinations are not

routinely a symptom of vascular dementia, Alzheimer's disease, or dementia associated with Parkinson disease.

18. **a.** Atherosclerotic coronary artery disease is by far the number one killer of women and men, not only in the United States but also in the world. It is estimated that every minute 1 person in the United States dies of coronary artery disease. The number of women who die from cardiovascular disease is 10 times that from breast cancer.

19. **d.** Dietary therapy should be the first line of treatment in reducing serum cholesterol. Regular aerobic exercise and limited alcohol intake have a beneficial effect on serum cholesterol by increasing HDL cholesterol. Medications are used after other modalities such as diet and exercise have not lowered cholesterol adequately. Weight loss can be associated with a lowering of cholesterol; however, in and of itself, it is not the first line of treatment for reducing serum cholesterol.

20. **c.** Statins are the first choice for medical therapy in virtually all patients whose LDL goals cannot be achieved by therapeutic lifestyle changes alone.

21. **a.** The glare phenomenon and disturbances of color vision are the most striking and the most common adverse ocular reactions seen with the use of digoxin. Corneal microdeposits occur with use of chloroquine and amiodarone. Keratoconjunctivitis sicca is not a specific side effect of digoxin but may be observed in patients using β-blockers. Bull's-eye maculopathy may be a side effect of chloroquine.

22. **b.** If a patient is not expected to survive at least 1 year with good functional status, an implantable cardioverter-defibrillator (ICD) is not recommended under current ACC/AHA guidelines. Survival and functional status are improved with an ICD in the setting of a previous cardiac arrest, hemodynamically unstable ventricular tachycardia episode, or inducible ventricular arrhythmias on electrophysiologic testing. ICDs are not indicated for chronic atrial fibrillation.

23. **a.** Statins are the first choice for medical therapy in patients who have not achieved LDL goals through therapeutic lifestyle changes (TLC) alone. The role of statins in relation to the risk of age-related macular degeneration (AMD) is unclear, but multiple studies suggest a decreased risk, particularly in late stages of AMD. The JUPITER study suggests that patients with an elevated C-reactive protein and no hyperlipidemia have a reduced risk of stroke and coronary artery disease when statins are used.

24. **d.** Patients with the metabolic syndrome have 3 or more of the following: a decreased HDL, increased abdominal obesity, elevated triglycerides, hypertension, and an elevated fasting glucose. Elevated HDL is generally a protective factor, reducing the risk of cardiovascular events.

25. **d.** In many states, reporting suspected elder abuse is mandatory. You should be aware of your state's rules and regulations. Trauma to the eyes can be seen in elder abuse. If you suspect elder abuse, you need to report this immediately and not wait until a follow-up appointment. Sometimes the caregiver may be the abuser, and examining and interviewing the patient alone may alert you to the abuse situation.

26. **a.** Depression is a very frequent problem in the older population, and loss of vision often leads to depression. The role of ophthalmologists is to understand the effects that loss of vision and blindness will have on patients. Be aware of community resources, such as a vision rehabilitation center, to which the patient can be referred. Having a staff member in the office who can help the patient contact such resources can be an invaluable first step.

27. **b.** Traumatic brain injury in older adults is commonly caused by falls. Fall-related direct expenses for those over age 65 totaled over $19 billion in 2000 in the United States. Vision disorders are responsible for 4% of falls. After a fall in an older adult, he or she may experience depression and loss of mobility, self-confidence, and independence.

28. **c.** Ideal diseases to screen for are the ones that are reliably detectable, treatable, or preventable, progressive (especially if untreated), and generally asymptomatic. A high, rather than low, prevalence argues in favor of screening. For a rare disease, screening may not prove cost-effective.

29. **a.** Evidence suggests that hypertension in the young is more common than previously recognized and has substantial long-term health consequences. It is recommended that children older than 3 years who are seen in a medical setting have their blood pressure measured.

30. **c.** Carotid endarterectomy is beneficial for symptomatic patients with recent nondisabling carotid artery ischemic events and ipsilateral 70%–99% carotid artery stenosis. It is not beneficial for symptomatic patients with 0%–29% or 100% stenosis, and its potential benefit for symptomatic patients with 30%–69% stenosis is uncertain.

31. **b.** All suspected cases of stroke and threatened stroke should prompt computed tomography (CT) of the brain. Computed tomography is very sensitive to the presence of intracranial hemorrhage. Magnetic resonance imaging (MRI), however, is often more sensitive than CT in detecting an evolving stroke within hours of its onset and an early cerebral infarction; CT results may be negative for up to several days after an acute cerebral infarct.

32. **d.** Smoking cessation is the single most effective intervention to reduce the risk of chronic obstructive pulmonary disease or slow its progression. Ophthalmologists should not underestimate the impact of discussing the harmful effects of smoking with their patients.

33. **b.** Heparin therapy is monitored by the partial thromboplastin time (PTT). Prothrombin time, or the international normalized ratio (INR), is used to monitor oral warfarin therapy. Bleeding time reflects platelet count and function. Platelet abnormalities do not affect the PTT.

34. **d.** Risk difference is the difference between 2 risk measures and has dimensions, so the correct answer is option d because 1% per year minus 0.01% per year is 0.99% per year.

35. **c.** Sensitivity refers to the proportion of those who have the disease who screen positive. If 80% of the 100 who have the disease screened positive, then 20% of those who have the disease, or 20 out of 100, screened negative.

Index

(*f* = figure; *t* = table)

radiation affecting, 238, 244
systemic drugs affecting, 300–302, 301–302*t*
in systemic malignancies, 244
Eye movements, disorders of
in Parkinson disease, 260
seizure activity and, 263
Eyelids
aging affecting, 221
disorders of, in Parkinson disease, 260
retraction of, seizures causing, 263–264
in scleroderma, 174
in systemic lupus erythematosus, 170
tumors of, in multiple endocrine neoplasia, 216, 217*f*

Factitious disorders, 249
Factive. *See* Gemifloxacin
Factor V Leiden, 147, 157
Factor VIII deficiency (hemophilia A/classic
hemophilia), 155
Factor VIII transfusions, 155
Factor Xa inhibitor, for non–ST-segment elevation acute
coronary syndrome, 111–112
Falls, in older patients, 231–232
Famciclovir, 55*t*, 66
for herpes simplex virus infections, 23, 66
for herpes zoster, 23, 66
Familial Alzheimer disease, 266
Family history/familial factors
in cancer, 237
osteoporosis risk and, 228
Famotidine, preoperative, 308
Famvir. *See* Famciclovir
Faropenem, 50*t*, 59
Fascicular blocks (cardiology), 122*t*
Fast hemoglobin (glycosylated hemoglobin/HbA₁/
HbA₁c), in glucose control/surveillance, 203, 203*f*, 204
Fasting, preoperative, 308
Fasting glucose
in diabetes diagnosis/screening, 193
impaired, 191*t*, 192–193
Fatty streak, 100
Fecal DNA testing, in cancer screening, 272*t*, 276
Fecal occult blood tests, in cancer screening, 272*t*, 276
Felbamate, 263*t*
Felbatol. *See* Felbamate
Feldene. *See* Piroxicam
Felodipine, 77*t*, 78*t*
Felty syndrome, 162
FENDrix. *See* Hepatitis B vaccine
Fenofibrate
diabetic retinopathy affected by, 205
for hypercholesterolemia/heart disease prevention, 137*t*
Fenoprofen, 183*t*
Fenoterol, 144
with ipratropium, 145*t*
Fentanyl, perioperative, 309*t*, 311
Ferritin levels, in iron deficiency anemia, 148
Fetal alcohol syndrome, 250
Fetal hydantoin syndrome, 264
Fetal radiation, effects/ocular manifestations of, 238
FEV₁ (forced expiratory volume in 1 second), 143
Fibric acid derivatives, for hypercholesterolemia/heart
disease prevention, 137*t*

Fibrillation
atrial, 124–125, 124*t*
heart failure and, 119, 120
stroke and, 92, 94
ventricular, 125, 126–127, 126*t*, 289, 292
Fibrinolytic system, 152
Fibrotic pulmonary disease, 142
Finasteride, ocular effects of, 301*t*
Fine-needle aspiration biopsy (FNAB), of thyroid gland,
210
First-degree atrioventricular block, 122*t*
Fishbone diagram, 346, 347*f*
Fitting (contact lens), trial, disinfection and, 41
Flagyl/Flagyl IV. *See* Metronidazole
Flecainide, 123*t*
ocular effects of, 302*t*
Flomax. *See* Tamsulosin
"Floor effect," 340
Flovent. *See* Fluticasone
Flow cytometry, in paroxysmal nocturnal
hemoglobinuria screening, 147, 150
Flowchart (system of care), 346, 347*f*
Floxin. *See* Ofloxacin
Flu. *See* Influenza
Fluconazole, 54*t*, 64–65
Flucytosine/5-fluorocytosine, 54*t*
Flumadine. *See* Rimantadine
Flumazenil, for benzodiazepine reversal, 310
FluMist. *See* Intranasal influenza vaccine
Flunisolide, for pulmonary diseases, 145*t*
Fluorescein, allergic reactions to, 295
Fluorescein angiography, allergic reactions to, 295–296
Fluorescent bronchoscopy, in cancer screening, 275
Fluorescent treponemal antibody absorption (FTA-ABS)
test, 13, 279
5-Fluorocytosine, 54*t*
Fluoroquinolones, 60–61. *See also* Quinolones
Fluorouracil, 240*t*
Fluoxetine, ocular effects of, 301*t*
Fluphenazine, 251
Flurbiprofen, 183*t*
Flutamide, 242*t*
Fluticasone, 145*t*
with salmeterol, 145*t*
Flutrimazole, 65
Flutter
atrial, 124*t*, 125
ventricular, 125, 126*t*
Fluvastatin, for hypercholesterolemia/heart disease
prevention, 137*t*
FNAB. *See* Fine-needle aspiration biopsy
Foam cells, 100
Folate/folic acid
antagonists of, in cancer chemotherapy, 240*t*
deficiency of, 149
Follicle-stimulating hormone, pituitary adenoma
producing, 215
Follicular carcinoma, of thyroid gland, 213–214
Follow-up, in case series, 322–323
Follow-up studies (cohort studies), 321*f*, 324*f*, 326–327
Fomivirsen, for cytomegalovirus retinitis, 24, 38
Fondaparinux, for non–ST-segment elevation acute
coronary syndrome, 111–112